Recent Developments in Magnetic Resonance Imaging

Recent Developments in Magnetic Resonance Imaging

Editor: Zachary Garcia

AMERICAN MEDICAL PUBLISHERS
www.americanmedicalpublishers.com

AMERICAN
MEDICAL PUBLISHERS
www.americanmedicalpublishers.com

Cataloging-in-Publication Data

Recent developments in magnetic resonance imaging / edited by Zachary Garcia.
p. cm.
Includes bibliographical references and index.
ISBN 978-1-63927-082-8
1. Magnetic resonance imaging. 2. Diagnostic imaging. 3. Imaging systems in medicine. I. Garcia, Zachary.
RC78.7.N83 R43 2022
616.075 48--dc23

American Medical Publishers,
41 Flatbush Avenue,
1st Floor, New York,
NY 11217, USA

ISBN 978-1-63927-082-8 (Hardback)

Contents

Preface

This book has been an outcome of determined endeavour from a group of educationists in the field. The primary objective was to involve a broad spectrum of professionals from diverse cultural background involved in the field for developing new researches. The book not only targets students but also scholars pursuing higher research for further enhancement of the theoretical and practical applications of the subject.

Magnetic Resonance Imaging (MRI) is a technique used in radiology. It is used in forming the pictures of the anatomy and the physiological processes of the body. MRI uses magnetic field gradients, strong magnetic fields and radio waves to generate an image of the organs in the body. Magnetic resonance imaging is different from a CT scan and PET scan as it does not involve X-rays and ionizing radiation. MRI is primarily used for medical diagnosis, staging of disease and monitoring without exposing the body to radiation. The major components of an MRI scanner are the main magnet, gradient system and shim coils. Main magnet is used to polarize the sample, whereas MR signal and the RF system are localized by the gradient system. Shim coils are the components used for correcting shifts in the homogeneity of the main magnetic field. This book provides comprehensive insights into the field of magnetic resonance imaging. It is a valuable compilation of topics, ranging from the basic to the most complex advancements in this field. This book is a vital tool for all researching and studying medical imaging.

It was an honour to edit such a profound book and also a challenging task to compile and examine all the relevant data for accuracy and originality. I wish to acknowledge the efforts of the contributors for submitting such brilliant and diverse chapters in the field and for endlessly working for the completion of the book. Last, but not the least; I thank my family for being a constant source of support in all my research endeavours.

Editor

1

The use of MRI apparent diffusion coefficient (ADC) in monitoring the development of brain infarction

Jian-Min Shen*, Xian-Wu Xia*, Wu-Gen Kang, Jian-Jun Yuan, Liang Sheng

Abstract

Background: To study the rules that apparent diffusion coefficient (ADC) changes with time and space in cerebral infarction, and to provide the evidence in defining the infarction stages.

Methods: 117 work-ups in 98 patients with cerebral infarction (12 hyperacute, 43 acute, 29 subacute, 10 steady, and 23 chronic infarctions) were imaged with both conventional MRI and diffusion weighted imaging. The average ADC values, the relative ADC (rADC) values, and the ADC values or rADC values from the center to the periphery of the lesion were calculated.

Results: The average ADC values and the rADC values of hyperacute and acute infarction lesion depressed obviously. rADC values in hyperacute and acute stage was minimized, and increased progressively as time passed and appeared as "pseudonormal" values in approximately 8 to 14 days. Thereafter, rADC values became greater than normal in chronic stage. There was positive correlation between rADC values and time ($P < 0.01$). The ADC values and the rADC values in hyperacute and acute lesions had gradient signs that these lesions increased from the center to the periphery. The ADC values and the rADC values in subacute lesions had adverse gradient signs that these lesions decreased from the center to the periphery.

Conclusion: The ADC values of infarction lesions have evolution rules with time and space. The evolution rules with time and those in space can be helpful to decide the clinical stage, and to provide the evidence in guiding the treatment or judging the prognosis in infarction.

Background

Brain infarction leads to high mortality and disability [1]. The post-infarction treatments available were largely dependent on the timing after infarction to determine the stages of brain damage [2]. The fast and accurate radiological diagnosis could provide important reference in judging the timing and development stages of brain infarction. In recent years, the diffusion weighted imaging (DWI) based on echo planar imaging (EPI) has emerged to be applicable in early diagnosis of brain infarction [3-9]. The present study investigated the changes of apparent diffusion coefficient (ADC) and relative ADC (rADC) values in different timing points after brain infarction as well as different brain regions to understand if ADC value could be instructive in clinical diagnosis of brain infarction progression and treatment.

* Correspondence: sjm_60@126.com; xu8858000@126.com
Department of Medical imaging, Taizhou municipal hospital, Taizhou Medical College, Taizhou 318000, PR China

Methods

Clinical data

98 cases (55 male, 43 female, ages 41-76 years with an average of 65) of brain infarction patients were diagnosed and verified with radiology data. 117 MRI and DWI examinations were performed: 12 hyperacute (< 6 hours post brain infarction), 43 acute (7-24 hours), 29 subacute (2-7 days), 10 steady (8-14 days), and 23 chronic (> 15 days) infarctions. The ethics approval was obtained by Taizhou Medical college committee of clinical research, and written form approvals were obtained from patients.

MRI and DWI scanning

Siemens NOVUS 1.5 superconducting MR scanning system was used. Routine MRI was firstly used to define T1W1 and T2W1: T1W1 was using spin echo sequences (SE) with TR/TE of 350 ms/8 ms; T2W1 was using turbo spin echo sequences (TSE) with TR/TE = 2500 ms/9 ms; the acquisition matrix is 218 × 256. For DWI scanning, single time activated SE-EPI sequences was used with following parameters: TR3300 ms, TE94 ms, acquisition matrix 128 × 128, FOV 230 mm × 230 mm, with diffusion gradient in x, y and z dimensions, and acquire images at b = 0 and 1000; the ADC pictures were automatically built. All scanning sections were 7 mm thick with 2 mm distance to each other.

Image analysis

Four regions of interest (ROI) were selected from central, near central, near edge, edge of infracted areas on ADC figures according to T1W1 and T2W1, with 5 pixels for each ROI to compute the average ADC value of the whole infracted region. The rADC value is given by: rADC = (average ADC value in infracted side/average ADC value in heath side) × 100%. Sulcus and ventricle were avoided in ADV value measurement.

Statistics

The statistics were performed with SPSS12.0 software. A significant difference was considered when $P < 0.01$ in T test.

Results

The average ADC and rADC in brain infracted regions change with time

The average ADC values in brain infracted area and contralateral (unaffected) areas as well as the average rADC values from 117 scanning were shown in table 1. The results suggested in the super acute and acute cases the average ADC values significantly decreased and is lower than the contralateral side (Figure 1); The average rADC values were 58% and 66% for super acute and acute cases, respectively, without significant difference ($P > 0.01$). In subacute cases, the average ADC and rADC values were higher in compared to hyper acute and acute cases ($P < 0.01$), with the average rADC value of 79%. The ADC value in the infracted area came back to normal range, showing the "false normal" phenomenon. In the chronic cases the average ADC values in infracted regions were higher than the contralateral side, with an average rADC value of 174%; both values were significant different from other three time periods ($P < 0.01$) (Table 1, Figure 2).

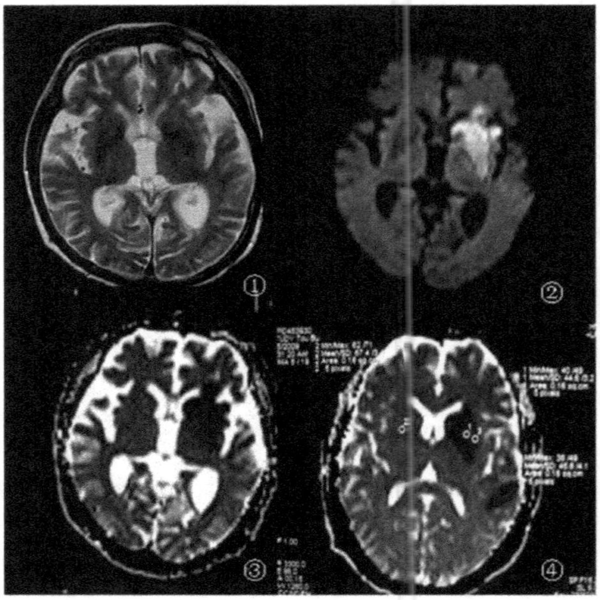

Figure 1 1-3 were taken from one super acute case patient, 4 hours after brain infarction. 1 showed the T2W1 image, which failed to diagnose the infracted region; 2 showed DWI images, with clear infracted region in basal ganglia; 3 is ADC image, showing lower ADC value in infracted region. 4 is acute case 7 hours after infarction, with lower ADC value in the center of infracted region.

Table 1 ADC and rADC value in different time points after brain infraction

Time phase	Number of cases	ADC valuen	rADC value ($x \pm s$) (%)
superacute(< 6 h)	12	30~63	58 ± 6.75
acute(7~24 h)	43	49~78	66 ± 5.36
subacute(2~7 d)	29	60~90	79 ± 4.83
steady (8~14 d)	10	87~108	100 ± 5.43
chronic (> 15 d)	28	110~219	174 ± 33.47

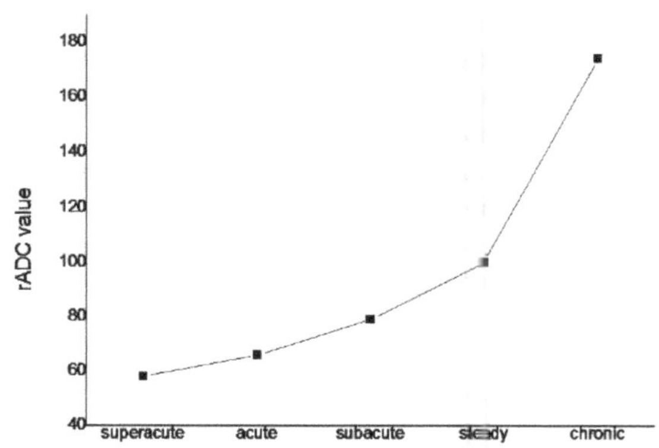

Figure 2 rADC values (%) change in different time period after brain infarction.

The ADC and rADC values vary within brain infracted region

In the infracted region of 12 super acute and 43 acute cases, the ADC and rADC values were unevenly distributed; they increase from the center to the edge, forming a "gradient" (Figure 1); for example, the average rADC value in the center is 61%, which was 78% in the edge. In contrast to this, the 29 subacute cases showed reversed gradient - that is, the ADC and rADC values decreased from center to the edge regions, which were 85% and 66%, respectively.

Discussion

DWI is currently the only imaging method to investigate diffusion activities of water molecules in vivo; ADC reflects the diffusion speed of water molecules, and the fast diffusion of water molecules could be revealed with a larger ADC value with lower signals of DWI images. Therefore the changes of ADC value could reflect the water molecule diffusion status in post brain infarction periods [8,10-12]. In superacute and acute brain infarction periods, the slowdown of water molecule diffusion could be explained by the cellular edema: following ischemia, the outflow of intracellular potassium ions and the inflow of calcium, sodium as well as water caused the swelling of the cells. The water molecules inside the cells were however bounded by cell membrane and organelles, and therefore diffuse much slower, causing the lower ADC values. Because of the relative balance in total amount of water in the acute phase after brain infarction, T2W1 often show no change even that the ADC value decreased, as found in 12 super acute cases in present manuscript - which suggested that the accuracy of using ADV value in diagnosis of brain infracted regions is 100% in our hand. This cannot be reach in routine MRI images. To normalize the ADC value and eliminate the individual differences, the present study measured the ADC value in the contralateral side to compute the rADC value [13,14], which could be useful in comparative studies, even among individuals across countries.

In present study we showed that the average ADC and rADC value change with time period post-brain infarction, which is caused by pathophysiological changes following brain damages. In superacute and acute cases the rADC reached the lowest point, and began to increase in subacute cases, and appeared to be "normal" between 10-14 days after brain infarction happened. This could be explained by two possibilities: first, vessel-sourced edema caused injury to endothelial cells 5-6 hours after brain infarction, and exacerbated in subacute phase, leading to enhanced permeability of blood brain barrier, and increased movement of many molecules including water molecules in extracellular spaces; second, the cell membrane broken and released intracellular water molecules [15]. In chronic phase the infracted brain tissues liquidize and were replaced by cerebrospinal fluid, which has a free movement of water molecules and the high ADC value when compared with brain tissues, leading to a rADC value more than 100%. Given the fact the ADC and rADC values vary during the post brain infarction period, we suggest that the combined analysis of ADC, rADC and routine MRI images could be important and useful in clinical diagnosis of the progression after brain infarction.

The other interesting point is the spatial distribution of ADC and rADC values within infracted region. In superacute and acute cases ADC values increase from the center to the side areas, suggesting that the decreases of ADC values could reflect the severity of the tissue damage. The surrounding regions of brain infarction area were considered to be plastic and could be re-perfused in proper conditions, or infracted if untreated [16]. The gradient of ADC value thus provided a chance to diagnose the surrounding sensitive regions, to follow the efficacy of treatment and prediction of the recovery. In subacute phase the reversed gradient suggested the liquidation of infracted tissues from the center, and brought the increased ADC value. The "false normal" phenomena would appear in the late phase of subacute patients, and during this period the reperfusion could not save the brain tissue from necrosis. Moreover, this would point the possibility to use ADC values to predict the recovery into normal tissue or final degeneration after the intervention in patients with brain infraction [17].

Conclusion

In summary, the present study showed that in brain infracted regions the ADC and rADC values change both temporally and spatially, reflecting the progression of infarction and tissue damage severity. The adoption of these values in clinical diagnosis and treatment of brain infarction patients could be helpful and instructive.

Acknowledgements

The study was supported by Taizhou Shujiang Scientific funding 6284.

Authors' contributions

all authors participated in the design of the experiment; JMS provided the funding and analyzed the data; all authors participated in the writing of the manuscript.

Competing interests

The authors declare that they have no competing interests.

References

1. Pantano P, Totaro P, Raz E: **Cerebrovascular diseases.** *Neurol Sci* 2008, **29(Suppl 3)**:314-318.
2. Venketasubramanian N, Chang HM, Chan BP: **Update in the management of stroke.** *Ann Acad Med Singapore* 2002, **31**:717-720, quiz 721.
3. Yanaka K, Shirai S, Kimura H, Kamezaki T, Matsumura A, Nose T: **Clinical application of diffusion-weighted magnetic resonance imaging to intracranial disorders.** *Neurol Med Chir (Tokyo)* 1995, **35**:648-654.
4. Maldjian JA, Grossman RI: **Future applications of DWI in MS.** *J Neurol Sci* 2001, **186(Suppl 1)**:S55-57.
5. Schaefer PW, Copen WA, Lev MH, Gonzalez RG: **Diffusion-weighted imaging in acute stroke.** *Neuroimaging Clin N Am* 2005, **15**:503-530, ix-x.
6. Warach S, Gaa J, Siewert B, Wielopolski P, Edelman RR: **Acute human stroke studied by whole brain echo planar diffusion-weighted magnetic resonance imaging.** *Ann Neurol* 1995, **37**:231-241.
7. Warach S, Chien D, Li W, Ronthal M, Edelman RR: **Fast magnetic resonance diffusion-weighted imaging of acute human stroke.** *Neurology* 1992, **42**:1717-1723.
8. Schlaug G, Siewert B, Benfield A, Edelman RR, Warach S: **Time course of the apparent diffusion coefficient (ADC) abnormality in human stroke.** *Neurology* 1997, **49**:113-119.
9. Weber J, Mattle HP, Heid O, Remonda L, Schroth G: **Diffusion-weighted imaging in ischaemic stroke: a follow-up study.** *Neuroradiology* 2000, **42**:184-191.
10. Srivastava AK, Mehrotra G, Bhargava SK, Agarwal S, Tripathi RP: **Studies on the time course of apparent diffusion coefficient and signal intensities on T2- and diffusion-weighted MR Imaging in acute cerebral ischemic stroke.** *J Med Phys* 2008, **33**:162-170.
11. Lansberg MG, Thijs VN, O'Brien MW, Ali JO, de Crespigny AJ, Tong DC, Moseley ME, Albers GW: **Evolution of apparent diffusion coefficient, diffusion-weighted, and T2-weighted signal intensity of acute stroke.** *AJNR Am J Neuroradiol* 2001, **22**:637-644.
12. Roberts TP, Rowley HA: **Diffusion weighted magnetic resonance imaging in stroke.** *Eur J Radiol* 2003, **45**:185-194.
13. Sotak CH: **The role of diffusion tensor imaging in the evaluation of ischemic brain injury - a review.** *NMR Biomed* 2002, **15**:561-569.
14. Schwamm LH, Koroshetz WJ, Sorensen AG, Wang B, Copen WA, Budzik R, Rordorf G, Buonanno FS, Schaefer PW, Gonzalez RG: **Time course of lesion development in patients with acute stroke: serial diffusion- and hemodynamic-weighted magnetic resonance imaging.** *Stroke* 1998, **29**:2268-2276.
15. Matsumoto K, Lo EH, Pierce AR, Wei H, Garrido L, Kowall NW: **Role of vasogenic edema and tissue cavitation in ischemic evolution on diffusion-weighted imaging: comparison with multiparameter MR and immunohistochemistry.** *AJNR Am J Neuroradiol* 1995, **16**:1107-1115.
16. Na DG, Thijs VN, Albers GW, Moseley ME, Marks MP: **Diffusion-weighted MR imaging in acute ischemia: value of apparent diffusion coefficient and signal intensity thresholds in predicting tissue at risk and final infarct size.** *AJNR Am J Neuroradiol* 2004, **25**:1331-1336.
17. Taleb M, Lövblad KO, El-Koussy M, Guzman R, Bassetti C, Oswald H, Remonda L, Schroth G: **Reperfusion demonstrated by ADC mapping after intra-arterial thrombolysis for human ischemic stroke confirmed by cerebral angiography.** *Neuroradiology* 2001, **43**:591-594.

2

Evaluation of the normal-to-diseased apparent diffusion coefficient ratio as an indicator of prostate cancer aggressiveness

Andrei Lebovici[1], Silviu A Sfrangeu[1], Diana Feier[1*], Cosmin Caraiani[2], Ciprian Lucan[3], Mihai Suciu[3], Florin Elec[3], Gheorghita Iacob[4] and Mircea Buruian[5]

Abstract

Background: We tested the feasibility of a simple method for assessment of prostate cancer (PCa) aggressiveness using diffusion-weighted magnetic resonance imaging (MRI) to calculate apparent diffusion coefficient (ADC) ratios between prostate cancer and healthy prostatic tissue.

Methods: The requirement for institutional review board approval was waived. A set of 20 standardized core transperineal saturation biopsy specimens served as the reference standard for placement of regions of interest on ADC maps in tumorous and normal prostatic tissue of 22 men with PCa (median Gleason score: 7; range, 6–9). A total of 128 positive sectors were included for evaluation. Two diagnostic ratios were computed between tumor ADCs and normal sector ADCs: the ADC peripheral ratio (the ratio between tumor ADC and normal peripheral zone tissue, ADC-PR), and the ADC central ratio (the ratio between tumor ADC and normal central zone tissue, ADC-CR). The performance of the two ratios in detecting high-risk tumor foci (Gleason 8 and 9) was assessed using the area under the receiver operating characteristic curve (AUC).

Results: Both ADC ratios presented significantly lower values in high-risk tumors (0.48 ± 0.13 for ADC-CR and 0.40 ± 0.09 for ADC-PR) compared with low-risk tumors (0.66 ± 0.17 for ADC-CR and 0.54 ± 0.09 for ADC-PR) ($p < 0.001$) and had better diagnostic performance (ADC-CR AUC = 0.77, sensitivity = 82.2%, specificity = 66.7% and ADC-PR AUC = 0.90, sensitivity = 93.7%, specificity = 80%) than stand-alone tumor ADCs (AUC of 0.75, sensitivity = 72.7%, specificity = 70.6%) for identifying high-risk lesions.

Conclusions: The ADC ratio as an intrapatient-normalized diagnostic tool may be better in detecting high-grade lesions compared with analysis based on tumor ADCs alone, and may reduce the rate of biopsies.

Keywords: Prostate cancer, Diffusion-weighted magnetic resonance imaging, Neoplasm grading

Background

The assessment of local aggressiveness of prostate cancer (PCa) is of key importance for appropriate management of this disease. The increase in life expectancy of the general population combined with efficient screening methods will lead to an increase in the number of new PCa cases [1]. These cases will tend to be more localized and at an earlier stage. Over the last few years, new focal methodologies have emerged for PCa treatment, such as high-intensity focused ultrasound, cryotherapy, focal laser ablation, intensity-modulated radiation therapy, radiofrequency ablation, and others. These relatively new therapeutic methods come as alternatives to existing treatment modalities such as radical prostatectomy or radiotherapy [2]. The diagnosis of PCa is based on physical (i.e., digital rectal) examination, prostate specific antigen (PSA) levels, and, when PSA levels are abnormal, blind biopsy. All of these assessments are of low diagnostic accuracy [3-5]. Multiparametric magnetic resonance imaging (MRI) has shown great potential, with significant improvement in detection, localization, and characterization of PCa [6,7].

* Correspondence: diana.feier@gmail.com
[1]Radiology Department, Emergency County Hospital, "Iuliu Hatieganu" University of Medicine and Pharmacy, Cluj-Napoca, Romania
Full list of author information is available at the end of the article

This is of great importance for the selection of precise treatment options, and for minimizing treatment-related morbidity. Patients with tumors rated with a Gleason score of 6 or greater represent an important target population for PCa detection and effective therapy [8,9].

According to recent guidelines [10], multiparametric MRI of the prostate includes three functional MR sequences: diffusion weighted imaging (DWI) [11], dynamic contrast enhancement-MR [12], and MR spectroscopy [13]. These sequences contribute to the PI-RADS scoring system of prostate lesions [10], with DWI as the main contributor. With a short acquisition time and high contrast resolution between tumor and normal prostatic tissue [14], DWI and apparent diffusion coefficient (ADC) mapping demonstrate an inverse and significant correlation with the Gleason score [7,14]. Although ADC can estimate tumor aggressiveness, there is still a large overlap between ADCs of different tumors with the same Gleason score [7]. The purpose of this study was to establish a simple method for PCa assessment of tumor aggressiveness using ADC ratios between prostate cancer and healthy prostatic tissue.

Methods

We analyzed the images of 43 men who underwent prostate MRI examinations with an endorectal coil in our institution between February 2011 and August 2012. Written informed consent had been obtained from patients prior to the MR examinations, as well as before all interventions, such as prostatic biopsy. The requirement to obtain written, informed consent for the retrospective analysis of the data was waived. To be included in our study, subjects needed to have biopsy-proven PCa from a standard 20-core transperineal saturation biopsy. We excluded five cases because of post-biopsy hemorrhage, five cases because of motion artifacts, and 11 cases because of unavailable or negative biopsy specimens. Thus, 22 cases (median age: 64.5 years; range: 52–75 years) were further selected in this retrospective single-center study. All subjects had undergone MRI with an endorectal coil including T2-weighted images (T2WI) and DWI 4–6 weeks after PCa confirmation by biopsy.

Saturation biopsy

Saturation biopsy was conducted under general anesthesia in the supine position. The biopsy needle was guided with transrectal ultrasound into the sectors (Figure 1) and 20 transperineal cores were obtained. Each biopsy core was numbered, assigned to a sector, and sent for histopathological analysis.

Histopathological analysis

Biopsy specimens were fixed in formaldehyde, embedded in paraffin, and stained with hematoxylin-eosin.

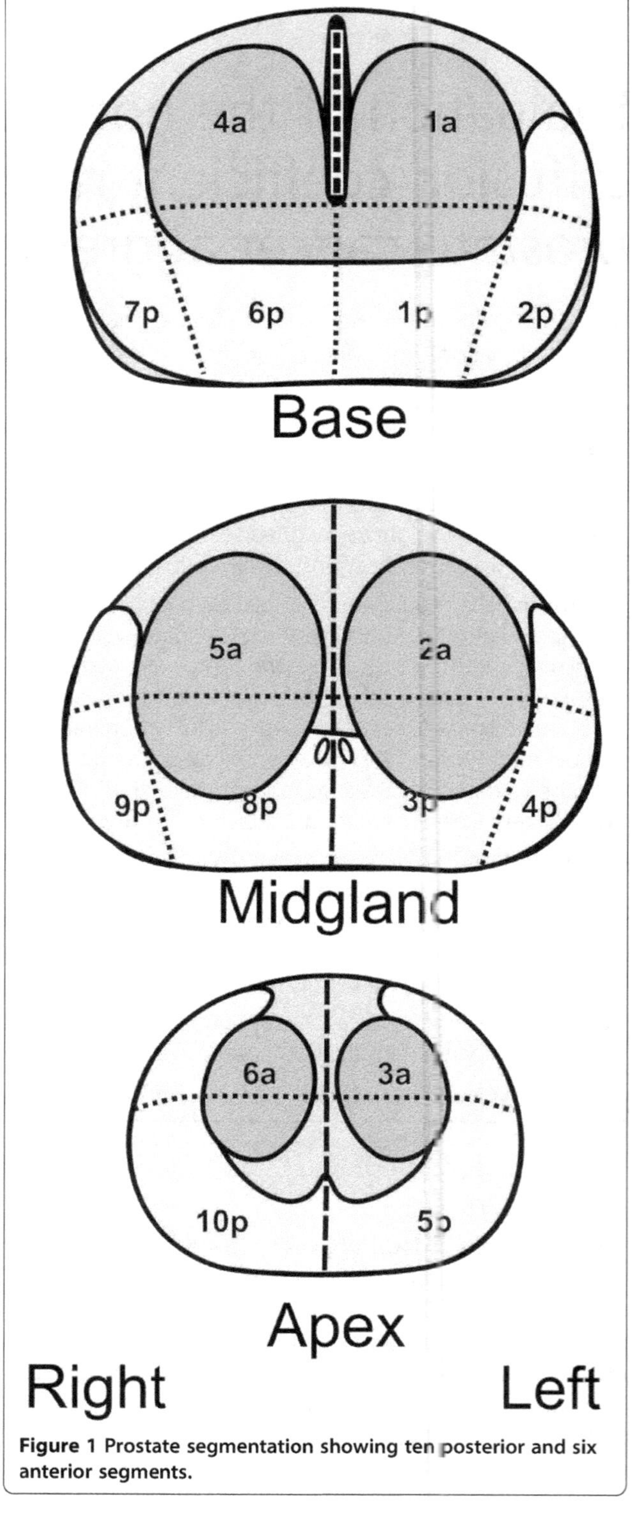

Figure 1 Prostate segmentation showing ten posterior and six anterior segments.

The diagnosis was confirmed with immunohistochemistry for basal cells (p63) and AMCAR expression (p504s). Results were reported as cancer with an assigned Gleason score or as benign tissue.

MRI technique and image interpretation

MRI was performed with a 1.5 T scanner (Symphony; Siemens AG, Erlangen, Germany) using an eight-channel phased array body coil combined with an endorectal coil (MEDRAD, Inc., Warrendale PA, USA). After digital rectal examination, the balloon of the endorectal coil was inflated with 60 mL of air. T2WI were obtained in axial, coronal, and sagittal planes using turbo spin echo sequences and the entire prostate was investigated. DWI was performed in the axial plane using echo-planar imaging (EPI) sequences at three b-values (0, 400, and 800 mm^2/s) and restriction of diffusion was quantified by ADC values. T2WI parameters and DWI parameters are shown in Table 1.

Image interpretation

Image interpretation was done on a PACS station (KODAK/Carestream Version 10.2; Carestream Health, Rochester, NY, USA) by two radiologists with 5 years' combined experience in uroradiology and prostate imaging and 3 years' combined experience interpreting DWI (L.A., C.C.). The readers were aware of the results of biopsy and clinical data. PCa-positive biopsy cores were assigned to a 16-region standardized prostate reporting scheme including ten posterior and six anterior glandular sectors (Figure 1) as recommended by Dickinson et al. [15]. ADC maps were generated from the DWI sequences, and regions of interest (ROIs) were placed according to biopsy results and the prostate reporting scheme. Lesions with low signal intensity compared with surrounding tissue on ADC were considered malignant. ROIs were drawn to occupy approximately 75% of the lesion in a given segment to be sure that normal tissue outside lesion margins would not be included. ROIs were drawn also in the tumor-free sectors, with a standard ROI size of 0.8 cm^2. The mean signal intensity was measured automatically by the PACS system. ADC ratios were calculated by dividing tumoral ADCs by tumor-free ADCs from the peripheral and the central zones of the gland (Figure 2A and B). The highest ADCs of normal sectors were taken as reference values. T2WI and T1-weighted images (T1WI) were assessed for post-biopsy hemorrhage.

Statistical analysis

The analysis was performed per patient and per tumor unit accordingly. Categorical variables were presented as numbers and percentages. Continuous variables were

Table 1 MRI parameters' description

	T2W-MRI	DW-MRI
Sequence	Fast spin echo	Spin echo EPI
TR (ms)	5500	3200
TE (ms)	104	90
Flip angle	150°	
FOV (mm^2)	180 × 180	300 × 300
Matrix	256 × 256	128 × 128
Voxel size (mm^3)	0.8 × 0.8 × 3	2.3 × 2.3 × 4
Slice thickness (mm)	3	4
Gap (mm)	0.3	0.3
Spectral suppression	No	Yes
b-values	-	0/400/800
NEX	1	2
TA (min:sec)	4:09	2:40

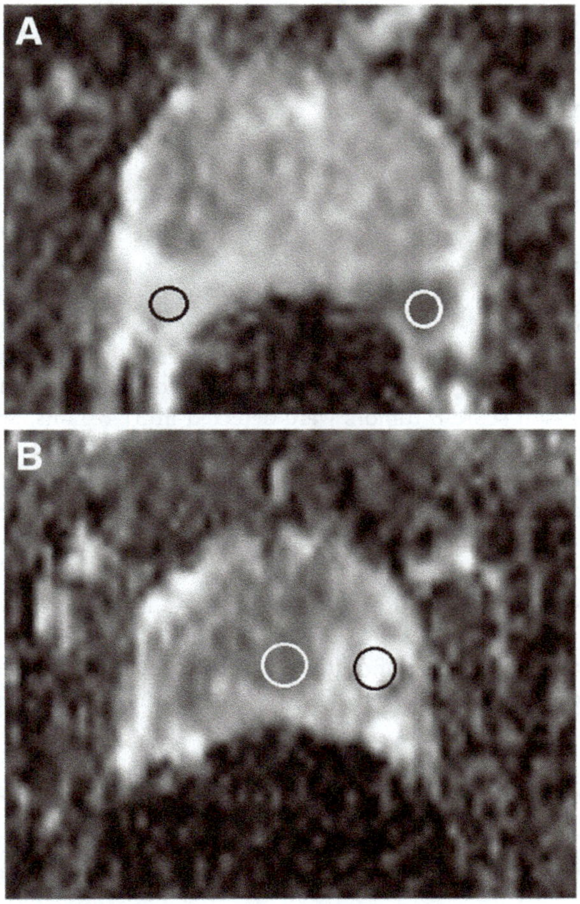

Figure 2 Placement of regions of interest (ROI) for (A) peripheral gland tumor (B) central gland tumor. A. Placement of regions of interest (ROI) for signal intensity measurements of Gleason 8 (4 + 4) peripheral tumor (white ROI = 0.78×10^{-3} mm^2/s) and normal peripheral zone (black ROI = 1.9×10^{-3} mm^2/s). The ADC-PR (white ROI/black ROI) is 0.41, which indicates a high-grade tumor. **B.** The white ROI is placed in the central gland (CG) portion of a Gleason 9 (4 + 5) lesion (0.82×10^{-3} mm^2/s) while the black ROI is located in tumor-free CG tissue (1.87×10^{-3} mm^2/s) The ADC-CR (white ROI/black ROI) is 0.43, which indicates a high-grade prostate tumor.

expressed as mean values and standard deviation or median and range, as appropriate. We used a linear multilevel model, so no linearity or normality assumptions were made. The discriminative capability of each ADC ratio was determined by calculating the area under the receiver operating characteristic curve (AUC). Optimal cut-off values were chosen to maximize the Youden index, and sensitivity (%) and specificity (%) were computed from the same data, without further adjustments. Discriminative capability was examined per tumor unit and not per patient, because of the low number of available patients. Comparisons were performed among different ADCs using the Student's *t*-test for continuous variables and $p < 0.05$ was considered statistically significant. The statistical analysis was performed using commercially available software (MedCalc version 12.4.0; MedCalc Software, Mariakerke, Belgium).

Results

Median PSA serum levels were 15.5 ng/mL (range, 6.8–100 ng/mL) and median prostate volume was 44 mL (range, 31–67 mL). On saturation biopsy, cancer was detected in 157 of the 440 cores (36%). After assigning the cancer-positive cores to the 16-region standardized prostate reporting scheme, 128 out of 352 regions were cancer positive (36%). The median Gleason score was 7 (range: 6–9). Gleason score 6 tumors were detected in 12 regions, Gleason score 7 tumors were detected in 38 regions, Gleason score 8 tumors were detected in 31 regions, and Gleason score 9 tumors were detected in 46 regions. From the positive tumor sectors, 86 (67%) were peripherally located, while 42 (33%) were centrally located.

ADC findings

Results of mean prostatic tumor ADC for lower-grade cores (Gleason 6 and 7) and higher-grade cores (Gleason 8 and 9) were significantly different ($p < 0.001$), as were the ADC-PR and ADC-CR ($p < 0.0001$), as presented in Table 2.

For a cut-off level $\leq 0.82 \pm 0.32 \times 10^{-3}$ mm^2/s, the tumor ADCs for Gleason 8 and 9 positive sectors showed a sensitivity and specificity of 72.7 and 70.6%, while the AUC was 0.75. Using a cut-off value ≤ 0.57, the ADC-CR showed more promising results with sensitivity = 82.2%, specificity = 66.7%, and AUC of 0.77 (Table 3). The best diagnostic performance was obtained for ADC-PR, with an AUC of 0.84, when applying a cut-off value ≤ 0.5.

When analyzing the performance for ADC-PR in detecting tumors with a high Gleason score (8 or 9) in relation to the lesion location, the ratio had robust accuracy in detecting central zone tumors (AUC = 0.81) and an excellent discriminatory ability to detect tumors located in the peripheral zone (AUC = 0.90) (Figure 3). The results are summarized in Table 4.

Discussion

Our study shows promising results in the assessment of PCa aggressiveness using tumor-to-normal ADC ratios. In this study, both central and peripheral ADC ratios demonstrated a better sensitivity, specificity, and AUC than the interpretation of ADCs alone, with the most promising results obtained for the ratios computed using normal ADCs measured in the periphery of the gland. It is not yet possible to find a cut-off value to delineate malignant tissue from benign because of the overlap of ADCs of PCa and those of normal prostatic tissue; even Gleason 9 tumors showed ADCs up to 1.27×10^{-3} mm^2/s. This finding is well known; Litjens et al. concluded in their study that tumor ADCs should not be considered absolute because of the influence of "background" variation of normal peripheral zone (PZ) tissue composition [16]. This statement is supported by the results of our study, in which we were able to demonstrate better AUC for ADC ratios in comparison with tumor ADCs alone. In our study, the ADCs of the PCa-positive biopsy cores showed statistically significant differences from the biopsy cores of normal PZ and central gland

Table 2 ADC and ADC-R characteristics of 128 prostatic sectors for low- and intermediate-risk group (Gleason 6 and 7) and high-risk group (Gleason 8 and 9)

Biopsy specimen characteristics	Gleason 6 and 7 (n = 51)	Gleason 8 and 9 (n = 77)	p
*Number of patients	14 (64%)	8 (36%)	
Age (years)	66 (56–76)	59 (46–76)	<0.001
PSA (ng/mL)	10.74 (3.5-25)	26 (14–100)	<0.001
ADC (mm^2/sec)	$0.88 \times 10^{-3} \pm 0.13$	$0.73 \times 10^{-3} \pm 0.17$	<0.001
Normal central zone ADC (mm^2/sec)	$1.38 \times 10^{-3} \pm 0.24$	$1.59 \times 10^{-3} \pm 0.22$	<0.001
Normal peripheral zone ADC (mm^2/sec)	$1.64 \times 10^{-3} \pm 0.19$	$1.90 \times 10^{-3} \pm 0.35$	<0.001
ADC-CR	0.66 ± 0.17	0.48 ± 0.13	<0.001
ADC-PR	0.54 ± 0.09	0.41 ± 0.09	<0.001

Note: Data are presented as mean and standard deviation or median and range, except where indicated. *: Data are presented as number and percentages. ADC-CR: ratio between tumor ADCs and healthy central gland tissue ADCs. ADC-PR: ratio between tumor ADCs and healthy peripheral zone tissue ADCs.

Table 3 DWI cut-off values and performance values of tumor ADC, ADC-CR, and ADC-PR in predicting Gleason 8 and 9

	Tumor ADC	ADC-CR	ADC-PR
Cut-off	≤ 0.82	≤ 0.57	≤ 0.5
Sensitivity	72.7	82.2	88.9
Specificity	70.6	66.7	64.7
AUROC	**0.75**	**0.77**	**0.84**
p value	**< 0.001**	**< 0.001**	**< 0.001**

Note: AUC: area under the receiver operating characteristic curve. ADC-CR: ratio between tumor ADCs and healthy central gland tissue ADCs. ADC-PR: ratio between tumor ADCs and healthy peripheral zone tissue ADCs.

Table 4 The cut-off values and diagnostic performance of ADC-Peripheral Ratio in predicting Gleason 8 and 9 stages, according to tumor location

	Central zone tumors	Peripheral zone tumors
Cut-off	≤ 0.42	≤ 0.50
Sensitivity	62.1	93.7
Specificity	92.7	80
AUC	**0.81**	**0.90**
p value	**< 0.001**	**< 0.001**

Note: AUC: area under the receiver operating characteristic curve.

(CG). These results are consistent with results previously published [17-19]. The mean ADC for positive PCa cores in our group ($0.79 \pm 0.18 \times 10^{-3}$ mm^2/s) was slightly higher than the one reported by Woodfield et al. [14] ($0.737 \pm 0.154 \times 10^{-3}$ mm^2/s, range, $0.108–1.263 \times 10^{-3}$) but lower than results published recently by Yamamura et al. [18] ($0.96 \pm 0.24 \times 10^{-3}$ mm^2/s), Rinaldi et al. [19] ($0.99 \pm 0.15 \times 10^{-3}$ mm^2/s) and Nagayama et al. [20] ($1.07 \pm 0.35 \times 10^{-3}$ mm^2/s) ($p > 0.5$). The lower ADCs for positive cores in our study group were probably because of the high number of Gleason score 8 and 9 biopsy-proven sectors, which exceeded 60% of all PCa positive biopsies. This large number of biopsy-proven, high-grade PCa is likely the consequence of larger tumors in this group of patients and a higher percentage of positive biopsy cores (for example, all 20 biopsy cores were tumor-positive in two patients).

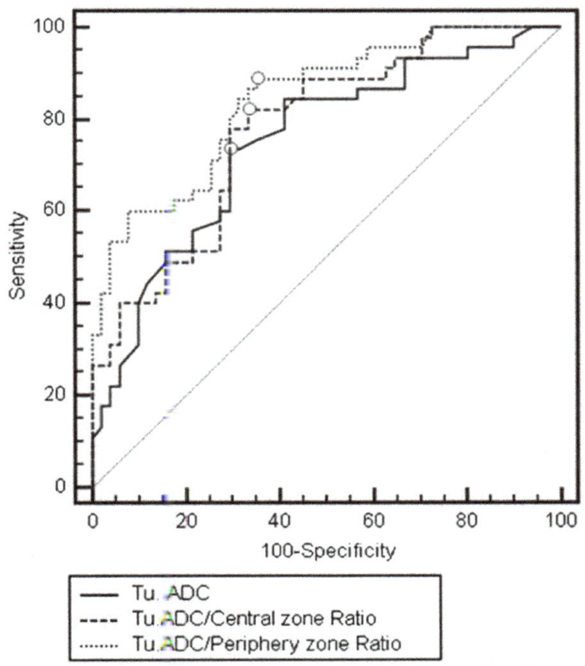

Figure 3 Comparison of receiver operating characteristic curves for tumor ADC, ADC-CR, and ADC-PR for cases with Gleason scores 8 and 9.

Healthy PZ prostatic tissue is rich in tubular structures, allowing water molecules to move easily. As a consequence, the ADCs of healthy PZ are high. Published ADC mean values for PZ have been $1.65 \pm 0.21 \times 10^{-3}$ mm^2/s and $1.73 \pm 0.27 \times 10^{-3}$ mm^2/s [15,18]. Our study of the normal PZ shows similar results, with a mean ADC of $1.71 \pm 0.32 \times 10^{-3}$ mm^2/s. Normal CG structure is composed of two different tissues, a glandular component with high signal intensity on T2WI and a stromal component with low signal intensity on T2WI, which can mimic PCa. The ADCs of normal CG should be lower than normal values from the PZ because of benign stromal hyperplasia changes taking place in the central gland. Oto et al. showed that there is a significant difference between ADCs of hyperplasic stromal nodules ($1.27 \pm 0.21 \times 10^{-3}$ mm^2/s) and hyperplastic glandular nodules ($1.73 \pm 0.28 \times 10^{-3}$ mm^2/s) [21]. Our measurements were done on the entire CG including both macroscopically stromal and glandular areas and the mean ADC was $1.44 \pm 0.22 \times 10^{-3}$ mm^2/s, which is lower than the PZ ADC and close to the results published by Oto et al. [22].

When comparing the Gleason scores, the ADC values in subjects with Gleason 6 and 7 were significantly lower than those with Gleason 8 and 9. As an additional observation, patients with Gleason 8 and 9 were significantly younger ($p < 0.0001$). We hypothesize that the ADC differences arise from natural variations in prostate physiology in younger patients, owing to less significant fibrotic and atrophic changes of prostate glandular structure that would tend to decrease the ADC measurements [17].

In the last several years, many authors have investigated the correlation between ADC and Gleason score. Woodfield et al. [14] demonstrated a statistically significant difference between ADCs of low-grade tumors (Gleason 6) and intermediate-grade tumors (Gleason 7) and between low-grade tumors and high-grade tumors (Gleason 8 and 9). Verma et al. [7], in a large study of 197 prostate tumors, concluded that ADCs negatively correlated with the Gleason score. Somford et al. [22] showed the capacity of ADC mapping to predict the presence of high-grade tumors in patients with Gleason 6 (3 + 3) findings on biopsy. Although there are promising results with DWI, there are still discrepancies between ADCs of PCa and the final Gleason score in the many papers published. The differences among ADCs can be explained by physiologic factors such as age and tumor size and by technical factors (e.g., acquisition parameters, software, and the use of endorectal coils). The results of our study are very encouraging; we demonstrated that there is a statistically significant difference between ADCs of low- and intermediate-grade tumors compared with high-grade tumors. Our results are consistent with those reported by Woodfield et al. [14].

PCa is a major health problem. The diagnostic methodology remains practically the same, with ultrasound-guided systematic biopsy as the main diagnostic modality. Systematic biopsy has important limitations; it can miss up to 35% of cancers [23], and the Gleason score resulting from systematic biopsy has to be upstaged in up to 50% of the patients after radical prostatectomy [24]. In addition, Nam et al. concluded in their extensive study that complications after TRUS-guided biopsy have increased dramatically in the last 10 years [25]. With, new less-invasive focal therapy techniques and the active surveillance approach (which is based only on biopsy results), it is of great importance to improve PCa detection, characterization, and staging while reducing biopsy-related morbidity as much as possible.

The results of this study show the potential of ADC mapping in estimating the aggressiveness of PCa. By analyzing the ADC ratios when applying DWI sequences in PCa imaging, we can detect high-grade tumors more accurately than when carrying out analysis based on ADC alone. From our point of view, ADC mapping has the potential to guide the biopsy needle into the most aggressive region of a malignant lesion, resulting in fewer and more accurate biopsies, better staging, and more information to select appropriate treatment options.

We have to state several limitations: (1) We used a systematic biopsy as the reference standard, even though it may miss a substantial percentage of prostate cancers. However, it is the method of choice for cancer detection. (2) Our study population was relatively small. Patients with Gleason 8 and 9 scores tend to be younger than patients with Gleason 6 and 7 scores, so the cases could not be age-matched. (3) We do not have data on intraobserver and interobserver variability. (4) Prostate biopsy was performed prior to MRI examination, which might have influenced the ADC measurements. The presence of microscopic hemorrhage undetectable on standard MRI sequences might have altered the ADC values and underestimated the diagnostic value of ADC ratios.

Conclusions

The ADC tumor-to-normal ratio may be more predictive of tumor grade than analysis based on ADCs alone.

Abbreviations

PCa: Prostate cancer; ADC: Apparent diffusion coefficient; ADC-PR: Ratio of tumor ADC to normal PZ ADC; PZ: Peripheral zone; CG: Central gland; ADC-CR: Ratio of tumor ADC to normal CG ADC; PSA: Prostate specific antigen; MRI: Magnetic resonance imaging; T2WI: T2-weighted images; T1WI: T1 weighted images; DWI: Diffusion weighted imaging; AUC: Area under receiver operating characteristic curve.

Competing interests

The authors declare that they have no financial or non-financial competing interests.

Authors' contributions

LA performed the study concept and design, acquisition of data, analysis and interpretation of data, and drafted the manuscript. SS supervised the study concept and design and helped draft the manuscript. FD formulated the study concept and design, analysis, and interpretation of data, and drafting of the manuscript. CC performed the imaging acquisition, interpretation of data, and helped draft the manuscript. LC performed the acquisition of data and drafting of the manuscript. SM performed analysis and interpretation of data and drafting of the manuscript. EF performed the acquisition of data and helped draft the manuscript. IG performed the histological studies and analysis of data. BM performed critical revision of the manuscript for important intellectual content. All authors read and approved the final manuscript.

Author details

[1]Radiology Department, Emergency County Hospital, "Iuliu Hatieganu" University of Medicine and Pharmacy, Cluj-Napoca, Romania. [2]Department of Imaging, Regional Institute of Gastroenterology and Hepatology, "Iuliu Hatieganu" University of Medicine and Pharmacy, Cluj-Napoca, Romania. [3]Department of Urology, Clinical Institute of Urology and Kidney Transplant, "Iuliu Hatieganu" University of Medicine and Pharmacy, Cluj-Napoca, Romania. [4]Department of Pathology, Clinical Institute of Urology and Kidney Transplant, "Iuliu Hatieganu" University of Medicine and Pharmacy, Cluj-Napoca, Romania. [5]Department of Radiology, County Emergency Hospital Mures, University of Medicine and Pharmacy, Targu-Mures, Romania.

References

1. Melnikow J, LeFevre M, Wilt TJ, Moyer VA: **Counterpoint: Randomized trials provide the strongest evidence for clinical guidelines: The US Preventive Services Task Force and Prostate Cancer Screening.** *Med Care* 2013, **51**:301–303.
2. Bozzini G, Colin P, Nevoux P, Villers A, Mordon S, Betrouni N: **Focal therapy of prostate cancer: energies and procedures.** *Urol Oncol* 2013, **31**:155–167.
3. Scardino PT, Weaver R, Hudson MA: **Early detection of prostate cancer.** *Hum Pathol* 1992, **23**:211–222.
4. Schröder FH, Carter HB, Wolters T, van den Bergh RC, Gosselaar C, Bangma CH, Roobol MJ: **Early detection of prostate cancer in 2007. Part 1: PSA and PSA kinetics.** *Eur Urol* 2008, **53**:468–477.
5. Gómez Veiga F, Ponce Reixa J, Barbagelata López A, Fernández Rosado E, Gonzalez MM: **Current role of PSA and other markers in the diagnosis of prostate cancer.** *Arch Esp Urol* 2006, **59**:1069–1082.
6. Bonekamp D, Jacobs MA, El-Khouli R, Stoianovici D, Macura KJ: **Advancements in MR imaging of the prostate: from diagnosis to interventions.** *Radiographics* 2011, **31**:677–703.
7. Verma S, Rajesh A, Morales H, Lemen L, Bills G, Delworth M, Gaitonde K, Ying J, Samartunga R, Lamba M: **Assessment of aggressiveness of prostate cancer: correlation of apparent diffusion coefficient with histologic grade after radical prostatectomy.** *Am J Roentgenol* 2011, **196**:374–381.
8. Gleason DF, Mellinger GT: **Prediction of prognosis for prostatic adenocarcinoma by combined histological grading and clinical staging.** *J Urol* 1974, **111**:58–64.

9. Bianco FJ Jr, Wood DP Jr, Cher ML, Powell IJ, Souza JW, Pontes JE: Ten-year survival after radical prostatectomy: specimen Gleason score is the predictor in organ-confined prostate cancer. *Clin Prostate Cancer* 2003, 1:242–247.
10. Barentsz JO, Richenberg J, Clements R, Choyke P, Verma S, Villeirs G, Rouviere O, Logager V, Fütterer JJ, European Society of Urogenital Radiology: ESUR prostate MR guidelines 2012. *Eur Radiol* 2012, 22(4):746–757.
11. Aigner F, Pallwein L, Pelzer A, Schaefer G, Bartsch G, Nedden D, Frauscher F: Value of magnetic resonance imaging in prostate cancer diagnosis. *World J Urol* 2007, 25:351–359.
12. Chen YJ, Chu WC, Pu YS, Chueh SC, Shun CT, Tseng WY: Washout gradient in dynamic contrast-enhanced MRI is associated with tumor aggressiveness of prostate cancer. *J Magn Reson Imaging* 2012, 36:912–919.
13. Boonsirikamchai P, Choi S, Frank SJ, Ma J, Elsayes KM, Kaur H, Choi H: MR Imaging of Prostate Cancer in Radiation Oncology: What Radiologists Need to Know. *Radiographics* 2013, 33:741–761.
14. Woodfield CA, Tung GA, Grand DJ, Pezzullo JA, Machan JT, Renzulli JF 2nd: Diffusion-weighted MRI of peripheral zone prostate cancer: comparison of tumor apparent diffusion coefficient with Gleason score and percentage of tumor on core biopsy. *Am J Roentgenol* 2010, 194:W316–W322.
15. Dickinson L, Ahmed HU, Allen C, Barentsz JO, Carey B, Futterer JJ, Heijmink SW, Hoskin PJ, Kirkham A, Padhani AR, Persad R, Puech P, Punwani S, Sohaib AS, Tombal B, Villers A, van der Meulen J, Emberton M: Magnetic resonance imaging for the detection, localisation, and characterisation of prostate cancer: recommendations from a European consensus meeting. *Eur Urol* 2011, 59(4):477–494.
16. Litjens GJ, Hambrock T, Hulsbergen–van de Kaa C, Barentsz JO: Interpatient variation in normal peripheral zone apparent diffusion coefficient: effect on the prediction of prostate cancer aggressiveness. *Radiology* 2012, 265:260–266.
17. Hosseinzadeh K, Schwarz SD: Endorectal diffusion-weighted imaging in prostate cancer to differentiate malignant and benign peripheral zone tissue. *J Magn Reson Imaging* 2004, 20:654–661.
18. Yamamura J, Salomon G, Buchert R, Hohenstein A, Graessner J, Huland H, Graefen M, Adam G, Wedegaertner U: Magnetic resonance imaging of prostate cancer: diffusion-weighted imaging in comparison with sextant biopsy. *J Comput Assist Tomogr* 2011, 35:223–228.
19. Rinaldi D, Fiocchi F, Ligabue G, Bianchi G, Torricelli P: Role of diffusion-weighted magnetic resonance imaging in prostate cancer evaluation. *Radiol Med* 2012, 117:1429–1440.
20. Nagayama M, Watanabe Y, Terai A, Araki T, Notohara K, Okumura A, Amoh Y, Ishimori T, Nakashita S, Dodo Y: Determination of the cutoff level of apparent diffusion coefficient values for detection of prostate cancer. *Jpn J Radiol* 2011, 29(7):488–494.
21. Oto A, Kayhan A, Jiang Y, Tretiakova M, Yang C, Antic T, Dahi F, Shalhav AL, Karczmar G, Stadler WM: Prostate cancer: differentiation of central gland cancer from benign prostatic hyperplasia by using diffusion-weighted and dynamic contrast-enhanced MR imaging. *Radiology* 2010, 257(3):715–723.
22. Somford DM, Hambrock T, Hulsbergen-van de Kaa CA, Fütterer JJ, van Oort IM, van Basten JP, Karthaus HF, Witjes JA, Barentsz JO: Initial experience with identifying high-grade prostate cancer using diffusion-weighted MR imaging (DWI) in patients with a Gleason score $\leq 3 + 3 = 6$ upon schematic TRUS-guided biopsy: a radical prostatectomy correlated series. *Invest Radiol* 2012, 47:153–158.
23. Djavan B, Ravery V, Zlotta A, Dobronski P, Dobrovits M, Fakhari M, Seitz C, Susani M, Borkowski A, Boccon-Gibod L, Schulman CC, Marberger M: Prospective evaluation of prostate cancer detected on biopsies 1, 2, 3 and 4: when should we stop? *J Urol* 2001, 166(5):1679–1683.
24. Cookson MS, Fleshner NE, Soloway SM, Fair WR: Correlation between Gleason score of needle biopsy and radical prostatectomy specimen: accuracy and clinical implications. *J Urol* 1997, 157(2):559–562.
25. Nam RK, Saskin R, Lee Y, Liu Y, Law C, Klotz LH, Loblaw DA, Trachtenberg J, Stanimirovic A, Simor AE, Seth A, Urbach DR, Narod SA: Increasing hospital admission rates for urological complications after transrectal ultrasound guided prostate biopsy. *J Urol* 2013, 189(1 Suppl):S12–S17. discussion S17-18.

3

3D-MRCP for evaluation of intra- and extrahepatic bile ducts: comparison of different acquisition and reconstruction planes

Kristina Imeen Ringe*, Dagmar Hartung, Christian von Falck, Frank Wacker and Hans-Jürgen Raatschen

Abstract

Background: Magnetic resonance cholangiopancreatography (MRCP) is an established technique for the evaluation of intra- and extrahepatic bile ducts in patients with known or suspected hepatobiliary disease. However, the ideal acquisition and reconstruction plane for optimal bile duct evaluation with 3D technique has not been evaluated. The purpose of our study was to compare different acquisition and reconstruction planes of 3D-MRCP for bile duct assessment.

Methods: 34 patients (17f/17 m, mean age 41y) referred for MRCP were included in this prospective IRB-approved study. Respiratory-triggered 3D-T2w-MRCP sequences were acquired in coronal and axial plane. Coronal and axial MIP were reconstructed based on each dataset (resulting in two coronal and two axial MIP, respectively). Three readers in two sessions independently assessed the MIP, regarding visualization of bile ducts and image quality. Results were compared (Wilcoxon test). Intra- and interobserver variability were calculated (kappa-statistic).

Results: In case of coronal data acquisition, visualization of bile duct segments was significantly better on coronal reconstructed MIP images as compared to axial reconstructed MIP ($p < 0.05$). Regarding visualization, coronal MIP of the coronal acquisition were equal to coronal MIP of the axial acquisition ($p > 0.05$). Image quality of coronal and axial datasets did not differ significantly. Intra- and interobserver agreement regarding bile duct visualization were moderate to excellent (κ-range 0.55-1.00 and 0.42-0.85, respectively).

Conclusions: The results of our study suggest that for visualization and evaluation of intra- and extrahepatic bile duct segments reconstructed images in coronal orientation are preferable. The orientation of the primary dataset (coronal or axial) is negligible.

Keywords: MRCP, MRC, Magnetic resonance cholangiopancreatography, Bile ducts, Common hepatic duct

Background

Magnetic resonance cholangiopancreatography (MRCP) is an established technique for the evaluation of intra- and extrahepatic bile ducts in patients with known or suspected hepatobiliary disease [1]. It is considered a reliable non-invasive alternative to diagnostic endoscopic retrograde cholangiopancreatography (ERCP) [2,3]. Since the first description by Wallner and colleagues in 1991 [4], different acquisition techniques have evolved.

Most current MRCP techniques are based on heavily T2-weighted fast spin echo (FSE) pulse sequences, which yield a luminal image of the bile ducts that is based on the inherent signal of slow-flowing or stationary bile. Both, single shot projections and multislice techniques are available [5], with the latter being distinguished into 2D [6] and 3D techniques [7]. Single shot projections are preferred in individuals who are unable to hold their breath, such as severely sick patients or small children [7]. 3D imaging techniques provide better image quality compared to 2D sequences [1,8,9], even though the combination of different MRCP sequences has proven to be valuable in the assessment of bile duct anatomy and pathology [10].

3D FSE sequences are usually acquired with the slab in coronal orientation. Maximum intensity projections

* Correspondence: ringe.kristina@mh-hannover.de
Department of Diagnostic and Interventional Radiology, Hannover Medical School, Carl-Neuberg Str. 1, Hannover 30625, Germany

(MIP) can then be obtained in any plane [7]. Previous studies have addressed the matter of optimal slice thickness for data acquisition [11] and different techniques regarding respiratory triggering [12]. However, to the best of our knowledge, the ideal acquisition and reconstruction plane, in practical terms meaning best suitable for optimal bile duct visualization with 3D techniques, has not been evaluated. The purpose of this study was to compare different acquisition and reconstruction planes of T2-weighted 3D-MRCP acquisitions for assessment of the intra- and extrahepatic bile ducts.

Methods

Patients

This HIPAA-compliant study was approved by the institutional review board of Hannover Medical School. Written informed consent from each patient was obtained. 34 patients (17 female, 17 male, mean age 41.5 years, range 18-79 years) who were referred for liver MRI and dedicated MRCP were included in this prospective study. Inclusion criteria were as follows: completion of the entire MR examination; patient age equal or greater than 18 years. Indications for performing MRI were as follows: primary sclerosing cholangitis (n = 16), status post liver transplantation (n = 7), tumor (n = 6), suspicion of Caroli's disease (n = 2), stone disease (n = 2) and recurrent pancreatitis (n = 1).

MR imaging technique

MR examinations were performed on a 1.5 T system (Magnetom Avanto, Siemens, Erlangen, Germany) using dedicated multichannel surface coils covering the abdomen. Prior to image acquisition, patients received 200 mL of a negative oral contrast agent (Lumirem®; Guerbet, Sulzbach, Germany) for suppression of gastroenteric fluid signal, as well as 20 mg butylscopolamine (Buscopan®; Boehringer Ingelheim, Ingelheim, Germany; administered as a bolus over approximately 20 s) i.v. for spasmolysis. All patients underwent a clinical routine imaging protocol of the liver, including a respiratory-triggered 3D MR cholangiography in the coronal (dataset A) as well as in the axial (dataset B) plane. MRCP-sequences were acquired prior to intravenous contrast injection. The specific MRCP sequences had sequential k-space filling with partial Fourier filling allowed, resulting in acquisition of central k-space lines approximately 3 minutes after the start of the sequence. MRCP sequence parameters are provided in detail in Table 1.

Table 1 Imaging parameters of the respiratory-triggered fat-saturated 3D T2-weighted MR cholangiographic sequence

Parameter	1.5 T Magnetom Avanto
Plane	Coronal, Axial
Respiratory triggering	Navigator based
Repetition time	Breathing cycle
Echo time (msec)	700-800
Refocusing pulse	140°
In-plane spatial resolution (mm)	1 × 1
Slab thickness (mm)	60-80
Partitions per slab	60-80
Type of k-space filling	Sequential
Partial Fourier factor	Allowed
Estimated total acquisition time (min)	Approximately 5

Image evaluation

Three readers (D.H., C.F., H.J.R.) independently performed image evaluation in terms of visibility of different bile duct segments up to the 3rd order and assessment of technical quality. All readers were board certified radiologists with at least eight years of experience in abdominal MR imaging. Readers were blinded to each patient's history and other imaging findings.

A single coronal and axial maximum intensity projection (MIP) covering the central, left, right and peripheral bile ducts was generated from each acquired MRCP dataset, resulting in two coronal and two axial MIP datasets, respectively. Care was taken to exclude the renal pelvis, ureter of both kidneys and spinal canal to allow for blinded reading. Each reader performed two reading sessions separated by an interval of two weeks, evaluating the reconstructed MIP in the following way: 1, Coronal reconstructed MIP of the coronal acquisition vs. coronal reconstructed MIP of the axial acquisition; 2, Axial reconstructed MIP of the coronal acquisition vs. axial reconstructed MIP of the axial acquisition. After each reading session the readers were asked to choose the preferred image dataset of any given comparison. The readers had no knowledge of initial MRCP dataset orientation.

Depiction of bile duct segments was assessed by using the following four-point scale proposed by Papanikolaou and colleagues [13]: 1, segment not seen; 2, segment faintly seen; 3, segment well seen but portion of the duct or the confluence not seen; and 4, excellent depiction including the proximal and distal portions. This scale was applied to the following sections (segments) of the biliary tract: the common bile duct (CBD), the right anterior bile duct, the right posterior bile duct, the left hepatic duct, and third-order biliary branches. Overall technical image quality was assessed using a four-point scale proposed by Lim and colleagues [14]: 1, poor quality with severe artifacts; 2, satisfactory quality with few artifacts; 3, good quality with minimal artifacts; and 4, excellent quality without artifacts.

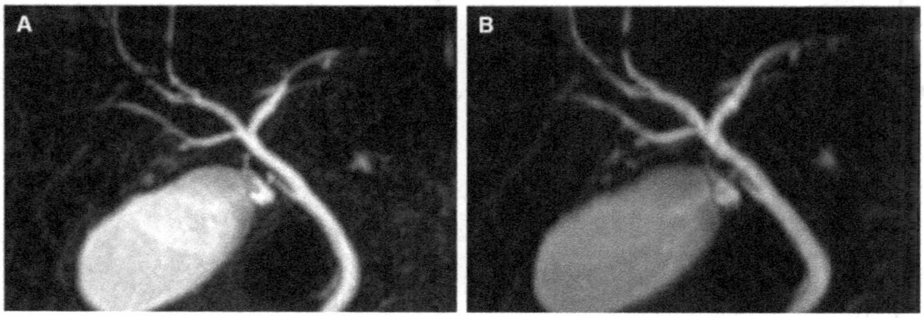

Figure 1 Comparison of coronal MIP reconstructions of coronal and axial acquired datasets. 35-year old male patient with diagnosis of primary sclerosing cholangitis (PSC). Coronal MIP of a coronal **(A)** and axial **(B)** acquired MRCP dataset. Bile duct visualization up to the 3rd order is equal on both datasets (see also Table 2), even though the image impression is more blurred on the MIP derived from the axial acquired dataset **(B)**.

In addition, a total score was defined as the sum of the visibility and quality scores for each dataset to determine which of the two acquired MRCP datasets (coronal or axial) yielded the most diagnostic information.

Statistical analysis

Statistical analysis was performed using GraphPad Prism software (version 6; GraphPad Software, Inc., La Jolla, CA).

Results regarding bile duct visualization and overall technical image quality were compared with a two-sided Wilcoxon signed-rank test (with a p-value <0.05 deemed significant) in the following way: 1, Coronal reconstructed MIP of the coronal acquisition vs. coronal reconstructed MIP of the axial acquisition; 2, Axial reconstructed MIP of the coronal acquisition vs. axial reconstructed MIP of the axial acquisition; 3, Coronal vs. axial reconstructed MIP of the coronal acquired dataset; 4. Coronal vs. axial reconstructed MIP of the axial acquired dataset. Intra- and interobserver agreement was assessed by means of a kappa-statistic and classified as follows: a K value of less than 0.20 indicated poor agreement; K values of 0.21-0.40, fair agreement; K values of 0.41-0.60, moderate agreement; K values of 0.61-0.80, good agreement; and K values of 0.80-1.00, excellent agreement [14].

Results

Bile duct visualization

In case of coronal data acquisition (dataset A), visualization of bile duct segments was significantly better on coronal reconstructed MIP as compared to axial reconstructed MIP ($p < 0.05$). This was true for visualization of the CBD, right anterior hepatic duct, left hepatic duct and third order biliary branches. In case of axial data acquisition (dataset B), a significant better visualization of the CBD and left hepatic duct on coronal reconstructed MIP as compared to axial reconstructed MIP was observed only by one reader.

Regarding bile duct visualization, coronal MIP of the coronal acquisition (dataset A) were equal to coronal MIP of the axial acquisition (dataset B) ($p > 0.05$) (Figure 1; Table 2). Axial MIP of the axial acquisition (dataset B) were significantly better than axial MIP of the coronal acquisition (dataset A) for visualization of third order biliary branches whereas lower order branches did not show a difference (Figures 2 and 3).

Intraobserver agreement regarding bile duct visualization was good to excellent (weighted K-range 0.63-1.0). Interobserver agreement was moderate to good, regarding bile duct visualization in both datasets (coronary acquisition: weighted K range 0.51-0.75; axial acquisition: weighted K range 0.42-0.67).

Technical image quality

Regarding overall technical image quality (including axial and coronal reconstructed MIP of a given dataset), there was no significant difference between the coronal and axial acquired dataset ($p > 0.05$). At detailed dataset analysis however, in case of coronal data acquisition (dataset A) technical image quality of the coronal MIP was significantly better as compared to the axial reconstructed MIP ($p < 0.05$). In case of axial data acquisition (dataset B), there was no significant difference regarding technical image quality of the reconstructed MIP ($p > 0.05$).

Table 2 P-values for each reader and biliary segment: comparison of coronal reconstructed MIP of coronal and axial acquired datasets regarding bile duct visualization

Reader No. (Session No.)	CBD	Right posterior bile duct	Right anterior bile duct	Left hepatic duct	2nd and 3rd order branches
1 (1)	0.424	0.923	0.499	0.685	0.305
1 (2)	0.766	0.309	0.236	0.783	0.790
2 (1)	1.000	1.000	0.536	0.358	0.145
2 (2)	1.000	0.609	0.400	0.891	0.393
3 (1)	0.174	0.943	0.305	0.266	0.627
3 (2)	0.345	0.898	0.143	0.627	0.608

P values were calculated with the two-sided Wilcoxon Test to compare depiction scores of coronal axial acquired datasets.

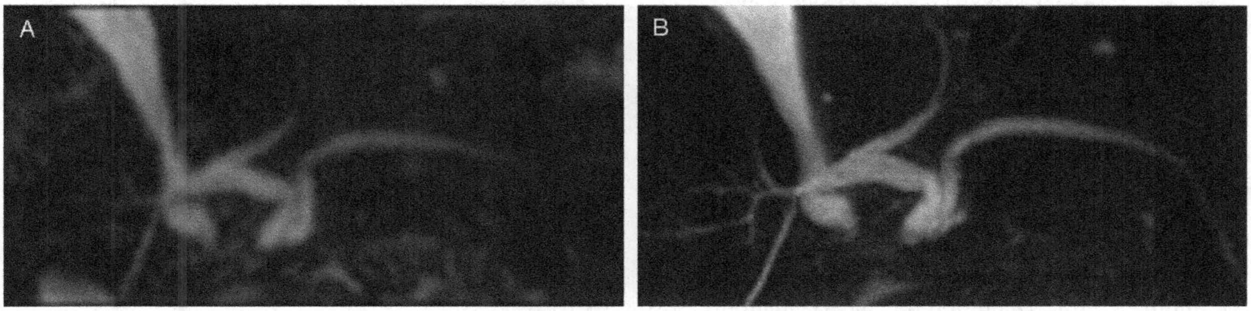

Figure 2 Comparison of axial MIP reconstructions of coronal and axial acquired datasets. 79-year old male patient status post radiofrequency ablation of a colorectal liver metastasis. Axial MIP of a coronal **(A)** and axial **(B)** acquired MRCP dataset. Bile duct visualization of 1st and 2nd order branches is equal on both datasets, whereas 3rd order branches are depicted significantly better on the axial dataset.

Intraobserver agreement regarding technical image quality was moderate to excellent (weighted K range 0.55-0.96); interobserver agreement was moderate (weighted K range 0.42-0.59).

Choice of preferred image dataset

When reading coronal reconstructed MIP, the readers preferred coronal acquisitions over axial acquisitions in 66% of the readings. Regarding axial MIP reconstruction, axial acquisitions were preferred over coronal acquisitions in 80% of the readings.

Intraobserver agreement regarding choice of the preferred image dataset was excellent (weighted K range 0.94-1.00); interobserver agreement was moderate to excellent (weighted K range 0.57-0.85).

Discussion

To the best of our knowledge the ideal acquisition and reconstruction plane for optimal bile duct evaluation with 3D techniques has not yet been evaluated. For single shot FSE techniques it has been suggested that straight coronal and initial left posterior oblique images clearly depict the common hepatic duct and the left hepatic duct, whereas the CBD and right hepatic ducts are seen better on a left posterior images obtained at a steeper angle [15]. Especially in children with segmental liver transplants sagittal oblique planes are preferred due to the more anteroposterior orientation of the neo-porta hepatis [16]. In a first approach towards projection cholangiography by means of MRI in 1991, Wallner and colleagues used a heavily T2-weighted gradient echo sequence for assessment of bile duct dilatation [4]. They concluded that imaging in the coronal plane provided a good view of the biliary system, whereas no additional information was found by imaging in the sagittal plane.

In this study we compared different acquisition and reconstruction planes of T2-weighted 3D-MRCP acquisitions for assessment of the intra- and extrahepatic bile ducts. In contrast to single shot techniques, 3D MRCP has the advantage to facilitate secondary reconstructions. Coronal reconstructions were preferred, regardless of the initial acquisition plane. These findings were supported by good intra- and interobserver agreement. One of the reasons for coronal image preference might be the fact that these images are similar to image impressions of ERCP and conventional cholangiograms.

There are other studies that evaluated secondary reconstruction techniques for MRCP. Schaible and

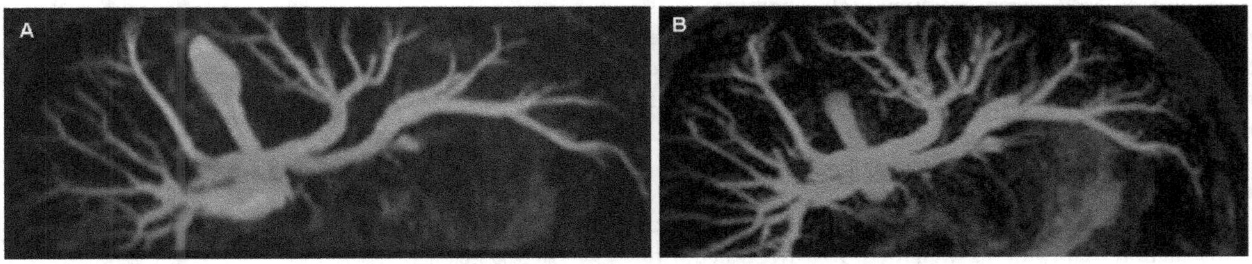

Figure 3 Comparison of axial MIP reconstructions of coronal and axial acquired datasets. 18-year old male patient with jaundice and suspicion of cholelithiasis. Axial MIP of a coronal **(A)** and axial **(B)** acquired MRCP dataset. Bile duct visualization up to the 3rd order is equal on both datasets, even though the image impression is more blurred on the MIP derived from the coronal acquired dataset **(A)**.

colleagues evaluated selective MIP reconstructions of respiratory-triggered 3D MRCP versus standard MIP reconstructions and single-shot MRCP [17]. Single-shot and standard MIP reconstructions of 3D MRCP were comparable in terms of anatomical bile duct visualization, whereas selective MIP postprocessing proved useful for detection of pathological alterations. In a retrospective study, Morita and colleagues compared volume rendering (VR) and MIP of 3D TSE MRCP sequences to define biliary anatomy mostly in patients without major biliary tract anomaly [18]. Definition of biliary anatomy was found to be more accurate using VR reformation than MIP. However, the assessment of VR images was not the purpose of the present study. One disadvantage of VR reconstructions is that the detection degree of each structure depends on the setting of display parameters, particularly on the lower threshold of the opacity curve. Therefore VR images need to be evaluated interactively [18].

Our study had some limitations. We did not perform quantitative SNR measurements of the MRCP datasets as the focus of our study was to qualitatively evaluate visualization of intra- and extrahepatic bile ducts using multiple readers. This seemed closer to the clinical reality than SNR values that are difficult to measure for small bile ducts. We did not evaluate the added value of acquisition or reconstruction planes. In 1999, Boraschi and colleagues compared axial and coronal 2D FSE sequences with 3D MIP projection images in patients with suspected hepatobiliary disease [19]. A higher global accuracy for axial and coronal FSE T2-weighted sequences was found regarding the diagnosis of the level and probable cause of biliary obstruction in depiction of small intraductal pathology such as calculi or neoplastic lesions.

We have limited our analysis to reconstructed rather thin-slice source images as the purpose of this specific was to directly compare acquisition and reconstruction planes for MIP assessment. A well-known limitation of MIP is that small filling defects may be obscured due to partial volume effects [20]. Further, overestimation of ductal narrowing and pseudostricture may result from the nature of MIP reconstruction [21]. Therefore it is important, that MIP reconstructions should not be appraised separately, but always in combination with the original acquired dataset and in combination with other morphological sequences.

Conclusions

In conclusion, we compared different acquisition and reconstruction planes of T2-weighted 3D-MRCP acquisitions for assessment of the intra- and extrahepatic bile ducts in patients with different hepatobiliary pathologies. The results of our study suggest that for visualization and evaluation of the bile ducts coronal reconstructions are preferred. In this context, the orientation of the primary dataset (coronal or axial) is negligible.

Competing interests

The authors declare that they have no competing interests.

Authors' contributions

KIR and DH conceived and designed the experiments, KIR, DH and CF performed the experiments and acquisition of data. KIR, DH, CF, FW and HJR analyzed and interpreted the data. FW and HJR contributed materials and analysis tools. All authors participated in drafting and revising the manuscript. All authors read and approved the final manuscript.

References

1. Sodickson A, Mortele KJ, Barish MA, Zou KH, Thibodeau S, Tempany CM: **Three-dimensional fast-recovery fast spin-echo MRCP: comparison with two-dimensional single-shot fast spin-echo techniques.** *Radiology* 2006, **238:**549–559.
2. Holzknecht N, Gauger J, Sackmann M, Thoeni RF, Schurig J, Holl J, Weinzierl M, Helmberger T, Paumgartner G, Reiser M: **Breath-hold MR cholangiography with snapshot techniques: prospective comparison with endoscopic retrograde cholangiography.** *Radiology* 1998, **206:**657–664.
3. Hekimoglu K, Ustundag Y, Dusak A, Erdem Z, Karademir B, Aydemir S, Gundogdu S: **MRCP vs. ERCP in the evaluation of biliary pathologies: review of current literature.** *J Dig Dis* 2008, **9:**162–169.
4. Wallner BK, Schumacher KA, Weidenmaier W, Friedrich JM: **Dilated biliary tract: evaluation with MR cholangiography with a T2-weighted contrast-enhanced fast sequence.** *Radiology* 1991 **181:**805–808.
5. Laubenberger J, Buchert M, Schneider B, Blum U, Hennig J, Langer M: **Breath-hold projection magnetic resonance-cholangio-pancreaticography (MRCP): a new method for the examination of the bile and pancreatic ducts.** *Magn Reson Med* 1995, **33:**18–23.
6. Bilgin M, Shaikh F, Semelka RC, Bilgin SS, Balci NC, Erdogan A: **Magnetic resonance imaging of gallbladder and biliary system.** *Top Magn Reson Imaging* 2009, **20:**31–42.
7. Chavhan GB, Babyn PS, Manson D, Vidarsson L: **Pediatric MR cholangiopancreatography: principles, technique, and clinical applications.** *Radiographics* 2008, **28:**1951–1962.
8. Yoon LS, Catalano OA, Fritz S, Ferrone CR, Hahn PF, Sahani DV: **Another dimension in magnetic resonance cholangiopancreatography: comparison of 2- and 3-dimensional magnetic resonance cholangiopancreatography for the evaluation of intraductal papillary mucinous neoplasm of the pancreas.** *J Comput Assist Tomogr* 2009, **33:**363–368.
9. Yun EJ, Choi CS, Yoon DY, Seo YL, Chang SK, Kim JS, Jy W: **Combination of magnetic resonance cholangiopancreatography and computed tomography for preoperative diagnosis of the Mirizzi syndrome.** *J Comput Assist Tomogr* 2009, **33:**636–640.
10. Kinner S, Dechene A, Ladd SC, Zöpf T, de Dechene EM, Gerken G, Lauenstein TC: **Comparison of different MRCP techniques for the depiction of biliary complications after liver transplantation.** *Eur Radiol* 2010, **20:**1749–1756.
11. Ikenoue H, Ito S, Yamada M, Takikawa Y, Yamamuro O: **Comparison MR cholangiopancreatography with 3D-fast recovery fast spin echo in several different slice thicknesses.** *Nihon Hoshasen Gijutsu Gakkai Zasshi* 2010, **66:**749–757.
12. Matsunaga K, Ogasawara G, Tsukano M, Iwadate Y, Inoue Y: **Usefulness of the navigator-echo triggering technique for free-breathing three-dimensional magnetic resonance cholangiopancreatography.** *Magn Reson Imaging* 2012, **31:**396–400.
13. Papanikolaou N, Karantanas AH, Heracleous E, Costa JC, Gourtsoyiannis N: **Magnetic resonance cholangiopancreatography: comparison between respiratory-triggered turbo spin echo and breath hold single-shot turbo spin echo sequences.** *Magn Reson Imaging* 1999, **17:**1255–1260.
14. Lim JS, Kim MJ, Myoung S, Park MS, Choi JY, Choi JS, Kim SI: **MR cholangiography for evaluation of hilar branching anatomy in transplantation of the right hepatic lobe from a living donor.** *AJR Am J Roentgenol* 2008, **191:**537–545.

15. Vitellas KM, Keogan MT, Spritzer CE, Nelson RC: **MR cholangiopancreatography of bile and pancreatic duct abnormalities with emphasis on the single-shot fast spin-echo technique.** *Radiographics* 2000, **20:**939–957.
16. Arcement CM, Meza MP, Arumanla S, Towbin RB: **MRCP in the evaluation of pancreaticobiliary disease in children.** *Pediatr Radiol* 2001, **31:**92–97.
17. Schaible R, Textor J, Kreft B, Neubrand M, Schild H: **Value of selective MIP reconstructions in respiratory triggered 3D TSE MR-cholangiography on a workstation in comparison with MIP standard projections and single-shot MRCP.** *Röfo* 2001, **173:**416–423.
18. Morita S, Saito N, Suzuki K, Mitsuhashni N: **Biliary anatomy on 3D MRCP: comparison of volume-rendering and maximum-intensity-projection algorithms.** *J Magn Reson Imaging* 2009, **29:**601–606.
19. Boraschi P, Braccini G, Gigoni R, Geloni M, Perri G: **MR cholangiopancreatography: value of axial and coronal fast Spin-Echo fat-suppressed T2-weighted sequences.** *Eur J Radiol* 1999, **32:**171–181.
20. Anderson CMSD, Tsuruda JS, Shapeero LG, Lee RG: **Artifacts in maximum-intensity-projection display of MR angiograms.** *AJR Am J Roentgenol* 1990, **153:**623–629.
21. David V, Reinhold C, Hochman M, Chuttani R, McKee J, Waxman I, Wang L, Li W, Kaplan R, Edelmann RR: **Pitfalls in the interpretation of MR cholangiopancreatography.** *AJR Am J Roentgenol* 1998, **170:**1055–1059.

4

Interactive neonatal gastrointestinal magnetic resonance imaging using fruit juice as an oral contrast media

Owen J Arthurs[1,2,3*], Martin J Graves[1], Andrea D Edwards[1], Ilse Joubert[1], Pat AK Set[1] and David J Lomas[1]

Abstract

Background: The objective was to evaluate the use of fruit juice with an interactive inversion recovery (IR) MR pulse sequence to visualise the gastrointestinal tract.

Methods: We investigated the relaxation properties of 12 different natural fruit juices in vitro, to identify which could be used as oral contrast. We then describe our initial experience using an interactive MR pulse sequence to allow optimal visualisation after administering pineapple juice orally, and suppressing pre-existing bowel fluid contents, with variable TI in three adult and one child volunteer.

Results: Pineapple juice (PJ) had both the shortest T_1 (243 ms) and shortest T_2 (48 ms) of the fruit juices tested. Optimal signal differentiation between pre-existing bowel contents and oral PJ administration was obtained with TIs of between 900 and 1100 ms.

Conclusion: The use of an inversion recovery preparation allowed long T_1 pre-existing bowel contents to be suppressed whilst the short T_1 of fruit juice acts as a positive contrast medium. Pineapple juice could be used as oral contrast agent for neonatal gastrointestinal magnetic resonance imaging.

Keywords: Neonatal, MRI, Bowel, Fruit juice

Background

Congenital abnormalities of gut rotation in neonates and infants are usually investigated by the upper gastrointestinal contrast study (UGI), using traditional X-ray fluoroscopy techniques. Malrotation is typically excluded on the basis of confidently identifying a normally positioned duodeno-jejunal (DJ) flexure, usually on the first pass of radio-opaque oral contrast medium through the duodenum at UGI [1]. However, these procedures require skilled interpretation, carry a significant radiation burden to the child, and may not always be diagnostic [2]. Optimal imaging of the neonatal GI tract is currently under review, with ongoing debate in the literature as to whether ultrasound or cross sectional imaging (such as CT) could replace the UGI series [3,4], although both have limitations, including ionising radiation doses in CT higher than that of UGI, and a significant false negative rate just as with UGI.

Recent advances in magnetic resonance imaging (MRI), particularly the development of interactive multi-contrast pulse sequences, may now provide an alternative imaging technique, thus avoiding ionising radiation. Interactive MRI allows real-time control over image plane location as well as a number of image acquisition parameters, including the development of an IR based Single Shot Fast Spin Echo (IR-SSFSE) sequence [5,6]. This could be useful in the setting of possible gut malrotation, just as interactive MRI has been used to visualise vesicoureteric reflux in the neonatal urinary tract [7]. However, in order to closely replicate the UGI series using MRI, an easily visualised contrast medium is needed.

The ideal medium should be easily tolerated, provide high positive signal enhancement, and help to distinguish the DJ flexure from pre-existing bowel contents in adjacent small bowel (likely to be a combination of milk or

* Correspondence: owen.arthurs@gosh.nhs.uk
[1]Department of Radiology, Cambridge University Hospitals NHS Foundation Trust, Cambridge CB2 0QQ, UK
[2]Department of Radiology, Great Ormond Street Hospital for Children NHS Foundation Trust, London, UK
Full list of author information is available at the end of the article

water-based material in neonates). There are several practical limitations in neonatal gut MRI, particularly regarding the choice of oral contrast agent. This is largely determined by their signal properties, the imaging modality used, the degree of gut distension required, and therefore the minimum volume of contrast agent required. Traditionally, barium sulphate is used in conventional radiographic gastrointestinal studies, but where there is a risk of spillage into the respiratory tract or perforation (particularly in paediatric studies) it has been replaced by non-ionic, low osmolality compounds (e.g. Iopamidol; Gastromiro, Bracco, High Wycombe, UK). High density barium has been used as a negative oral contrast agent for MR imaging of the gut [8], but typically requires high volumes of contrast medium to be ingested, which is not practical for neonates and small children.

Administering water (high contrast on T_2w images) may not allow confident identification of the DJ flexure separately from the pre-existing fluid in adjacent jejunal loops, a key diagnostic factor for the UGI series. Currently, there are no gadolinium-based contrast agents licensed for oral use in children, but several commercially available (i.e. commodity) fruit juices have been used as both positive and negative oral contrast agents. For example, the paramagnetic properties of fruit juices such as concentrated pineapple or blueberry juice have been used to suppress the signal from bowel fluid in paediatric magnetic resonance cholangio-pancreatography (MRCP) studies which employ heavily T_2 -weighted imaging [9,10]. As well as their T_2 effects, the T_1 shortening properties of these juices may also make them suitable positive contrast agents. However, they cannot be administered in high concentrations to neonates, due to the inability of the immature gut to deal with complex carbohydrate loads (of greater than 10%; [11]).

Administering an oral contrast medium with unknown positive signal properties, to an infant with unknown signal properties of small bowel content provides a wide range of variables. In this study, we first investigated the relaxation properties of several diluted fruit juices in vitro, to identify which could be used as oral contrast. We then describe our initial experience using an interactive MR pulse sequence, whereby real-time control over imaging parameters such as IR pulse timing could allow optimal contrast medium visualisation by suppressing pre-existing bowel fluid contents.

Methods

We optimised the interactive IR-SSFSE sequence as part of an ethically approved study into optimising gut imaging (Cambridgeshire 3 Research Ethics Committee formal approval 08/H0306/7). Three adult volunteers and one child participated, who were nil-by-mouth for 6 hours and 3 hours respectively prior to the MR examination. Full informed written consent was obtained from each participant and the child's parent. No sedation or anaesthesia was used. Ethical approval was not required for in-vitro studies.

Contrast agent testing

12 different contrast media were prepared, as follows: Tap water, standard infant formula milk (SMA Gold, SMA nutrition, Berkshire, UK), Iopamidol (Gastromiro, Bracco, High Wycombe, UK), and the following 9 commercially available (standard supermarket stock) fruit juices: orange juice, two examples of pineapple juice (one from juice; PJ, and one reconstituted from concentrate, PJ2), apple & beetroot juice, prune juice, blackcurrant juice, blueberry juice, raspberry juice, and blackberry juice. Three of these products (PJ2, prune, and blueberry juice) required further dilution to achieve a carbohydrate concentration of <10%, all other media were imaged undiluted (see Table 1). Estimated nutritional and paramagnetic agent contents of each juice are given (Table 2).

Each proposed contrast agent was placed within a multi-compartment phantom positioned inside an 8 channel brain array coil, and images acquired on a standard 1.5 T whole-body MR system (Signa HDx; GE Healthcare, Waukesha, WI; Figure 1).

The T_1 values were measured using a 2D inversion recovery (IR) prepared fast radiofrequency (RF) spoiled gradient echo (FSPGR) sequence with variable inversion times (TI) at nine different TIs (40, 80, 160, 320, 640 ms, and 1.28, 2.56, 5.12, 10.24 sec). Other imaging parameters

Table 1 Carbohydrate (COH) concentration, and measured T_1 and T_2 relaxation times of 12 different contrast media

	Solution	COH conc (per 100 ml)	T_1 (ms)	T_2 (ms)
1	Water	0	2831	1950
2	Milk	7.3%	930	148
3	Iopamidol	0	810	165
4	Orange	9.0%	1796	440
5	PJ	10.0% (12.7%*)	243	48
6	PJ2	8.6%	258	53
7	Apple/beetroot	9.6%	1679	518
8	Prune	10.0% (16.8%*)	1245	324
9	Blackcurrant	1.0%	2803	1480
10	Blueberry	10.0% (10.5%*)	573	80
11	Raspberry	0.3%	1055	146
12	Blackberry	0	831	103

COH concentration was provided from manufacturers packaging, and not tested directly.

3 juices (*) had too high a COH concentration, and so were diluted down to 10% prior to testing: the original concentrations are given in parentheses.

Table 2 Contents of each juice tested as provided by manufacturer

	Solution	Manufacturer	Description as purchased	Energy (kcal)	Protein (g)	COH (g)	Fat (g)	Iron (mg)	Manganese (mg)	Copper (mg)
2	Milk	SMA Gold	SMA Gold	67	1.9	7.3	3.3	0.64	0.09	0.06
4	Orange	Sainsburys	Pure orange juice (conc)	47	0.5	9.0	trace	0.12	0.04	0.02
5	PJ	Sainsburys	Pure pineapple juice (conc)	54	0.1	12.7	0.0	0.29	0.92	0.11
6	PJ2	Marks & Spencers	99% pineapple juice	35	0.5	8.6	0.1	0.29	0.92	0.11
7	Apple/beetroot	Marks & Spencers	Pressed apple & beetroot	40	0.3	9.6	0.1	0.12	0.07	0.01
8	Prune	Tesco	Pure prune juice	75	0.7	16.8	0.1	1.18	0.15	0.07
9	Blackcurrant	Disney	Blackcurrant with sweetener	2	trace	1.0	trace	1.54	0.26	0.08
10	Blueberry	Sainsburys	Blueberry juice drink (conc)	44	0.1	10.5	trace	0.28	0.33	0.06
11	Raspberry	Sainsburys	Juice	30	0.4	0.3	0	0.35	0.33	0.04
12	Blackberry	Twinings tea	2% blackberry flavouring, 10% blackberry leaves	0	0	0	0	0.31	0.32	0.08

Water and Iopamidol have been excluded from the table as no nutritional information is provided. All values are given per 100 ml from concentrate. Estimated iron, manganese and copper content of standard juices were obtained from the USDA National Nutrient Database (http://ndb.nal.usda.gov/).

were: field of view (FOV) 25×25 cm, slice thickness 5 mm, matrix 256 × 256, TR 7.2, TE 3.3 ms.

The T_2 values were measured using an 8-echo spin echo sequence. Eight different echo times (TE) were used, 30, 60, 90, 120, 150, 180, 210, 240 ms. Other imaging parameters were: FOV 25×25 cm, slice thickness 5 mm, matrix 256 × 256, TR 2000 ms.

We then measured the signal intensity of each contrast medium using the IR-SSFSE sequences at variable TI times (0–4000 ms), to simulate the in-vivo environment, and subtracted the signal intensity of milk to predict the possible optimal TI times in vivo.

Interactive IR-SSFSE

Interactive MRI in-vivo was performed using an IR-SSFSE pulse sequence. This modified pulse sequence has been custom developed to operate within a proprietary interactive imaging interface (i/Drive Pro Plus; GE Healthcare) which allows interactive control over many imaging parameters such as image plane location, phase encode ordering, and the use of a 180° inversion pulse that can be interactively toggled on and off prior to the SSFSE readout. The inversion time (TI) between the 180° inversion pulse and the SSFSE readout could also be interactively controlled during imaging, by inputting different IR times in ms. Initial imaging parameters for the SSFSE sequence were: FOV 25×25 cm, matrix 256×256, TR 2500 ms, TE 50.1 ms, single slice thickness of 10 mm. No motion suppression or breathing suppression technique was used.

In volunteer imaging, initial localiser images and non-interactive axial and coronal FIESTA and SSFSE sequences

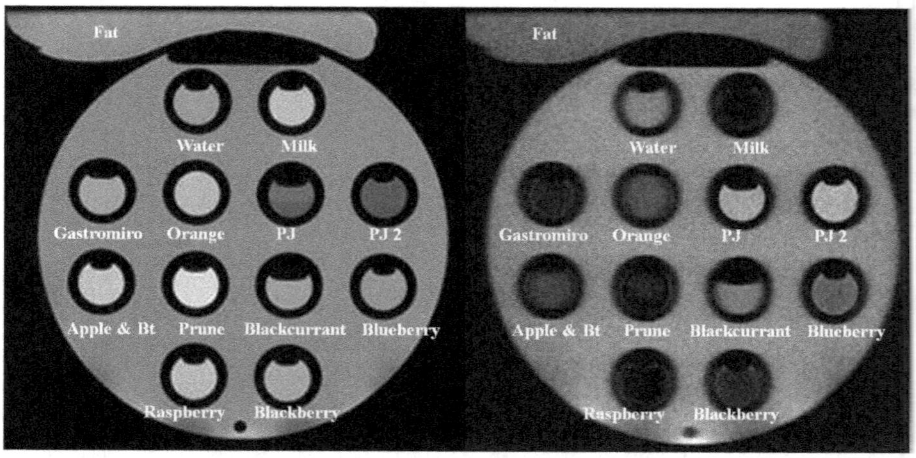

Figure 1 12 different contrast media assessed in-vitro. Pineapple juice (PJ and PJ2) have the lowest signal on T2w imaging (left : PDw SSFSE; TR 2500), but highest signal recovery on T1w imaging (right: IR-FSPGR with TI = 640 ms).

were obtained in a supine position to outline upper gastrointestinal anatomy and localise pre-existing small bowel contents. Coronal interactive IR-SSFSE was then used during free breathing to vary the TI at 100 ms intervals (between 0 and 2000 ms), and signal intensities were measured in 3 regions of interest (ROIs): stomach, proximal small bowel (duodenum) and mid-small bowel (jejunum; Figure 2), in order to characterise the signal properties of pre-existing bowel contents.

We then repeated the study with increasing TIs within 10 minutes of the oral administration of 200 ml pineapple juice to three adult volunteers, and after 20 ml pineapple juice administration to a single neonatal infant (2 week old 3 kg male infant). We did not use any form of respiratory or cardiac gating.

Results

In vitro testing

Figure 1 demonstrates the phantom used for in-vitro testing. The T_1 and T_2 relaxation times for the contrast media tested are reported in Table 1: pineapple juice from juice (PJ) was found to have both the shortest T_1 (243 ms) and T_2 (48 ms) relaxation times.

Assuming that milk was likely to be the main constituent of pre-existing bowel contents in pre-weaned infants, a representative graph of the relative difference in signal intensity between PJ and formula milk is shown in Figure 3, demonstrating that maximal differences are seen in-vitro with TIs between 500 – 900 ms.

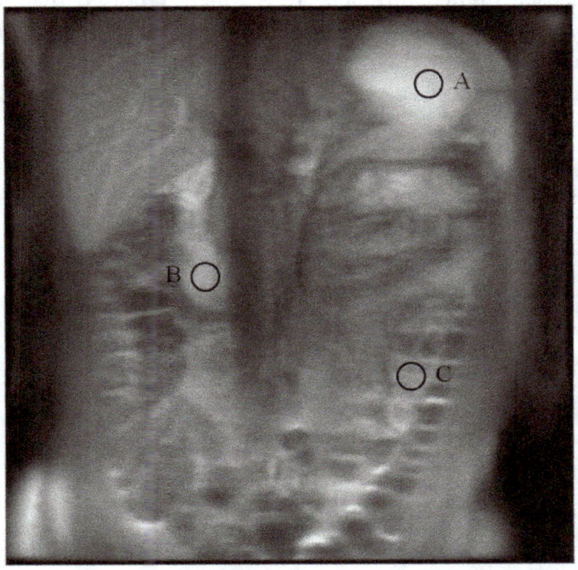

Figure 2 Coronal IR-SSFSE images through the abdomen in an adult following oral pineapple juice administration. Signal intensity was measured in 3 regions of interest: the stomach **(A)**, proximal small bowel (duodenum; **B**) and mid-small bowel (jejunum; **C**).

In vivo strategy

We subsequently tested pineapple juice as an in vivo contrast agent using the IR-SSFSE sequence: we measured signal intensity in three different ROIs (Figures 2), with increasing T1 at 100 ms intervals (0 – 2000 ms; Figure 4) before and after oral PJ administration. By subtracting the signal intensity of distal (jejunal) small bowel contents, we plotted differences in signal intensity (Figure 5) and showed that maximum differences between stomach and jejunum contents were observed at TIs of 1000 ms, 1100 ms, and 900 ms in the three adult volunteers respectively (Figure 6). We were unable to obtain good images of every TI in the neonate following 20 ml PJ administration due to patient motion, but maximal signal differences were seen at 1000 ms (Figure 7).

Discussion

This study demonstrates that pineapple juice could be used as a positive contrast agent for the proximal neonatal gut. By tailoring an IR-SSFSE sequence to null the signal from existing bowel fluid and thereby optimise the signal from PJ, we have developed a strategy for bowel visualisation using MRI which could be used in a similar fashion to the traditional UGI series in children. The true diagnostic performance of an interactive MRI strategy under these conditions remains to be evaluated.

IR-SSFSE sequences have previously been used for MR imaging of the abdomen [12], but not with interactive control. Our strategy used the IR-SSFSE sequence to effectively suppress bowel fluid signal where its properties were unknown, and to optimally tune the IR timing to provide optimal signal from a contrast agent with known signal properties. Several vendors may offer an IR-prepared sequence, such as T1-scout series or modified look-locker inversion recovery (MOLLI) sequences, where changes in inversion recovery time can be used to null myocardium during delayed enhanced imaging, for instance. However they do not allow for on-the-fly adjustment of the TI, which is necessary for rapid optimisation in a paediatric setting. Our strategy helps to tailor the examination to the individual, and has the potential to reduce overall examination time, although this remains to be evaluated in clinical practice.

One of the advantages of using the T_1 shortening properties of fruit juices are that smaller volume can be used as gut distension is not a requirement. Here, we were able to administer 200 ml to an adult, less than some studies using blueberry juice in adults (400–600 ml) [9,13,14]. Using only 20 ml in a neonate is comparable to that used in an UGI and is less than normal meal intakes. The majority of other substances used for MR gut imaging are typically combined with gut-distending agents such as mannitol, known to give gastrointestinal side effects such as flatulence

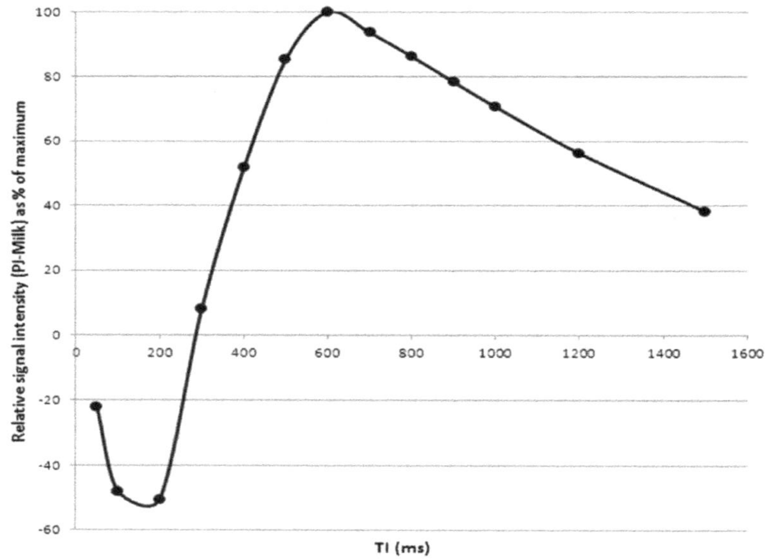

Figure 3 By subtracting the signal intensity of PJ and milk, we were able to plot the relative differences in signal (plotted as a % of maximum) between the two contrast media at different TIs. Maximal contrast differences are seen with TI between 500 – 900 ms.

and bloating, but still widely used for small bowel MR studies in older children and adults.

Despite differences in commercial products and dilutions, our measurements closely mirror those found in other studies, particularly regarding the short T_1 and T_2 of PJ [15]. We included formula milk in our evaluation and obtained similar values to the range previously measured (640–1750 ms) [16]. Several other fruit juices have been proposed as good gut contrast agents, but have only been evaluated in adults, including concentrated blueberry juice and blackberry juice [13,17,18].

The main difference between our phantom study and some previous experiments is likely to relate to the dilutions used; several previous studies measured the signal characteristics of concentrated fruit juices, or indeed fruit pulp itself [17]. Concentrated fruit juices can stimulate gut transit in non-weaned infants, causing diarrhoea and nappy irritation, which can be both uncomfortable and distressing for the child and care-giver, which is why we used diluted products. It is widely reported that the signal suppression effect is due to T_2 relaxation caused by their inherently high iron (blackberry) or manganese (pineapple, beet juice, green tea) content, although the

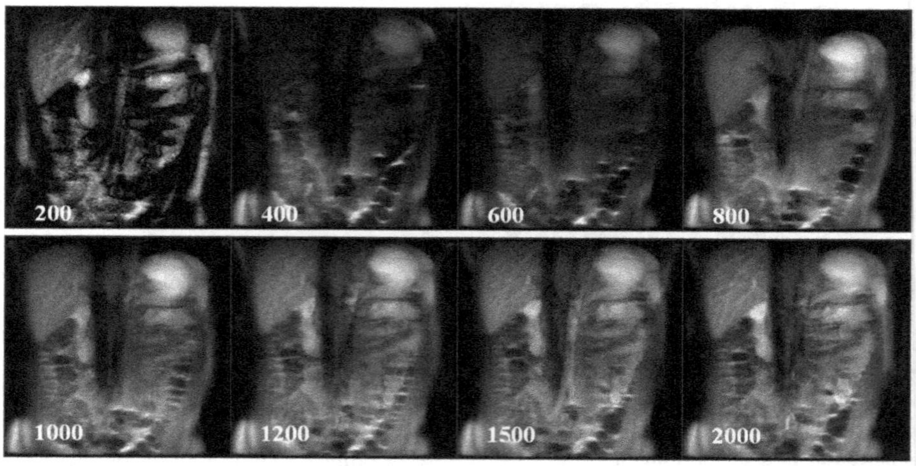

Figure 4 Coronal IR-SSFSE images (TI = 1200 ms) through the abdomen in an adult following oral pineapple juice administration. Examples of different TI times (200 – 2000 ms) are given. Relative signal intensity from this study is given in Figure 5.

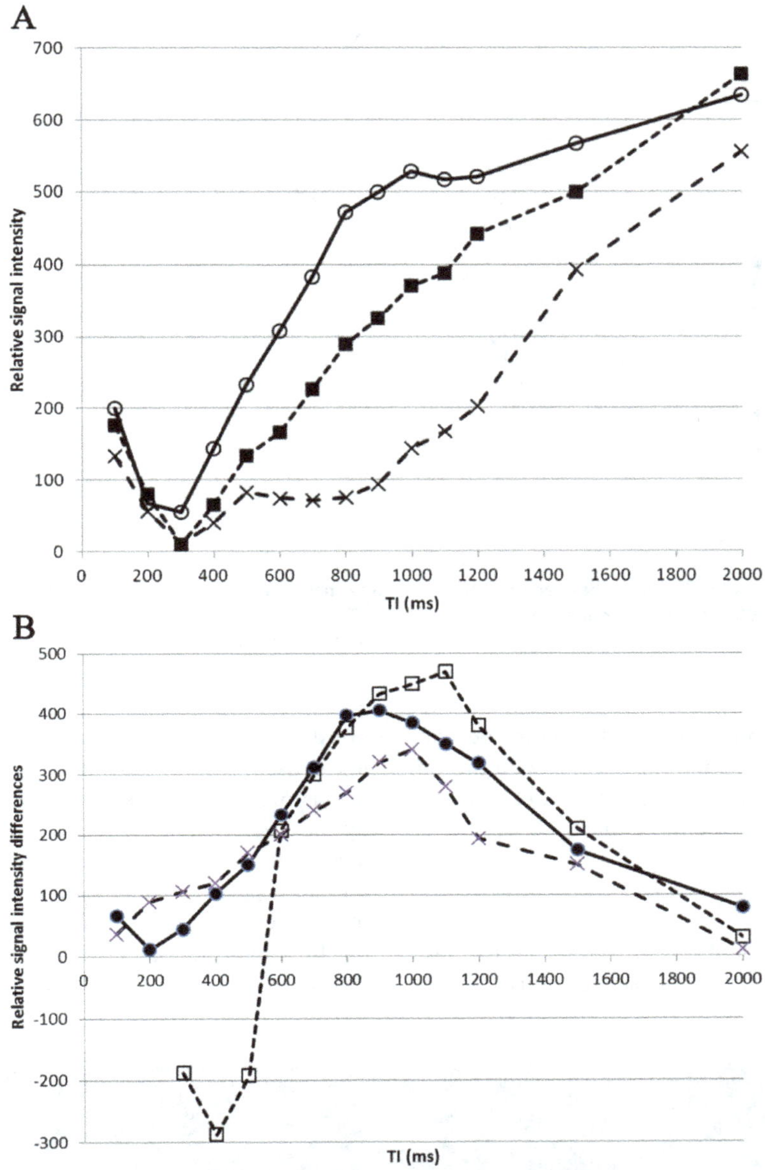

Figure 5 A. Relative signal intensity in three gut regions (A, B and C in Figure 2) following oral pineapple juice administration. ROIs were A: stomach (open circles, solid line), B : proximal small bowel (filled squares, dashed line), and C: more distal small bowel (cross, dotted line). **B.** Relative signal intensity *differences* (as a % of maximum) between stomach and distal small bowel (A – C; filled circles, solid line), and between proximal and more distal small bowel (B – C; open squares, dashed line).

exact contents of different commercial fruit juices vary widely, and the precise paramagnetic component (iron, copper or manganese) that gives the relaxation shortening property is debatable. We estimated the paramagnetic agent contents of each of our fruit juices (Table 2) and hypothesise that it may be the manganese content of pineapple juice which gave favourable properties in this study.

Several other oral agents have been developed and have been comprehensively reviewed elsewhere [19]. These can be grouped into predominantly *positive* gastrointestinal MR imaging contrast media, typically gadolinium-based compounds e.g. Magnevist Enteral® (Schering AG, Berlin, Germany) or Gadolinium zeolite (Gadolite®; Pharmacyclics, Sunnyvale, CA, now GlaxoSmithKline Ltd, Brentford, UK), or *negative* gastrointestinal MR imaging contrast agents, particularly iron-containing solutions such as Perflubron® (Imagent GI®, Alliance Pharma), or Abdoscan® (Nycomed-Amersham, Oslo, Norway). Most of these are not commercially available, and are not licensed for children. Carbon dioxide gas has also been used as a negative contrast agent

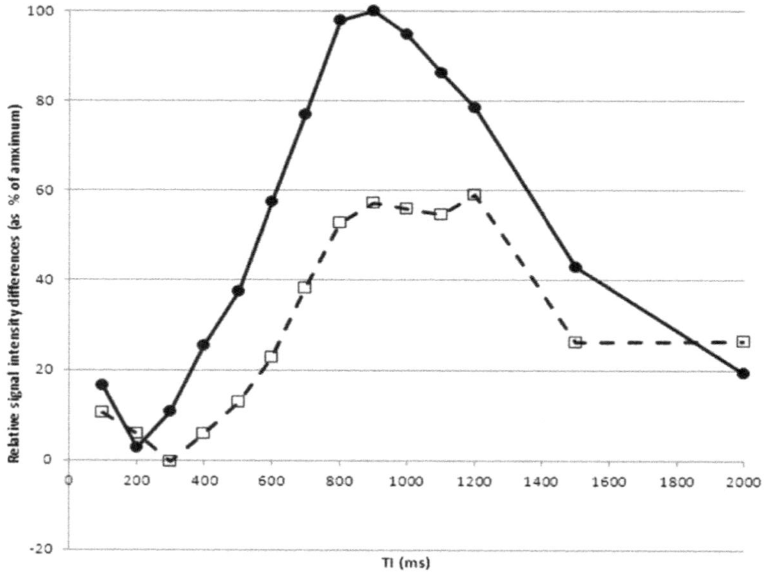

Figure 6 Relative signal intensity *differences* between stomach and proximal small bowel, with maximum differences observed at TIs of 1000 ms, 1100 ms, and 900 ms in three individual adult volunteers. The shape of each graph was similar, with signal brighter in small bowel than stomach in one individual, which may suggest rapid transit time. The consistent maximum differences at TI of 900 – 1100 ms are roughly in keeping with the in-vitro results.

for proximal gut MR imaging and early studies demonstrated acceptable visualisation of the duodenum but were limited in the jejunum and small bowel [20], but this remains to be investigated in neonates.

Limitations of this study

One limitation of this feasibility study could be the variable content of commercially available fruit juice. We did not determine the exact constituents of the different fruit juices used in this study, but relied on the manufacturers details provided on the packaging and estimated provided by the USDA National Nutrient Database (http://ndb.nal.usda.gov). Since the concentrations of fruit pulp and therefore paramagnetic properties of diluted commercial fruit juices may vary, the ability to interactively optimise the IR timing becomes even more important as a way to compensate for these variations.

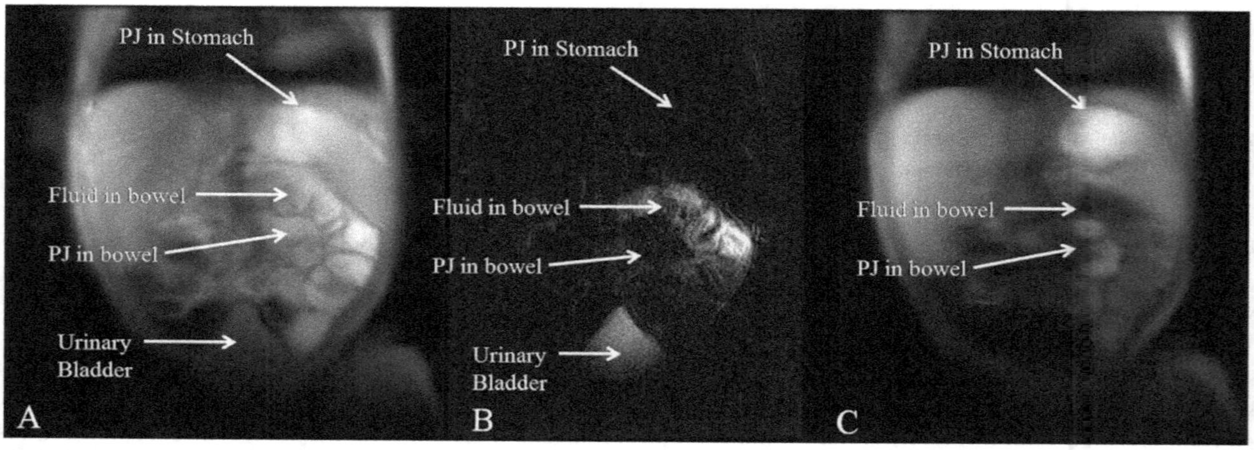

Figure 7 Coronal IR-SSFSE of neonatal GI tract. A 2 week old 3 kg male infant underwent MRI following PJ administration. **A.** Conventional SSFSE (TR 2500 ms) imaging. It is not possible to differentiate between PJ in the stomach and proximal small bowel from fluid already in the small bowel on conventional T2w imaging. **B.** T_2w hydrographic SSFSE image (TR of 4000 ms) demonstrating location of pre-existing bowel fluid. The short T_2 PJ in the stomach and proximal bowel is low signal. **C.** IR-SSFSE PDw (TI = 1000 ms) that nulls the signal from pre-existing bowel fluid, and demonstrates PJ as high signal in stomach and proximal bowel.

We acknowledge that we did not include any patients in this volunteer feasibility study, and have tested only a limited number of volunteers. The full diagnostic potential of this technique now needs to be evaluated in a larger patient population.

Conclusion

In conclusion, this work indicates that pineapple juice is the most promising natural commercially available short T_1 contrast medium suitable for neonatal GI tract imaging using an interactively adjusted inversion-recovery SSFSE strategy. This allows for pre-existing longer T_1, bowel contents to be suppressed, whilst the short T_1 of the PJ acts as a positive contrast medium to delineate the gut. This approach allows individual tailoring of the examination, to give optimal discrimination of an orally administered contrast agent from the background signal of gut contents. Further work is required using this strategy in a larger cohort of neonates and infants to evaluate both technical and diagnostic performance.

Competing interests
The authors declare that they have no competing interests, financial or non-financial

Authors' contributions
OA, MJG, IJ and ADE carried out the in-vitro studies, and OA, MJG, IJ and PS carried out the in-vivo interactive MRI studies. All authors participated in the design of the study and helped to draft the manuscript. All authors read and approved the final manuscript.

Acknowledgements
OJA was funded by a Medical Research Council/Royal College of Radiologists Clinical Research Training Fellowship. The views expressed in this publication are those of the author(s). The project was supported by the Addenbrookes Charitable Trust, and the NIHR comprehensive Biomedical Research Centre award to Cambridge University Hospitals NHS Foundation Trust in partnership with the University of Cambridge. None of the funding bodies had any role in analysis of data, results or conclusions of the study.

Author details
[1]Department of Radiology, Cambridge University Hospitals NHS Foundation Trust, Cambridge CB2 0QQ, UK. [2]Department of Radiology, Great Ormond Street Hospital for Children NHS Foundation Trust, London, UK. [3]UCL Institute of Child Health, London, UK.

References
1. Long FR, Kramer SS, Markowitz RI, Taylor GE: **Radiographic patterns of intestinal malrotation in children.** *Radiographics* 1996, **16**:547–556.
2. Sizemore AW, Rabbani KZ, Ladd A, Applegate KE: **Diagnostic performance of the upper gastrointestinal series in the evaluation of children with clinically suspected malrotation.** *Pediatr Radiol* 2008, **38**:518–528.
3. Daneman A: **Malrotation: the balance of evidence.** *Pediatr Radiol* 2009, **39**:S164–S166.
4. Taylor GA: **CT appearance of the duodenum and mesenteric vessels in children with normal and abnormal gut rotation.** *Pediatr Radiol* 2011, **41**:1378–1383.
5. Graves MJ, Wong P, Black RT, Lomas DJ: **MR fluoroscopy employing interactive pulse sequence switching.** *Proc ISMRM* 2007, **15**:1654.
6. Makki M, Graves MJ, Lomas DJ: **Interactive body MR fluoroscopy using SSFSE RARE with multiparameter control.** *J MRI* 2002, **16**:85–93.
7. Arthurs OJ, Edwards AD, Joubert I, Graves MJ, Set PAK, Lomas DJ: **Interactive magnetic resonance voiding cystourethrography (iMRVC) for vesicoureteric reflux (VUR) in unsedated infants: a feasibility study.** *Eur Radiol* 2011, **21**:1874–1881.
8. Li KCP, Tart RP, Fitzsimmons JR, Storm BL, Mao J, Rolfes RJ: **Barium sulfate suspension as a negative oral MRI contrast agent: In vitro and human optimization studies.** *MRI* 1991, **9**:141–150.
9. Riordan RD, Khonsari M, Jeffries J, Maskell GF, Cook PG: **Pineapple juice as a negative oral contrast agent in magnetic resonance cholangiopancreatography: a preliminary evaluation.** *Br J Radiol* 2004, **77**:991–999.
10. Darge K, Anupindi S: **Pancreatitis and the role of US, MRCP and ERCP.** *Pediatr Radiol* 2009, **39**:S153–7.
11. Baker SS on behalf of the Committee on Nutrition: **The use and misuse of fruit juice in paediatrics.** *Paediatrics* 2001, **107**:1210–1213.
12. Lauenstein TC, Sharma P, Hughes T, Heberlein K, Tudorascu D, Martin DR: **Evaluation of optimized inversion-recovery fat-suppression techniques for T2-weighted abdominal MR imaging.** *J Magn Reson Imaging* 2008, **27**:1448–54.
13. Hiraishi K, Narabayashi I, Fujita O, Yamamoto K, Sagami A, Hisada Y, Saika Y, Adachi I, Hasegawa H: **Blueberry juice: preliminary evaluation as an oral contrast agent in gastrointestinal MR imaging.** *Radiology* 1995, **194**:119–23.
14. Papanikolaou N, Karantanas A, Maris T, Gourtsoyannis N: **MR cholangiopancreatography before and after oral blueberry juice administration.** *J Comput Assist Tomogr* 2000, **24**:229–234.
15. Asbach P, Breitwieser C, Diederichs G, Eisele S, Kivelitz D, Taupitz M, Zeitz M, Hamm B, Klessen C: **Cine magnetic resonance imaging of the small bowel: comparison of different oral contrast media.** *Acta Radiol* 2006, **47**:899–906.
16. Balzarini L, Aimeb S, Barberob L, Ceglia E, Petrillo R: **Magnetic resonance imaging of the gastrointestinal tract: investigation of baby milk as a low cost contrast medium.** *Eur Radiol* 1992, **15**:171–174.
17. Karantanas AH, Papanikolaou N, Kalef-Ezra J, Challa A, Gourtsoyiannis N: **Blueberry juice used per os in upper abdominal MR imaging: composition and initial clinical data.** *Eur Radiol* 2000, **10**:909–13.
18. Espinosa MG, Sosa M, De León-Rodríguez LM, Córdova T, Bernal-Alvarado J, Avila-Rodríguez M, Reyes-Aguilera JA, Ortíz JJ, Barrios FA: **Blackberry (Rubus spp.): a pH-dependent oral contrast medium for gastrointestinal tract images by magnetic resonance imaging.** *Magn Reson Imaging* 2006, **24**:195–200.
19. Giovagnoni A, Fabbri A, Maccioni F: **Oral contrast agents in MRI of the gastrointestinal tract.** *Abdom Imaging* 2002, **27**:367–375.
20. Lomas DJ, Habib SH, Joubert IJ, Sala E, Graves MJ: **CO2 as a distending medium for gastric and small bowel MRI: a feasibility study.** *Eur Radiol* 2005, **15**:672–6.

5

Magnetic resonance imaging of penile paraffinoma

Luigi Cormio[1*], Giuseppe Di Fino[1], Carmen Scavone[2], Oscar Selvaggio[1], Paolo Massenio[1], Francesca Sanguedolce[3], Luca Macarini[2] and Giuseppe Carrieri[1]

Abstract

Background: Penile paraffinoma is a well-known delayed complication of paraffin oil injection into the penis for penile girth augmentation but its MRI features have not been previously described.

Case presentation: A 35-year-old Ukraine man presented with erectile dysfunction, voiding difficulty and an irregular, hard and painful penile mass that had progressively grown over the last year. He reported having received, seven years before, several penile injections of paraffin oil for penile girth augmentation. On physical examination, the mass was tender, poorly delimited, and involved the whole penile shaft and the cranial part of the scrotum. Preoperative MRI, performed to determine the extent of tissue to be removed and the possibilities of penile reconstruction, showed a newly-formed homogeneous tissue, compressing but not infiltrating Buck's fascia, iso-hypointense relative to muscle on T1-weighted sequences, and with a low signal intensity at T2-weighted sequences. On T1-weighted fat suppressed sequences, it did not enhance with contrast administration. MRI data were confirmed by surgical findings, as the newly-formed scar tissue did not infiltrate Buck's fascia. Pathology confirmed the diagnosis of penile paraffinoma.

Conclusion: MRI seems to provide an adequate imaging of the histological events occurring after injection of paraffin oil in the subcutaneous tissues. Penile paraffinoma remains a clinical diagnosis, but MRI features may be helpful in planning an adequate surgical strategy and, in selected cases, establishing the differential diagnosis with other penile diseases, including cancer.

Keywords: Lipogranuloma, Penis, Mineral oils, Diagnosis, MRI

Background

In the first half of the 20th century, subcutaneous injection of liquid paraffin has widely been used worldwide [1] for cosmetic purposes such as filling of wrinkles or cheeks, facial deformities, baldness [2], as well as to produce an artificial augmentation of muscle, breast [3] and penile shaft [4]. The potential destructive complications of such practice, however, have been reported since 1906 [5]. The most relevant acute complication is infection; delayed complications, conversely, are linked to a granulomatous foreign body reaction named paraffinoma [4,6].

Penile paraffinoma may present with penile scarring and deformity, abscess formation, ulceration, erectile dysfunction, painful intercourse, and voiding problems [4] up to acute urinary retention [7]. Although all such problems are well known, penile injection of paraffin remains a common means of increasing penile girth for Eastern Europe and Eastern Asia people. Reasons for this unreasonable practice include, on one hand, the fact that it is easily available and easily performed by non-medical personnel or the patient himself, on the other hand, lack of standardized medical or surgical techniques for penile girth enhancement.

Most reported cases of penile paraffinoma focused on disease clinical presentation or on techniques for surgical excision and penile reconstruction [8,9]. To our knowledge, the imaging features of penile paraffinoma have not been previously described. Therefore, we describe herein MRI findings in a case of penile paraffinoma and discuss their potential implications on differential diagnosis and surgical planning.

* Correspondence: luigicormio@libero.it
[1]Department of Urology and Renal Transplantation, University of Foggia, Via Luigi Pinto, 71122 Foggia, Italy
Full list of author information is available at the end of the article

Case presentation

A 35-year-old man emigrated from Ukraine presented to our Emergency Department with an irregular penile mass associated with erectile dysfunction and voiding difficulty. The patient reported that the penile mass had progressively grown over the last year up to become, in the last month, hard and painful. Physical examination revealed a tender, poorly delimited, subcutaneous indurated mass that extended on the whole surface of the penile shaft, from the coronal sulcus to the cranial part of the scrotum whereby the granulation tissue was palpable under the skin. The mass had no adherence to the overlying planes and was painful on palpation. There was no ulceration or inguinal lymphadenopathy.

There were no relevant findings in patient's medical history and he reluctantly admitted that 7 years before he had received 6 injections of paraffin oil into the penis, performed by an untrained person, for penile enlargement purposes; therefore, penile paraffinoma was diagnosed. He was scheduled for definite surgical treatment involving complete removal of the newly-formed penile mass and penile shaft reconstruction. In view of the extent of tissue to be removed and the risk of scrotal tissue as well being involved by scarring, thus leading to its removal rather than its use for reconstruction, the patient underwent preoperative penile MRI to properly plan surgery.

Penile MRI was performed with a 1.5 T whole body MR unit (Philips Achieva) with the patient supine. The penis was flexed dorsally against the lower abdomen and taped in position to reduce motion of the organ during the examination. A SENSE Torso coil (8 elements) was positioned on the pelvis. First, axial T2-weighted TSE (Turbo Spin Echo) images (TR/TE, 10111/120 ms; ETL, 20) and axial T1-weighted TSE images (889/12) were acquired. Then, coronal FFE T2-weighted images (500/13), sagittal and coronal TSE T2-weighted (6009/120) were acquired. Finally, axial T1-weighted GRE images (10,9/5,4) were acquired with fat suppression before and after a bolus injection of gadopentate dimegluine (0.5 mmol/mL; 0.2 mL/Kg). During all pulse sequences we used the following common parameters: a field of view of 260 mm, a slice thickness of 4 mm, and a matrix of 320 × 224. MRI showed a 18 mm thick lesion in the subcutaneous tissues of the penile shaft, surrounding the cavernous bodies up to spraining them in some points, causing a minimal distortion of the glans and a moderate narrowing of the bulbar urethra (Figure 1). Such lesion showed a homogeneous signal, iso-hypointense relative to muscle on T1-weighted sequences, and a low signal intensity at T2-weighted sequences (Figure 2). On T1-weighted fat suppressed sequences, it did not enhance with contrast administration. MRI features were therefore consistent with a fibrotic scar-tissue between dartos and Buck's fascia, attached but not infiltrating the latter, which remained visible as a thin line hypointense in all pulse sequences. MRI also showed, in the cranial part of the scrotum, a granulation tissue with high signal intensity on T2-weighted turbo spin-echo sequence, low signal intensity on T1-weighted turbo spin-echo sequence, and significant homogeneous contrast enhancement (Figure 3).

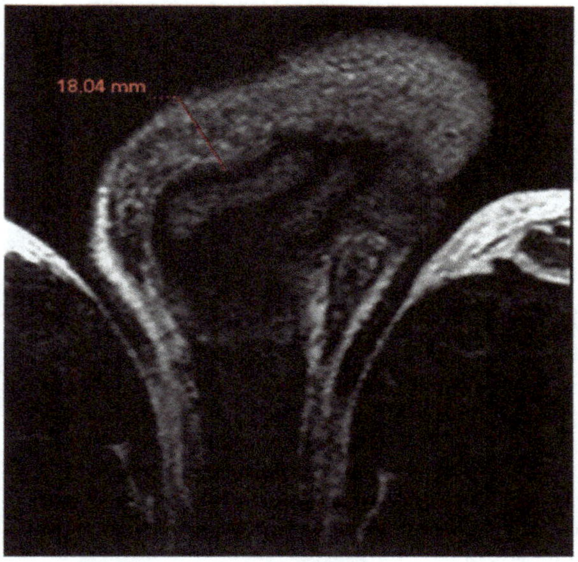

Figure 1 Axial T1-weighted TSA MR imaging shows iso-hypointense 18 mm tissue (red line) surrounding the corpora cavernosa of the penis.

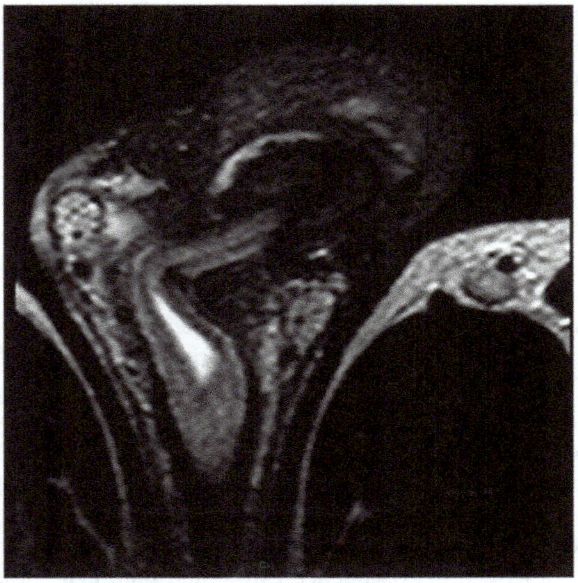

Figure 2 Axial T2-weighted TSA MR imaging showing the fibrotic tissue that leads to a severe narrowing of the penile urethra with dilatation of the upstream tract.

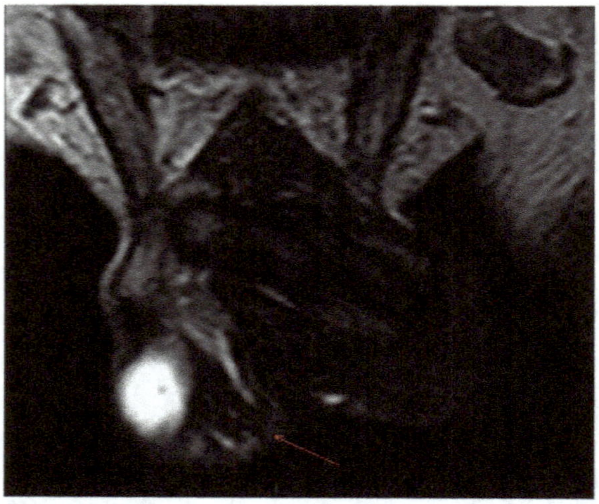

Figure 3 Coronal T2-weighted TSA MR imaging showing fibrotic reaction (red arrow) extended in the connective tissue of the scrotal sac.

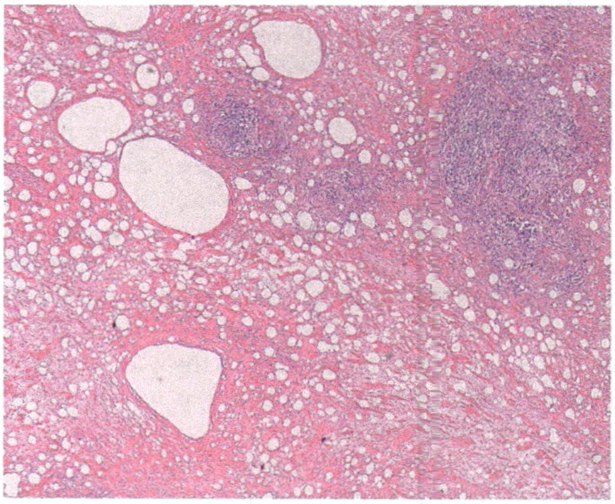

Figure 4 Histological image of the removed tissue showing optical empty spaces indicative of the presence of large fat globules dissolved during the staining process, along with a heavy inflammation mainly consisting of lymphocytes and histiocytes, throughout the whole specimen.

On the basis of these findings the patient was scheduled for surgical removal of the lesion, taking care to preserve Buck's fascia and the underlying dorsal penile neurovascular bundle and to reconstruct with vital tissue the penile shaft. Postoperative course was uneventful; the urethral catheter was removed on the following morning and the patient discharged. At six weeks follow-up, he reported to be very satisfied with the cosmetic result as well as with his sexual function. Histological examination of the removed tissue confirmed the diagnosis of paraffinoma, showing optical empty spaces indicative of the presence of large fat globules dissolved during the staining process, along with a heavy inflammation mainly consisting of lymphocytes and histiocytes, throughout the whole specimen (Figure 4).

Conclusion

There is clinical and histological evidence [10,11] that injection of paraffin oil into penile subcutaneous tissue promotes a slow foreign-body granulomatous reaction leading to conversion of the liquid mineral oil into a solid, fibrous-like tissue. The "early" MRI appearance of paraffin oil into penile shaft has been described by Picozzi et al. [12] who reported that, shortly (48 hours) after injection, the oil displays hyperintensity on both T1- and T2-weighted sequences. Herein we provide the first description of MRI findings in case penile paraffinoma, a "late" event following paraffin oil injection into the penis. Using the described MRI sequences, we found that, like fibrous tissue, penile paraffinoma displayed low to intermediate intensity on both T1- and T2- weighted sequences, with no contrast enhancement. Taking these findings together, it can be stated that MRI provides an adequate imaging of the histological events occurring after injection of paraffin in the penile subcutaneous tissue.

An interesting finding of our report is that, in case of paraffinoma, the newly-formed fibrotic tissue does not jeopardizes the ability of MR imaging to evaluate the normal penile structures, particularly Buck's fascia and neurovascular bundle. As a matter of fact, surgical exploration confirmed our MRI findings of paraffinoma fibrotic tissue attached but not infiltrating Buck's fascia, which was visible as a thin line hypointense in all pulse sequences. This information is of great clinical relevance in planning the surgical strategy and in counseling patient's about cosmetic and functional results of surgery.

Another interesting point is that, although penile paraffinoma remains a clinical diagnosis based on patient's admittance of such practice, diseases such as thrombosis of dorsal penile vein, syphilis, herpes genitalis, Behcet and, last but not least, tumors [13] may occur independently on injection of paraffin into the penis. Therefore, further validation of the reported MRI findings of penile paraffinoma could provide valuable clues in the differential diagnosis with all such diseases.

Finally, our MRI findings of penile paraffinoma were consistent with MRI findings of paraffinomas in the cervico-facial area [14] as well as of breast paraffinoma [1,15] somehow confirming the efficacy of MRI in providing an adequate imaging of the human body reaction to the injection of such oil.

In conclusion, though penile paraffinoma remains a clinical diagnosis, the MRI features described herein may be helpful in planning an adequate surgical strategy and, in selected cases, establishing the differential diagnosis with other penile diseases, including cancer.

Consent

Written informed consent was obtained from the patient for publication of this report and any accompanying images. A copy of the written consents is available for review by the Editor-in-Chief of this journal.

Abbreviations

MRI: Magnetic Resonance Imaging; TSE: Turbo Spin-Echo; T1W: T1-weighted; T2W: T2-weighted; TR: Repetition time; TE: Echo time; ETL: Echo train length.

Competing interests

The authors declare that they have no competing interests.

Authors' contributions

LC: manuscript conception and critical revision. GDF and CS: manuscript drafting. OS and PM: data analysis. FS: pathology review. LM and GC: supervision and manuscript final approval. All authors read and approved the final manuscript.

Acknowledgements

The study received no funding.

Author details

[1]Department of Urology and Renal Transplantation, University of Foggia, Via Luigi Pinto, 71122 Foggia, Italy. [2]Department of Radiology, University of Foggia, Foggia, Italy. [3]Department of Pathology, University of Foggia, Foggia, Italy.

References

1. Erguvan-Dogan B, Yang WT: **Direct injection of paraffin into the breast: mammographic, sonographic and MRI features of early complications.** *AJR Am J Roentgenol* 2006, **186:**888–894.
2. Klein JA, Cole G, Barr RJ, Bartlow G, Fulwinder C: **Paraffinomas of the salp.** *Arch Dermatol* 1995, **21:**382–385.
3. Alagaratnam TT, Ng WF: **Paraffinomas of the breast: an oriental curiosity.** *Aust N Z J Surg* 1996, **66:**138–140.
4. Cohen JL, Keoleian CM, Krull EA: **Penile paraffinoma: self-injection with mineral oil.** *J Eur Acad Dermatol Venereol* 2001, **45:**S222–S224.
5. Lee T, Choi HR, Lee YT, Lee YH: **Paraffinoma of the penis.** *Yonsei Med J* 1994, **35:**344–348.
6. Santos P, Chaveiro A, Nunes G, Fonseca J, Cardoso J: **Penile paraffinoma.** *J Eur Acad Dermatol Venereol* 2003, **17:**583–584.
7. De Siati M, Selvaggio O, Di Fino G, Liuzzi G, Massenio P, Sanguedolce F, Carrieri G, Cormio L: **An unusual delayed complication of paraffin self-injection for penile girth augmentation.** *BMC Urol* 2013, **13:**66.
8. Rosemberg E, Romanowsky I, Asali M, Kaneti J: **Three case of penile paraffinoma: a conservative approach.** *J Urol* 2007, **70:**372.e9–372.e10.
9. Shin YS, Zhao C, Park JK: **New reconscructive surgery for penile paraffinoma to prevent necrosis of ventral penile skin.** *J Urol* 2012, **81:**437–441.
10. Hohaus K, Bley B, Kostler E, Schonlebe J, Wollina U: **Mineral oil granuloma of the penis.** *J Eur Acad Derm Vener* 2003, **17**(5):585–587.
11. Pehlivanov G, Kavaklieva S, Kazandjieva J, Kapnilov D, Tsankov N: **Foreign-body granuloma of the penis in sexually active individuals (penile paraffinoma).** *J Eur Acad Derm Vener* 2008, **22**(7):845–851.
12. Picozzi SCM, Carmignani L: **Paraffinoma of the penis.** *Int J Emerg Med* 2010, **3:**507–508.
13. Pònyai K, Marschalkò M, Hàrsing J, Ostorhàzy E, Kelemen Z, Nyiràdy P, Vàrkonyi V, Kàrpàti S: **Paraffinoma.** *JDDG* 2010, **9:**686–688.
14. Gu DH, Yoon DY, Chang SK, Lim KJ: **CT features of foreign body granulomas after cosetic paraffin injection into the cervicofacial area.** *Diagn Interv Radiol* 2010, **4261:**1305–1825.
15. Khong PL, Ho LWC, Chan JHM, Leong LLY: **MR Imaging of breast paraffinomas.** *AJR* 1999, **173:**929–932.

6

Concomitant septic arthritis and osteomyelitis of the hip in young children; a new pathophysiological hypothesis suggested by MRI enhancement pattern

Laura Merlini[1*], Mehrak Anooshiravani[1] and Dimitri Ceroni[2]

Abstract

Background: In children, septic arthritis (SA) of the hip is either primary or concomitant with acute haematogenous osteomyelitis (AHO). However, seldom, patients with isolated SA at presentation, may later show osteomyelitis in the metaphysis. The aim of this study was to elaborate a physiopathological hypothesis based on the peculiar MRI findings to explain the onset of AHO after SA.

Methods: Cases of acute infection of the hip admitted between January 2010 and December 2013 were retrospectively reviewed to assess radiographic and MRI features, as well as bacteriological findings. Only children with isolated SA were included in this study, whereas cases of concomitant SA and AHO at presentation were excluded.

Results: Ten patients met the inclusion criteria. Six (1–11 months) demonstrated, on the initial MRI, decreased perfusion on gadolinium enhanced fat-suppressed T1-weighted sequence of the femoral epiphysis and developed one month later metaphyseal AHO. Four (5–14 years) did not show decreased perfusion and did not develop AHO on follow-up. The type of germ involved influenced neither the type of enhancement pattern nor the outcome.

Conclusions: Age under one year and decreased perfusion of the affected femoral epiphysis increases the risk of secondary AHO. Our study is the first report in human medicine supporting the physiopathological hypothesis described by Alderson et al. in an animal model: primary infection can originally affect the joint, then penetrate the epiphyseal cartilage, and finally spread into the metaphyseal region through transphyseal vessels present only in the first 12/18 months of life.

Background

Early diagnosis of hip septic arthritis (SA) is paramount to prevent immediate joint damage and to avoid late devastating complications in infants, especially in newborns. [1–5]. Children with concomitant SA and AHO have statistically less favorable outcome, and require both more surgical procedures and longer antibiotic therapy than patients with isolated SA or AHO [6–8].

In the literature, SA is reported as a frequent complication of AHO in children [9–11] and not the other way round. According to the classical pathogenetic theory, bone sepsis in the early stages of osteomyelitis typically arises in the metaphyseal side of the growth plate of long tubular bones favoured by a peculiar aspect of vessels beneath the physeal plate: in fact they present a dilated turning point with low velocity flow allowing bacterial development [12]. In addition, the endothelium wall of the metaphyseal capillaries has gaps that allow the passage of bacteria and, moreover, phagocytic cells are absent in this region of the bone [13]. Translocated pathogens then find locally favourable conditions to proliferate due to the absence of phagocytic cells in this region of the bone. Furthermore, infection easily spreads to the articular cavity due to the low attachment of capsular structures in young children, extensively involving the metaphyseal region [12, 14].

* Correspondence: laura.merlini@hcuge.ch
[1]Unit of Pediatric Radiology Geneva University Hospital HUG, 6 Willy-Donzé, Geneva 1205, Switzerland
Full list of author information is available at the end of the article

In recent years, MRI has gained interest to establish the diagnosis of osteoarticular infection of the hip, especially for excluding concomitant SA with AHO [15–18].

However, in few situations, the classical MRI signs of AHO are lacking at presentation and bone infection manifests later. This study attempts to suggest a physio-pathological hypothesis to explain the onset of AHO after SA and to identify early MRI signs predicting which patients are at risk secondary AHO.

Methods

After approval by the Institutional Review Board (University Hospital of Geneva 09-029R, Mat-Ped 09-008R), medical charts of all children admitted to our tertiary care hospital from January 2010 to December 2013 for suspicion of osteoarticular infection of the hip were retrospectively reviewed. Analyses were based on clinical records, demographics (age and gender), body temperature, and laboratory data including bacterial cultures (from blood and bone samples), white blood cell count (WBC), platelet count, erythrocyte sedimentation rate (ESR) and serum C-reactive protein (CRP). Since 2007, all samples are also analyzed using either a broad range PCR assay or a new, real-time PCR assay specific to *K. kingae*. Radiological studies of the hip were available for all patients, and included plain radiographs, and MRIs.

For children less than 5 years, MRI was performed under general anesthesia whereas the examination was realized without sedation in older children. MRI studies were performed on a 1.5-T Avanto (Siemens) machine and the protocol included coronal turbo spin echo T1-weighted sequences (TR/TE = 500/ 12), axial turbo spin echo T2-weighted images (TR/ TE =6420/99), 3 days T2 STIR SPACE images (TR/ TE =2000/201, thickness = 1,3–1,5 mm, isometric), and coronal (TR/ TE = 639/13) and axial (TR/TE = 350/8,8) fat-suppressed spin-echo T1-weighted images after intravenous administration of gadopentetate dimeglumine (Dotarem) at a dose of 0.1 mmol/kg body weight. Contrast enhanced images were obtained directly after contrast injection and no dynamic sequences were obtained. Then children were transferred under general anesthesia to the operating room where joint fluid or bone aspirate specimen were taken and sent to the laboratory for Gram staining and immediate inoculation onto Columbia blood agar (incubated under anaerobic conditions), CDC anaerobe 5 % sheep blood agar (incubated under anaerobic conditions), chocolate agar (incubated in a CO_2-enriched atmosphere), and brain-heart broth. Incubation time was 10 days. All samples were also analyzed using either a broad range PCR assay or a new, real-time PCR assay specific to *K. kingae*.

MRI studies were anonymized, coded and transferred to a dedicated computer station and stored in random order. Two senior pediatric radiologists (LM and MA) independently reviewed MR images. Only patients with MR signs of isolated SA were included in this study, whereas children with concomitant SA and AHO at initial investigation were excluded from the study. According to the literature, we analyzed the images as follows:

1. AHO was diagnosed when there was focally decreased marrow signal intensity on T1-weighted images and focally increased marrow signal intensity on fluid-sensitive images (fat-suppressed T2-Weighted and STIR sequences). On enhanced, fat- suppressed T1-weighted images, osteomyelitis usually presents as focal abnormal bone marrow enhancement [17, 19] and sometimes, in children, as focal enhancement defects of the epiphyseal cartilage [20].
2. We considered isolated SA when there was joint effusion with or without soft tissue involvement. Joint effusion was quantified as mild if there was only a small hyperintense line on T2-Weighted sequences, moderate if there was a more significant effusion and important if the femoral head was eccentric.
3. The enhancement pattern of the femoral epiphyseal head cartilage and bone nucleus was qualitatively compared to the contralateral side on substraction images, and on slices with the most intense enhancement.

On the Fat SAT T1 enhanced sequence, the normal cartilaginous femoral epiphysis appears uniformly hyperintense (Fig. 1a arrow) before the appearance of femoral head ossification centers. With the appearance of ossification centers, normal cartilaginous femoral epiphysis presents a « striate » aspect due to enhanced vessels (Fig. 2a arrows). Ossification centers are uniformly enhanced in comparison with the pre-contrast appearance and surrounded by a thin hyperintense line (Fig. 2a arrowhead). The cartilaginous part reduces with age and this « striate » aspect usually disappears by the second year of life.

In our study, decreased perfusion was considered when the pathological femoral epiphysis was uniformly hypointense in comparison to the contralateral side (Fig. 1a arrowhead) if the ossification centers were not present. If present, when they were hypointense, the surrounding line did not enhance and the "striate" aspect of the cartilaginous part was absent (Fig. 3a arrows). We did not measure enhancement ratios.

Conventional X ray studies of the hip were performed in all cases one month after the MRI and images were reviewed by the same two radiologists: signs of AHO sequelae (lytic lesions, sclerosis, or disappearing of ossification centers) were reported if present.

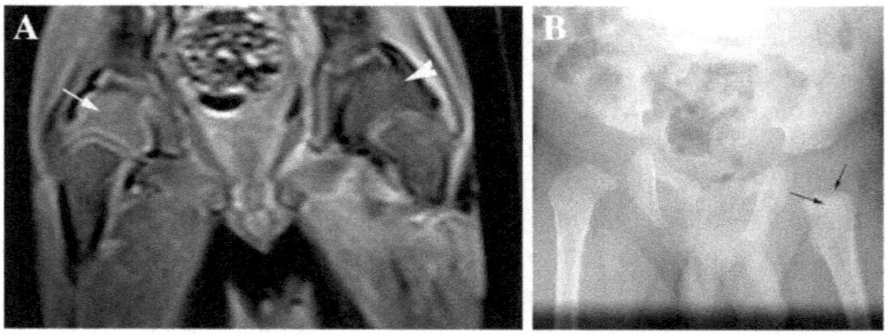

Fig. 1 a and **b** - 1 month-old boy. **a**) coronal contrast-enhanced fat-suppressed T1W: on the left femoral epiphysis hypointensity (arrowhead) in comparison to a homogeneously enhanced right femoral epiphysis (arrow). Epiphyseal nuclei are not yet present. **b**) X Ray study performed one month later showing a small lytic lesion (arrows) on the left side

Results

From January 2010 to December 2013, 22 patients were investigated with MRI in our tertiary care hospital for suspicion of osteoarticular acute infection of the hip. Twelve MRIs initially demonstrated either concomitant SA and AHO or isolated AHO; these cases were excluded of the present study. In 10 cases (45 % of all cases) MRI showed isolated SA without MRI signs of AHO at presentation and these patients were included in the study. The duration of symptoms ranged between 2 and 7 days at the time of the MRI . Body temperature (fever) was between 38.5 and 39.2 °C for 8 patients whereas 2 patients had 37 and 37.6 °C. CRP measurements also ranged between 12 and 180 mg/L (normal range 0–5 mg/L) and erythrocyte sedimentation rate test (ESR) between 19 and 100 mm/h and leucocytes between 9300 and 23.000 cells/μL. Clinical and biological inflammatory responses to *K.kingae* infection were mild-to-moderate in comparison with cases of Gram-positive bacilla infections.

Four patients (3 girls and one boy, mean age 7 years, range 5–14 years) had joint effusion of the hip and did not show decreased perfusion MRI pattern of the femoral epiphysis on fat-suppressed gadolinium-enhanced coronal T1-weighted MRI. The joint fluid effusion was mild in all four cases. The causative organism was *Streptococcus agalactae* in one case, *Streptococcus pneumonia* in two others and was unknown in the fourth. None of the children without this enhancement pattern (4 out of 10) later developed osteomyelitis sequela. Six patients (4 boys and 2 girls, mean 6.3 months, range 1–11 months) presented joint effusion and decreased perfusion of the femoral epiphysis on fat-suppressed gadolinium-enhanced coronal T1-weighted MRI (Fig. 1a, Fig. 2a, and Fig. 3a). In two patients, the causative organism was *Kingella kingae*, in three Gram Positive germs (one *Streptococcus pneumoniae*, one *Streptococcus agalactae* and one *Staphylococcus aureus*) and in one patient bacterial investigation was negative. The joint fluid effusion was mild in five cases and moderate in one. All patients (6 out of 10) with decreased enhancement of gadolinium in the affected hip compared to the contralateral hip, developed metaphyseal small lytic lesions on follow-up (one month later) X rays (Fig. 1b, Fig. 2b and Fig. 3b arrows) and in one case the ossification center disappeared. All of them were younger than one year. The type of germ involved influenced neither the type of enhancement pattern nor the outcome.

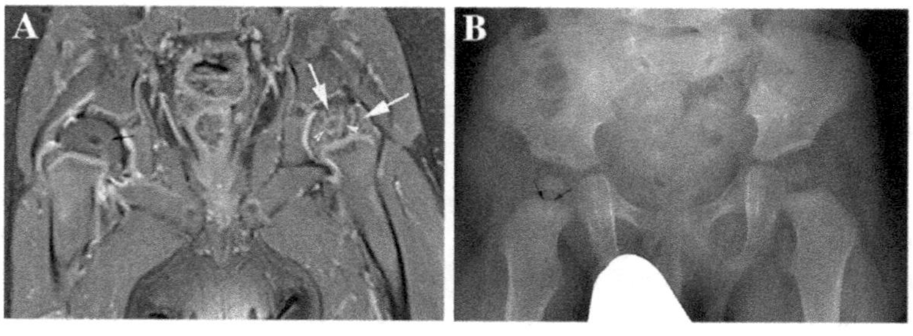

Fig. 2 a and **b** - 10 month-old boy **a**) coronal contrast-enhanced fat-suppressed T1W : femoral epiphyseal nuclei are present. The pathological right femoral cartilage lacks the « striate » normal aspect (white arrows on the left side), the nucleus is uniformly hypointense (red arrow on the right side) in comparison with the normal side (arrowheads) and the surrounding ring does not enhance. Metaphyseal right region shows no abnormalities. **b**) X Ray study performed one month later. A small lytic lesion is visible on the metaphyseal side of physis (arrows) on the right side

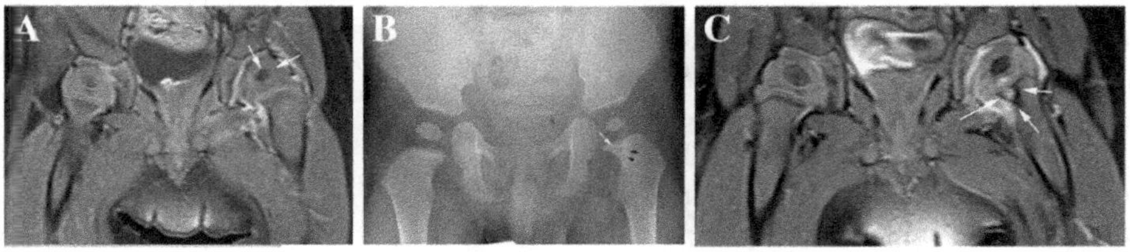

Fig. 3 a, **b** and **c** - 6 month-old boy **a**) Contrast-enhanced fat-suppressed spin-echo T1- weighted coronal image shows hypoperfusion of the left femoral epiphysis. **b**) X Ray study performed one month later showed a small lytic area on the metaphyseal side of the physis (white arrow) with a sclerotic halo (black arrows): the epiphyseal nucleus was also smaller on the pathological side (left). **c**) Contrast-enhanced fat-suppressed spin-echo T1-weighted coronal sequences performed one month later showing metaphyseal bone lesion on the left side. The left femoral nucleus showed hypointensity and was smaller in comparison to the right side

In one case with decreased enhancement, a second MRI performed one month later, clearly showed morphological and signal abnormalities of the growth plate and a round abscess in the metaphysis (Fig. 3c): decreased enhancement of the femoral cartilaginous head was no more visible but there was persistent relative hypointensity of the femoral nucleus which was also smaller in comparison to the contralateral side.

Discussion

The findings of the present study suggest that patients with isolated SA at presentation may later show bone lesions in the metaphysis suggestive of secondary osteomyelitis. A direct correlation seems to exist between a decreased perfusion of the femoral epiphysis on MRI in children below the age of 12 months and the later onset of osseous lesions in the metaphysis consistent with AHO on follow-up. In our experience, the type of germ involved influences neither the enhancement pattern nor the outcome. According to the recent literature, decreased perfusion of the femoral epiphysis on enhanced fat- suppressed T1-weighted MRI has already been described, but it was until now considered as a usual finding of SA [9–11], and in no case interpreted as a sign suggestive of a bone infection of the epiphysis. One study reported that epiphyseal cartilage enhancement defects may occur in the setting of AHO, but its significance was not investigated and remained uncertain. [20] In fact, SA is classically reported as a very common complication of AHO in little children due to the peculiar anatomy of the immature hip and the pathophysiology of pediatric AHO.

The cases reported in our study demonstrate that SA clearly preceded metaphyseal bony infectious lesions and not the opposite. In the literature, SA is classically reported as a frequent complication of AHO and not the other way round [12] as in our findings. We have thus considered two hypothesis in order to explain our findings. The first is that, at presentation, AHO had already started in the metaphysis but MRI was not yet able to visualize the concomitant bone lesion. This explanation would be in agreement with the classical pathophysiological theory of AHO in children [12, 14], where infection typically arises in the metaphysis of long tubular bones due to its rich vascular supply in young children. However, it would be difficult to explain why MRI did not detect any initial signs of metaphyseal bone infection. The second and more rational hypothesis can be formulated on the basis of the observations of Alderson et al. [20]: they investigated concurrent acute childhood osteomyelitis and septic arthritis using avian models which closely resemble human disease. They observed that, after intra-articular injection, bacteria penetrated the deeper epiphyseal cartilage and within 24 h occluded blood vessels. Furthermore, once bacteria were established in the epiphysis, spread occurred across the growth plate into the metaphyseal region due to the presence of transphyseal vessels [12, 14]. This vascular pattern seems to be specific of children in the first 12 to 18 months of life and we can assume, as suggested by Alderson and al, that these vessels may allow the translocation of bacteria in both directions from or to the epiphysis. According to this theory, the explanation of reduced enhancement of the femoral epiphysis and the lack of the normal "striate" aspect is the early thrombosis of epiphyseal cartilage vessels.

According to this theory, it would be more likely that AHO develops first in the epiphysis and then in the metaphysis. In our cases, however, no signal anomalies were detected in the epiphysis on the initial basic T1 and T2 sequences. The reason why may be that, unlike metaphyseal vessels, epiphyseal vessels have a linear morphology, providing much less favourable conditions for bacteria to proliferate.

The present study is a case-series with low-evidence level and has the limitations of being retrospective and including a small population. However we think that our findings deserve to be further investigated by prospective studies with follow-up investigations in patients with isolated SA at presentation.

Conclusion

Infants below the age of one year, with isolated septic joint effusion and decreased perfusion of the femoral epiphysis on enhanced fat- suppressed T1-weighted MRI at presentation, will likely develop metaphyseal AHO and should be treated accordingly. In children after the age of one we did not observe this enhancement pattern, and AHO was less likely.

On the basis of our observations we suggest a new physiopathological hypothesis, already suggested in the literature on the basis of avian models which closely resemble human disease. Finally, we would recommend to perform a contrast-enhanced MR in pediatric hip infection.

Competing interests
The authors declare that they have no competing interests.

Authors' contributions
LM wrote the majority of the original draft of the article. LM and DC were responsible for the design and conceptualization of the study. All authors gathered and interpreted the data and participated in writing the article. All the authors approved the final version of this article. LM guarantees that all individuals who meet the journal's authorship criteria are included as authors of this article.

Author details
[1]Unit of Pediatric Radiology Geneva University Hospital HUG, 6 Willy-Donzé, Geneva 1205, Switzerland. [2]Unit of Pediatric Orthopedics, University Hospital, Geneva, Switzerland.

References

1. Forlin EE, Milani CC. Sequelae of septic arthritis of the hip in children: a new classification and a review of 41 hips. J Pediatr Orthop. 2008;28:524–8.
2. Morrey BF, Bianco AJ, Rhodes KH. Septic arthritis in children. Orthop Clin North Am. 1975;6:923–34.
3. Fabry G, Meire E. Septic arthritis of the hip in children: poor results after late and inadequate treatment. J Pediatr Orthop. 1983;3:461–6.
4. Berberian GG, Firpo W, Soto AA, Lopez MÒ, Julio Torroija J, Cecilia Castro C, et al. Osteoarthritis in the neonate: risk factors and outcome. Braz J Infect Dis. 2010;14:413–8.
5. Rutz EE, Spoerri MM. Septic arthritis of the paediatric hip - a review of current diagnostic approaches and therapeutic concepts. Acta Orthop Belg. 2013;79:123–34.
6. Tetzlaff TR, McCracken GH, Nelson JD. Oral antibiotic therapy for skeletal infections of children. II. Therapy of osteomyelitis and suppurative arthritis. J Pediatr. 1978;92:485–90.
7. Unkila Kallio L, Kallio MJ, Peltola H. The usefulness of C-reactive protein levels in the identification of concurrent septic arthritis in children who have acute hematogenous osteomyelitis. A comparison with the usefulness of the erythrocyte sedimentation rate and the white blood-cell count. J Bone Joint Surg (Am Vol). 1994;76:848–53.
8. Goergens ED, McEvoy A, Watson M, Barrett IR. Acute osteomyelitis and septic arthritis in children. J Paediatr Child Health. 2005;41:59–62.
9. Kwack KK-S, Cho JHJ, Lee JHJ, Oh K, Ki K, Kim S, et al. Septic arthritis versus transient synovitis of the hip: gadolinium-enhanced MRI finding of decreased perfusion at the femoral epiphysis. AJR Am J Roentgenol. 2007;189:437–45.
10. Yang WJW, Im SAS, Lim GG-Y, Chun H, Ho J, Jung N, et al. MR imaging of transient synovitis: differentiation from septic arthritis. Pediatr Radiol. 2006;36:1154–8.
11. Lee SK, Suh KJ, Kim YW, Ryeom HK, Lee JM, Chang Y, et al. Septic arthritis versus transient synovitis at MR imaging: preliminary assessment with signal intensity alterations in bone marrow. Radiology. 1999;211:459–65.
12. Trueta J. The 3 types of acute hematogenous osteomyelitis. Schweiz Med Wochenschr. 1963;93:306–12.
13. Ceroni DD, Kampouroglou GG, Valaikaite RR, Anderson Della Llana R, Salvo D, et al. Osteoarticular infections in young children: what has changed over the last years? Swiss Med Wkly. 2014;144:w13971.
14. Ogden JA. Pediatric osteomyelitis and septic arthritis: the pathology of neonatal disease. Yale J Biol Med. 1979;52:423–48.
15. Saigal GG, Azouz EMG, Abdenour GG. Imaging of osteomyelitis with special reference to children. Semin Musculoskelet Radiol. 2004;8:255–65.
16. Averill LWL, Hernandez AA, Gonzalez LL, Pea AHA, Jaramillo D. Diagnosis of osteomyelitis in children: utility of fat-suppressed contrast-enhanced MRI. AJR Am J Roentgenol. 2009;192:1232–8.
17. Dangman BC, Hoffer FA, Rand FF, O'Rourke EJ. Osteomyelitis in children: gadolinium-enhanced MR imaging. Radiology. 1992;182:743–7.
18. Montgomery COC, Siegel EE, Blasier RDR, Suva LJL. Concurrent septic arthritis and osteomyelitis in children. J Pediatr Orthop. 2013;33:464–7.
19. Johnson DPD, Hernanz Schulman MM, Martus JEJ, Lovejoy SA, Yu C, Kan JH, et al. Significance of epiphyseal cartilage enhancement defects in pediatric osteomyelitis identified by MRI with surgical correlation. Pediatric radiology. 2010;41:355–61.
20. Alderson M, Speers D, Emslie K, Nada S. Acute haematogenous osteomyelitis and septic arthritis-a single disease. An hypothesis based upon the presence of transphyseal blood vessels. J Bone Joint Surg Br Vol. 1986;68:268–74.

7

Cardiovascular magnetic resonance assessment of the aortic valve stenosis: an *in vivo* and *ex vivo* study

Stefan Buchner[1*], Kurt Debl[1], Franz-Xaver Schmid[3], Andreas Luchner[1] and Behrus Djavidani[2]

Abstract

Background: Aortic valve area (AVA) estimation in patients with aortic stenosis may be obtained using several methods. This study was undertaken to verify the cardiovascular magnetic resonance (CMR) planimetry of aortic stenosis by comparing the findings with invasive catheterization, transthoracic (TTE) as well as tranesophageal echocardiography (TEE) and anatomic CMR examination of autopsy specimens.

Methods: Our study was performed in eight patients with aortic valve stenosis. Aortic stenosis was determined by TTE and TEE as well as catheterization and CMR. Especially, after aortic valve replacement, the explanted aortic valves were examined again with CMR *ex vivo* model.

Results: The mean AVA determined in vivo by CMR was 0.75 ± 0.09 cm^2 and ex vivo by CMR was 0.65 ± 0.09 cm^2 and was closely correlated ($r = 0.91$, $p < 0.001$). The mean absolute difference between AVA derived by CMR *ex vivo* and *in vivo* was -0.10 ± 0.04 cm^2. The mean AVA using TTE was 0.69 ± 0.07 with a significant correlation between CMR ex vivo ($r = 0.85$, $p < 0.007$) and CMR *in vivo* ($r = 0.86$, $p < 0.008$). CMR *ex vivo* and *in vivo* had no significant correlation with AVA using Gorlin formula by invasive catheterization or using planimetry by TEE.

Conclusion: In this small study using an ex vivo aortic valve stenosis model, the aortic valve area can be reliably planimetered by CMR *in vivo* and *ex vivo* with a well correlation between geometric AVA by CMR and the effective AVA calculated by TTE.

Keywords: Aortic valve, Aortic stenosis, Magnetic resonance imaging, Anatomy

Background

Aortic valve stenosis is the most common cardiac valve disease resulting in valve therapy [1]. Exact determination of the severity of stenosis is essential to guide therapy [2]. Standard methods, such as cardiac catheterization and transthoracic echocardiography (TTE) have to calculate the effective orifice area by measurement of the transvalvular pressure gradient [3, 4], as they do not allow a direct and precise measurement of the geometric orifice area. Therefore it seems desirable to directly determine the geometric orifice area by a flow independent technique such as planimetry. Several cardiologists take the view that TTE using the Doppler-technique is now the best reference ("gold standard") whereas the Gorlin-formula is the historical reference.

Cardiovascular magnetic resonance (CMR) is a noninvasive method that allows visualization of cardiac function, structure and valves [5, 6]. Recently, we and others have reported the success of planimetry by CMR in aortic valve [7–14].

However, to date, no studies have been published describing *ex vivo* CMR stenotic aortic valves. It therefore seemed useful to compare anatomic data with CMR imaging.

We hypothesized that direct planimetry of the stenotic aortic valve in an autopsy human valve as a standard of reference using CMR corresponds to the planimetry of the stenotic aortic valve *in vivo* using CMR. To address this hypothesis, we performed a head-to-head comparison between aortic valve area (AVA) planimetry preoperatively

* Correspondence: stefan.buchner@ukr.de
[1]Klinik und Poliklinik für Innere Medizin II, Universitätsklinikum Regensburg, Franz-Josef-Strauss-Allee 11, 93042 Regensburg, Germany
Full list of author information is available at the end of the article

by CMR and postoperatively of the explanted aortic valve by CMR in a series of eight patients with aortic valve stenosis. In addition, CMR measurements were compared with TTE and transesophageal echocardiography (TEE) as well as catheterization data

Methods

Patients

Eight patients referred to our institution for evaluation of aortic valve stenosis and were prospectively included in the study undergoing aortic valve replacement. All diagnostic procedures and measurements were performed by experienced observers, who were blinded to the results of the other imaging modalities. Informed consent was obtained in all patients. The study approved by local ethics committee of the Universität Regensburg.

Clinical characteristics of the patients

Clinical data of the eight patients are summarized in Table 1. Mean age was 76 ± 6 (62 to 82) years. The majority of patients presented with clinical symptoms of severe aortic stenosis, such as systolic murmur, dyspnea, chest pain or syncope. Concomitant aortic regurgitation was present in 5 patients and was defined as mild/trivial ($n = 4$) or moderate ($n = 1$) by CMR and echocardiography. TEE planimetry of AVA was not possible in one patient because of heavy calcifications. Planimetry of AVA was possible in all patients undergoing CMR. An impaired image quality was observed in one patient due to trigger problems by cardiac arrhythmia.

Transthoracic echocardiography

Standardized transthoracic echocardiography was performed with measurements of the left ventricular outflow tract diameter, the velocity of across the aortic valve and flow data of the left ventricular outflow tract to calculate the AVA using the continuity equation [15].

Table 1 Patient characteristics

Patient	Age	Sex	Rhythm	HR	SBP	NYHA	CCS	Syncope
1	80	female	SR	71	130	4	0	0
2	82	female	AF	77	158	3	1	0
3	74	female	SR	91	125	2	0	0
4	75	female	SR	67	115	3	0	1
5	79	female	SR	83	120	3	2	0
6	75	male	AF	97	116	4	3	0
7	62	female	SR	63	130	3	4	0
8	77	female	SR	80	130	3	2	0

SR, sinus rhythm; AF, atrial fibrillation; HR, heart rate; SBP, systolic blood pressure; NYHA, New York Heart Association, CCS, Canadian Cardiovascular Society

Transesophageal Echocardiography

Multiplane TEE was performed using a 5-Mhz annular phased array probe. For examination of the aortic valve, the imaging plane was rotated from 0° to 180° until the best image of the aortic valve opening in the short axis view was obtained (usually around 60°). Minimal probe manipulation was performed to ensure that the smallest orifice of the aortic valve at the leaflet tips was identified. Planimetry of the smallest orifice at the time of maximum opening in early systole (triggered by the electrocardiogram) was performed. At least three consecutive measurements were averaged

Catheterization

A standard cardiac catheterization procedure was performed via the percutaneous femoral approach, including right and left heart pressure measurement. Peak to peak and mean pressure gradients were determined between left ventricle and ascending aorta. Cardiac output was measured by thermodilution, averaging at least 3 measurements. AVA was estimated using the Gorlin formula [16].

Surgery and autopsy

The description of the aortic valve was obtained from one surgeon. We obtained human valves from patients with aortic valve stenosis at the time of surgical valve replacement. Despite the heavy calcification, all valves could be explanted totally. Specimens were originally preserved in formaldehyde solution.

Cardiovascular magnetic resonance studies – *in vivo*

All patient studies were performed on a 1.5 T scanner (Sonata, Siemens Medical Solutions, Erlangen, Germany). CMR studies were performed in supine position with a phased-array receiver coil and breath-hold acquisitions prospectively gated to the ECG. Cine images were acquired in multiple short axis and long axis views with fast imaging with steady state free precession (trueFISP, slice thickness 8 mm, echo time 1.53 ms, readout bandwidth 1.085 Hz/pixel, repetition time 3.14 ms, matrix 256*202).

Image analysis was performed off-line using the semi-automatic ARGUS evaluation program (Siemens Medical Solutions, Erlangen, Germany), which is a part of the commercially available cardiac package of the scanner software.

The imaging plane of the aortic valve was defined by acquiring a systolic 5-chamber view parallel to the long axis of the left ventricular outflow tract and a long axis view of the left ventricular outflow tract and the proximal aorta, perpendicular to the 5-chamber view, as described previously [7]. In brief, the subsequent slices were defined parallel to the valvular plane and, additionally, in cases of orifices with an eccentric outlet, perpendicularly to the direction of the jet. At least 4 slices (range 4–7) at different levels of the aortic valve were acquired and the imaging plane with the smallest orifice was chosen. Planimetry of the smallest orifice at the time of maximum opening in early systole in the acquisitions prospectively triggered to the electrocardiogram was performed by two independent observers, who were unaware of the echocardiographic, catheterization and ex vivo results. We placed our traces at the point of the bright pixels. Three measurements were performed and average for calculating the AVA. Intraobserver and interobserver variabilities regarding AVA were 3 % and 6 % for *in vivo* CMR, respectively.

Cardiovascular magnetic resonance studies – *ex vivo*

All specimens were examined on a 1.5 T scanner (Magnetom Sonata, Siemens Medical Solutions, Erlangen, Germany). The CMR imaging protocol included a 3D-CISS protocol (TR/TE/flip angle 17/8.08 ms/70° ms, band width 130 Hz/pixel, effective slice thickness 1 mm pixel size 0.6 × 0.45 mm). The aortic valve was placed on a rack into a water container. Then the container with the aortic valve was placed in the gantry. Slices in the orthogonal planes (transverse, coronal and sagittal) were obtained (Fig. 1). Serial angulated-axis views from the base to tip of the valve were acquired with 3D sequence (Fig. 2). Planimetry of the smallest orifice was performed by two independent observers, who were unaware of the echocardiographic, catheterization and in vivo results. We placed our traces at the edge of the bright pixels. Three measurements were performed and average for calculating the AVA. Intraobserver and interobserver variabilities were 1 % and 4 % for *ex vivo* CMR, respectively.

Statistical analysis

Data expressed as mean ± standard deviation. Linear regression analysis was performed to describe correlations between the different techniques. The mean AVA of the different techniques was compared by student's t-Test for paired samples. Intra- and interobserver variability ($n = 8$) were expressed as the percentage of variability (absolute value of the difference between 2 measurements divided by the mean of 2 measurements). Agreement between the different techniques was assessed as described by Bland and Altman. A level of significance of below 0.05 was defined as statistically significant. SPSS version 21 (SPSS Institute, Chicago) was used for statistical analysis.

Results

CMR planimetry of AVA *in vivo* and *ex vivo*

The measurements of all patients by the various modalities are depicted in Table 2. Six valves were tricuspid and two valves were bicuspid. Images of aortic valve specimen, in vivo and ex vivo CMR are depicted in Fig 3.

The mean AVA determined *ex vivo* by CMR was 0.65 ± 0.09 cm^2. Mean AVA determined *in vivo* by CMR was 0.75 ± 0.09 cm^2. The mean absolute difference between AVA derived by CMR *ex vivo* and *in vivo* was 0.10 ± 0.04 cm^2 ($p < 0.001$, Fig. 4 and Table 3). The AVA *in vivo* and *ex vivo* by CMR was closely correlated (r = 0.91, $p < 0.001$).

The mean absolute difference between AVA derived by CMR ex vivo and calculated using the continuity equation by TTE was −0.04 ± 0.05 cm^2 ($p = 0.066$). The mean absolute difference between AVA derived by CMR *in vivo* and calculated using the continuity equation by

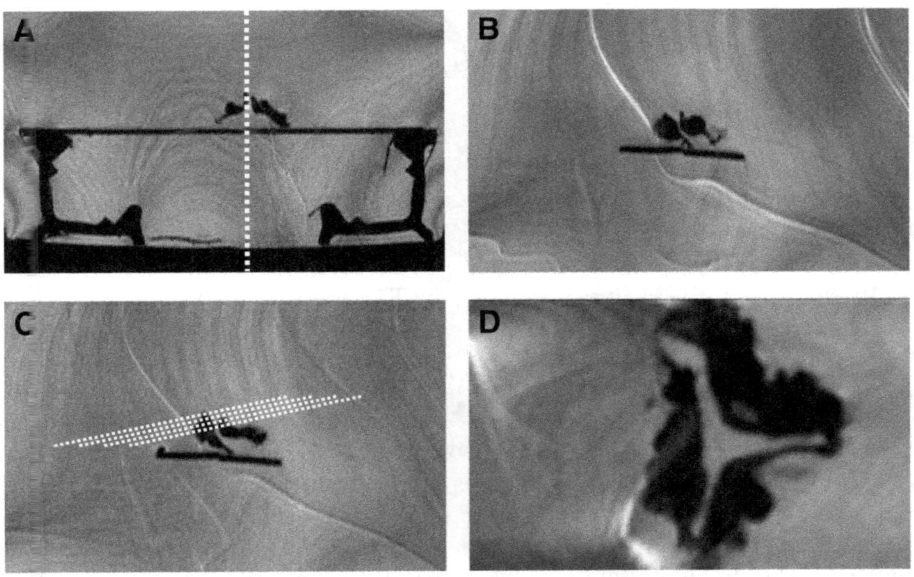

Fig. 1 Position of the *ex vivo* aortic valve fixed in a water container and planning the slices. **a**, overview; **b**, coronar view; **c**, angulation for planning the orthograd view; **d**, the resulting orthograd view

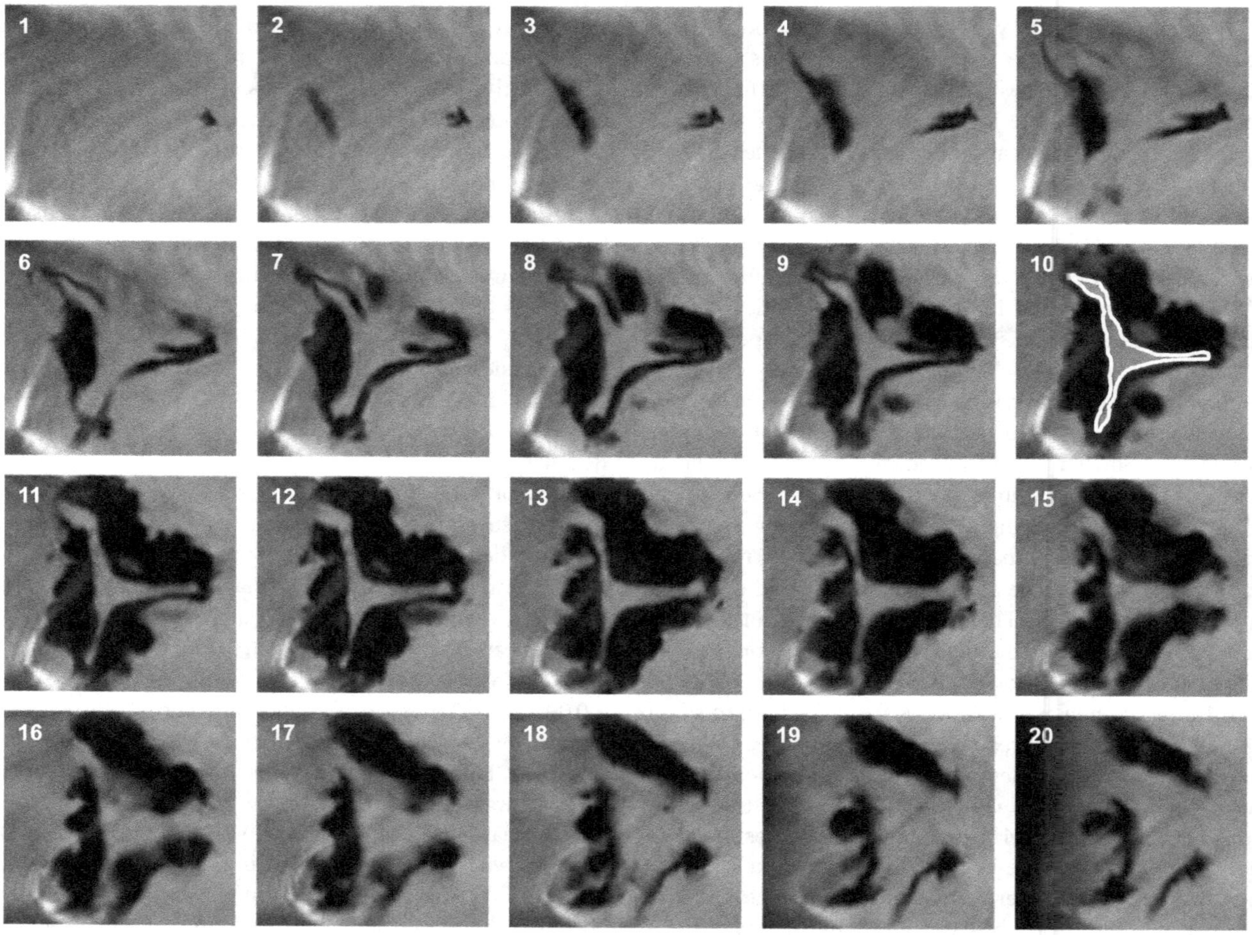

Fig. 2 To avoid assessing the aortic valve area beyond or above the leaflet tips, the imaging plane was moved shift wise in one mm steps in an orthograd direction. Planimetry was chosen on the slice where the smallest orifice was surrounded totally by the edge of the valve

TTE was +0.07 ± 0.04 cm^2. In linear regression analysis the correlation between CMR ex vivo and TTE (r = 0.85, $p < 0.007$) was similar to that between CMR *in vivo* and TTE (r = 0.86, $p < 0.008$).

The mean absolute difference between aortic valve area derived by CMR ex vivo and TEE was +0.12 ± 0.09 cm^2 ($p = 0.012$). The mean absolute difference between aortic valve area derived by CMR *in vivo* and TEE was −0.02 ± 0.10 cm^2 ($p = 0.75$). In linear regression analysis the correlation between CMR ex vivo and TEE was r = 0.44, $p = 0.323$) and between CMR *in vivo* and TEE r = 0.28, p = 0.551.

The mean absolute difference between AVA derived by CMR ex vivo and calculated using the Gorlin formula by catheterization was +0.07 ± 0.26 cm^2 ($p = 0.498$). The mean absolute difference between AVA derived by CMR *in vivo* and calculated using the Gorlin formula by catheterization was +0.17 ± 0.27 cm^2 ($p = 0.117$). In linear regression analysis the correlation between CMR *ex vivo* and Gorlin formula by catheterization was r = 0.09, $p = 0.835$ and between CMR *in vivo* and Gorlin formula by catheterization was r = −0.03, $p = 0.952$.

AVA with other methods

The mean of the aortic valve area calculated using the Gorlin formula by catheterization was 0.60 ± 0.27 cm^2. The mean aortic valve area determined by TEE was 0.79 ± 0.15 cm^2. The mean of the aortic valve area calculated by TTE was 0.69 ± 0.07 (Table 3).

The mean absolute difference between AVA derived calculated using the Gorlin formula by catheterization and calculated using the continuity equation by TTE was −0.11 ± 0.25 cm^2 ($p = 0.278$). The mean absolute difference between AVA using the Gorlin formula by catheterization and TEE was −0.13 ± 0.19 cm^2 ($p = 0.122$). The mean absolute difference between AVA calculated using the continuity equation by TTE and TEE was −0.08 ± 0.10 cm^2 ($p = 0.97$). In linear regression analysis the correlation between Gorlin formula by catheterization and TEE was r = 0.71, $p = 0.073$ and between Gorlin

Table 2 Results

Patient	Aortic valve type CMR	Aortic valve type surgery	AVA *in vivo* by CMR (cm^2)	AVA *ex vivo* by CMR (cm^2)	AVA by TEE (cm^2)	AVA by TTE (cm^2)	AVA by CATH (cm^2)	PG mean by Doppler (mmHg)	PG mean by CATH (mmHg)	LV EF by CMR (%)	LV Mass by CMR (g)	LV SV by CMR (ml)
1	BAV	BAV	0.84	0.76	-	0.74	0.29	65	77	50	151	61
2	TAV	TAV	0.70	0.55	0.65	0.65	0.36	59	65	41	126	36
3	TAV	TAV	0.84	0.73	0.70	0.75	0.64	53	45	81	177	81
4	TAV	TAV	0.86	0.70	0.80	0.75	0.52	76	76	59	178	73
5	TAV	TAV	0.62	0.50	0.70	0.55	0.34	44	46	19	134	40
6	BAV	BAV	0.76	0.69	1.10	0.65	0.85	40	35	45	210	72
7	TAV	TAV	0.72	0.68	0.75	0.73	0.67	49	55	77	113	57
8	TAV	TAV	0.71	0.59	0.80	0.69	1.08	30	20	71	120	50

AVA, aortic valve area; BAV, bicuspid aortic valve; CMR, cardiovascular magnetic resonance; CATH, cardiac catheterization; TEE, transesophageal echocardiography; TTE, transthoracic echocardiography; LV EF, left ventricular ejection fraction; LV mass, left ventricular mass; LV SV, left ventricular stroke volume; PG, pressure gradient; TAV, tricuspid aortic valve

formula by catheterization and the continuity equation by TTE was $r = 0.17$, $p = 0.639$ and between TEE and catheterization and the continuity equation by TTE was $r = 0.15$, $p = 0.748$.

Discussion

The results of this study demonstrate that aortic valve stenosis can be accurately planimetered by using CMR *in vivo* compared with ex vivo model. Precise assessment of aortic valve area in aortic stenosis is crucial for optimal patient treatment [17]. However, no comparison of planimetry of the aortic valve area has made with *in vivo* and *ex vivo* aortic valves by CMR or other modality. The present study is the first to validate the ability of CMR to accurately and precisely planimetry aortic valve stenosis in vivo comparing by *ex vivo* CMR.

Characterization of the severity of aortic stenosis is among the most difficult problems in valvular heart disease. Exact determination of the severity of stenosis is essential to guide therapy [18]. In evaluating the severity of the aortic valve stenosis, it is ideally desirable to determine geometric orifice area On the other hand, the opening of the aortic valve is though highly dependent of the flow and gradient. Because planimetry only provides geometric orifice area and does not characterize the flow property, this could be a challenge in low-flow/low-gradient aortic stenosis [19–21]. The guidelines allow various methods to determine the AVA. However, the

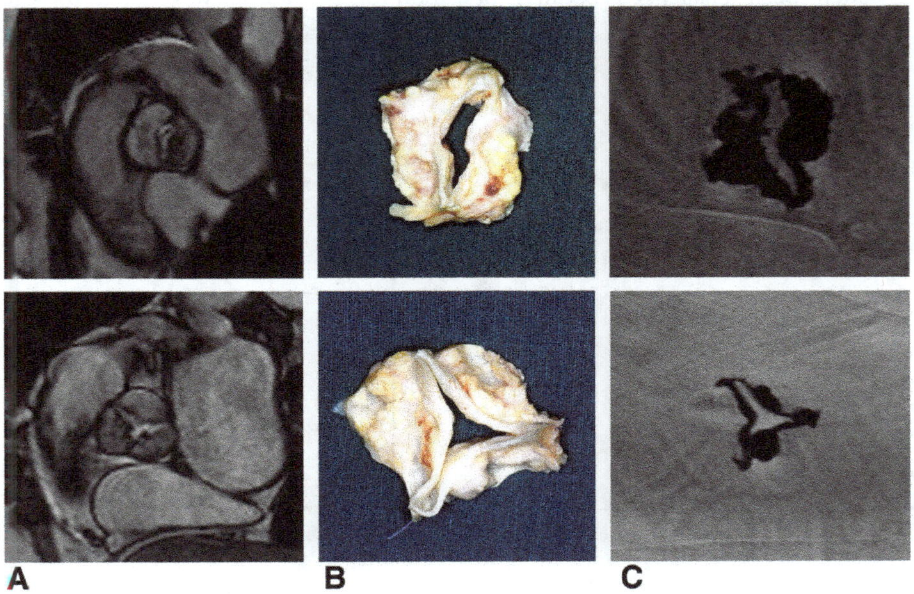

Fig. 3 Images derived from the in vivo CMR (**a**), from the aortic valve specimen (**b**) and from the ex vivo CMR (**c**) in a bicuspid stenotic valve (top) and in a tricuspid stenotic valve (bottom)

Table 3 Comparison of methods of planimetry and calculation of aortic valve area

	Aortic valve area (cm^2)	
Method	Mean	Range
CMR *ex vivo*	0.65 ± 0.09	0.50 – 0.76
CMR *in vivo*	0.75 ± 0.09	0.62 – 0.86
TEE	0.80 ± 0.16	0.65 – 1.10
TTE	0.69 ± 0.07	0.50 – 0.70
CATH	0.59 ± 0.27	0.29 – 1.08

CMR, cardiovascular magnetic resonance; CATH, cardiac catheterization; TEE, transesophageal echocardiography; TTE, transthoracic echocardiography

different available techniques often might lead to discrepancy results. This could demonstrate in the current study and previous studies which show that the planimtery of the AVA was systematically higher than the calculated AVA by Gorlin in catheterization or continuity equation in TTE. This is due to the fact that direct planimetry reflects the anatomical orifice while the calculated valve area reflects the effective orifice area. Despite the different available techniques for the assessment of the AVA all available techniques have their limitations and this should be keep in mind. In TTE, the inexact measurement of the diameter of the left ventricular outflow tract or missed peak transvalvular velocity might lead to a false AVA. In TEE, heavily calcification of the aortic valve could lead to impaired image quality e.g. by the acoustic shadowing, thus exact delineation of the cusps and planimetry of the AVA are impossible or the potential inability to identify the accurate imaging plane for planimetry. Hemodynamic assessment of the aortic valve area by invasive cardiac catheterization has often been challenged because of potential imprecision introduced by the hemodynamic parameters. Finally, CMR has its limitation in valve motion and exact slice orientation or in contraindication for CMR (e.g. claustrophia or metallic implants).

Prior to our study, several other investigators have determined the accuracy of several methods for CMR and cardiac computed tomography planimetry of the aortic valve using an angiographic reference standard or Doppler derived data [7–9, 22, 23]. However, the ultimate test of the value of the method seems to be comparison with anatomy. The current study extends these findings as it demonstrates that CMR allows to accurately visualizing the anatomic valve area *in vivo* compared to *ex vivo*.

To date, most CMR studies for the quantification of stenotic aortic valves have focused on direct planimetry [24], although the dimensions of CMR voxels relative to the size and shape of stenotic orifices sometimes influence this approach. Therefore, an *ex vivo* study was deemed as an essential intermediate study for assessing sources of errors in CMR aortic valve estimation prior to *in vivo* experiments. Ex vivo estimates eliminate errors due to motion blurring, which includes errors resulting from irregular heart rates and images acquired during motion. Furthermore, ex vivo determinations also minimize uncertainties due to edge definition and produced high-contrast edges in which the aortic valve boundary is defined to be pixel values above background. The results of this study should, therefore, be interpreted as the minimum errors which can be achieved using CMR.

Despite the close correlation between *ex vivo* and *in vivo* planimetry by CMR, we observed an underestimation of the aortic valve area by CMR *ex vivo*. The

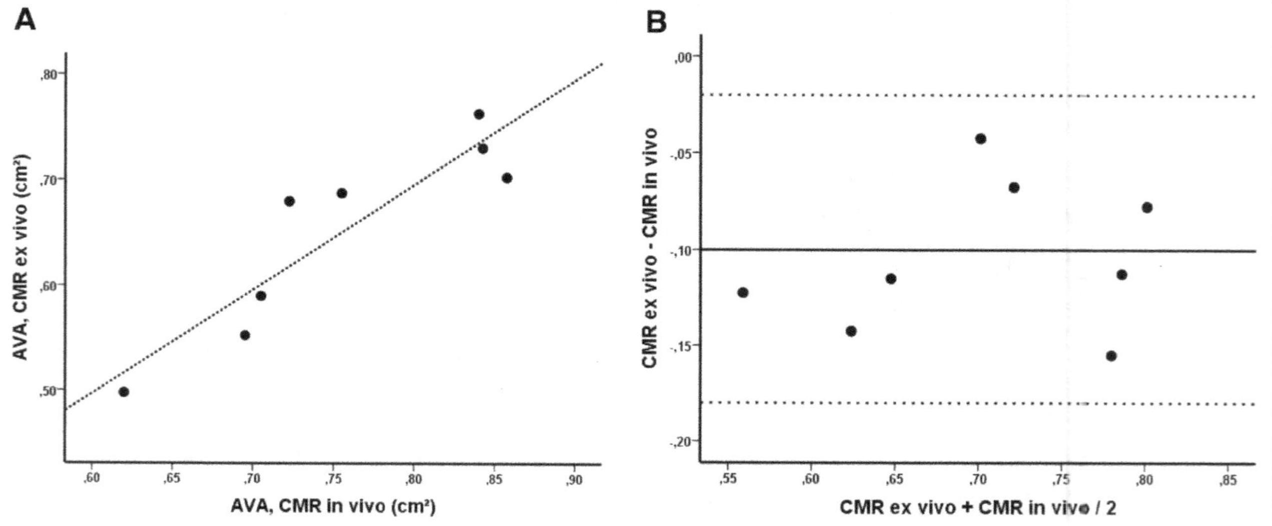

Fig. 4 Agreement between aortic valve area assessed by CMR in vivo and by CMR ex vivo (**a**). According to Bland-Altman (**b**), the difference between the two comparative measurements is plotted against their mean. The continuous line represents the mean difference and dashed lines represent the limits of agreement (mean difference ± 2SD)

underlying reason for underestimation of the aortic valve area by CMR may be related to valve motion and slice orientation. Specifically, transplanar valve motion during systole might lead to overestimation of valve area when the imaging plane misses the smallest orifice area. Taking measurement from CMR, one has to make sure that the plane is orthogonal and on the edge of the leaflets. *Ex vivo* imaging, however, eliminates potential errors caused by cardiac and respiratory motion.

Limitations

Several limitations of our study should be noted. The sample size of the current study was small. Most of the patients had been diagnosed with high-grade aortic valve stenosis, resulting in a selection bias. However, because we decided to use combined left and right heart catheterization and study the explanted aortic valve, we were unable to include patients with mild aortic stenosis, because, in these patients these would not be justified. Furthermore, only the static area of the aortic valve was measured and do not reflect the hemodynamic conditions *in vivo*. However, it is difficult to assess the dynamic change of stenotic aortic valve area in ex vivo specimens. In this study only due to the heavy calcification of the aortic valve, it was possible to explant the valve as a unit and we presume that the shape of the valve represent the maximum opening of the valve in systole. Consequently, the aortic valve area of the explanted aortic valve corresponds by the calcification the smallest maximal orifice may merely influenced by ejection and diastolic valve closing.

Conclusion

In conclusion, this is the first study to validate planimetry in aortic valve stenosis using CMR in an *ex vivo* model. CMR *in vivo* slightly overestimates the valve area in aortic stenosis compared to CMR ex vivo. Furthermore, planimetry of AVA using CMR *in vivo* and *ex vivo* model correlated well with calculated AVA by TTE, in contrast to TEE and invasive measurements of AVA. These certain methodical discrepancies between these methods must be taken into account when grading the severity of aortic stenosis by AVA.

Abbreviations

AVA: Aortic valve area; CMR: Cardiac magnetic resonance; TEE: Transoseophageal echocardiography.

Competing interests

The authors declare that they have no competing interests.

Authors' contributions

SB: study design, acquisition of the data, image analysis, statistical analysis, manuscript drafting. KD, AL: study design, image analysis, manuscript revising. FS: acquisition of the data, manuscript revising. BD: study design, acquisition of the data, image analysis, manuscript drafting.

Acknowledgment

The authors thank Marion Merdian and Heike Koitsch for excellent technical assistance.

Author details

[1]Klinik und Poliklinik für Innere Medizin II, Universitätsklinikum Regensburg, Franz-Josef-Strauss-Allee 11, 93042 Regensburg, Germany. [2]Institut für Röntgendiagnostik, Universitätsklinikum Regensburg, Regensburg, Germany. [3]Klinik und Poliklinik für Herz-, Thorax- und herznahe Gefäßchirurgie, Universitätsklinikum Regensburg, Regensburg, Germany.

References

1. Selzer A. Changing aspects of the natural history of valvular aortic stenosis. N Engl J Med. 1987;317:91–8.
2. Vahanian A, Alfieri O, Andreotti F, Antunes MJ, Baron-Esquivias G, Baumgartner H, et al. Guidelines on the management of valvular heart disease (version 2012): The joint task force on the management of valvular heart disease of the european society of cardiology (esc) and the european association for cardio-thoracic surgery (eacts). Eur J Cardiothorac Surg. 2012;42:S1–44.
3. Leborgne L, Tribouilloy C, Otmani A, Peltier M, Rey JL, Lesbre JP. Comparative value of doppler echocardiography and cardiac catheterization in the decision to operate on patients with aortic stenosis. Int J Cardiol. 1998;65:163–8.
4. Garcia D, Dumesnil JG, Durand LG, Kadem L, Pibarot P. Discrepancies between catheter and doppler estimates of valve effective orifice area can be predicted from the pressure recovery phenomenon: Practical implications with regard to quantification of aortic stenosis severity. J Am Coll Cardiol. 2003;41:435–42.
5. Schmidt M, Crnac J, Dederichs B, Theissen P, Schicha H, Sechtem U. Magnetic resonance imaging in valvular heart disease. Int J Card Imaging. 1997;13:219–31.
6. Lee SC, Ko SM, Song MG, Shin JK, Chee HK, Hwang HK. Morphological assessment of the aortic valve using coronary computed tomography angiography, cardiovascular magnetic resonance, and transthoracic echocardiography: Comparison with intraoperative findings. Int J Cardiovasc Imaging. 2012;28 Suppl 1:33–44.
7. Debl K, Djavidani B, Seitz J, Nitz W, Schmid FX, Muders F, et al. Planimetry of aortic valve area in aortic stenosis by magnetic resonance imaging. Invest Radiol. 2005;40:631–6.
8. John AS, Dill T, Brandt RR, Rau M, Ricken W, Bachmann G, et al. Magnetic resonance to assess the aortic valve area in aortic stenosis: How does it compare to current diagnostic standards? J Am Coll Cardiol. 2003;42:519–26.
9. Friedrich MG, Schulz-Menger J, Poetsch T, Pilz B, Uhlich F, Dietz R. Quantification of valvular aortic stenosis by magnetic resonance imaging. Am Heart J. 2002;144:329–34.
10. Kupfahl C, Honold M, Meinhardt G, Vogelsberg H, Wagner A, Mahrholdt H, et al. Evaluation of aortic stenosis by cardiovascular magnetic resonance imaging: Comparison with established routine clinical techniques. Heart. 2004;90:893–901.
11. Garcia J, Pibarot P, Capoulade R, Le Ven F, Kadem L, Larose E. Usefulness of cardiovascular magnetic resonance imaging for the evaluation of valve opening and closing kinetics in aortic stenosis. Eur Heart J Cardiovasc Imaging. 2013;14:819–26.
12. von Knobelsdorff-Brenkenhoff F, Rudolph A, Wassmuth R, Bohl S, Buschmann EE, Abdel-Aty H, et al. Feasibility of cardiovascular magnetic resonance to assess the orifice area of aortic bioprostheses. Circ Cardiovasc Imaging. 2009;2:397–404. 392 p following 404.
13. Buchner S, Hulsmann M, Poschenrieder F, Hamer OW, Fellner C, Kobuch R, et al. Variable phenotypes of bicuspid aortic valve disease: Classification by cardiovascular magnetic resonance. Heart. 2010;96:1233–40.
14. Buchner S, Debl K, Haimerl J, Djavidani B, Poschenrieder F, Feuerbach S, et al. Electrocardiographic diagnosis of left ventricular hypertrophy in aortic valve disease: Evaluation of ecg criteria by cardiovascular magnetic resonance. J Cardiovasc Magn Reson. 2009;11:18.
15. Baumgartner H, Hung J, Bermejo J, Chambers JB, Evangelista A, Griffin BP, et al. Echocardiographic assessment of valve stenosis: Eae/ase recommendations for clinical practice. Eur J Echocardiogr. 2009;10:1–25.

16. Gorlin R, Gorlin SG. Hydraulic formula for calculation of the area of the stenotic mitral valve, other cardiac valves, and central circulatory shunts. I Am Heart J. 1951;41:1–29.
17. Baumgartner H. Aortic stenosis: medical and surgical management. Heart. 2005; 91(11):1483–1488.
18. Vahanian A, Alfieri O, Andreotti F, Antunes MJ, Baron-Esquivias G, Baumgartner H, et al. Guidelines on the management of valvular heart disease (version 2012). Eur Heart J. 2012;33:2451–96.
19. Minners J, Allgeier M, Gohlke-Baerwolf C, Kienzle RP, Neumann FJ, Jander N. Inconsistencies of echocardiographic criteria for the grading of aortic valve stenosis. European Heart Journal. 2008;29:1043–8.
20. Hachicha Z, Dumesnil JG, Bogaty P, Pibarot P. Paradoxical low-flow, low-gradient severe aortic stenosis despite preserved ejection fraction is associated with higher afterload and reduced survival. Circulation. 2007;115:2856–64.
21. Jander N, Minners J, Holme I, Gerdts E, Boman K, Brudi P, et al. Outcome of patients with low-gradient "severe" aortic stenosis and preserved ejection fraction. Circulation. 2011;123:887–95.
22. Feuchtner GM, Muller S, Bonatti J, Schachner T, Velik-Salchner C, Pachinger O, et al. Sixty-four slice ct evaluation of aortic stenosis using planimetry of the aortic valve area. *AJR*. AJR Am J Roentgenol. 2007;189:197–203.
23. Ropers D, Ropers U, Marwan M, Schepis T, Pflederer T, Wechsel M, et al. Comparison of dual-source computed tomography for the quantification of the aortic valve area in patients with aortic stenosis versus transthoracic echocardiography and invasive hemodynamic assessment. Am J Cardiol. 2009;104:1561–7.
24. Ko SM, Song MG, Hwang HK. Evaluation of the aortic and mitral valves with cardiac computed tomography and cardiac magnetic resonance imaging. Int J Cardiovasc Imaging. 2012;28 Suppl 2:109–27.

8

A case of meningococcal meningitis with multiple cerebellar microbleeds detected by susceptibility-weighted imaging

Keita Miyazaki[1†], Hidetada Fukushima[1*], Youhei Kogeichi[2†], Tomoo Watanabe[3†], Kazunobu Norimoto[1†], Toshiaki Taoka[4†] and Kazuo Okuchi[1†]

Abstract

Background: Bacterial meningitis is a fatal infectious disease of the central nervous system complicating intravascular involvements. Multiple microbleeds are rarely identified as complications because of the limited detection threshold of conventional imaging modalities. We report the first case of meningococcal meningitis with successful identification of multiple microbleeds in the cerebellum by susceptibility-weighted imaging.

Case presentation: A 19-year-old Japanese female was brought to our emergency department because of fever and coma. A spinal tap was performed and turbid yellow fluid was collected. A diagnosis of bacterial meningitis was established and the patient was admitted to an intensive care unit. Dexamethasone and Antibiotics were administered and *Neisseria meningitides* was cultured from the spinal fluid. On day 10, postcontrast magnetic resonance imaging identified enhanced subarachnoid space in the cerebellum. Susceptibility-weighted imaging showed spotty low-intensity signals in the cerebellar tissue, indicating microbleeds. The patient made a full recovery from coma and was discharged without neurological sequelae on day 24.

Conclusion: Meningococcal meningitis can cause multiple microbleeds in the cerebellum. In this report, we successfully identified microbleeds by susceptibility-weighed imaging. Using this imaging modality, further investigations will clarify its clinical incidence and significance.

Keywords: Bacterial meningitis, Magnetic resonance imaging, Susceptibility-weighted imaging, Bleeding

Background

Bacterial meningitis is a fatal infectious disease of the central nervous system with an annual incidence of 4–6 cases per 100,000 adults (patients older than 16 years of age). The most common pathogens are *Streptococcus pneumoniae*, *Neisseria meningitides*, and *Haemophilus influenzae*. Even with advanced medical care, mortality remains high between 10 and 40 % and severe neurological damage affects 30–52 % of survivors [1, 2].

Among the complications of bacterial meningitis, intracranial vascular involvement is well known, i.e., ischemic infarction, sinus thrombosis, and hemorrhagic complications [3]. According to both animal experiments and a human autopsy study, bacterial meningitis can also cause microbleeds [4–6]. However, microbleeds are not commonly identified in clinical practice because of the limited detection threshold of head computed tomography (CT) scans and conventional magnetic resonance imaging (MRI). Therefore, microbleeds, as a complication of bacterial meningitis, are rarely recognized.

In this report, we present a case of bacterial meningitis due to *N. meningitides* with successful identification of microbleeds in the cerebellum by susceptibility-weighted imaging (SWI), a sensitive method that can be used to detect microbleeds in brain tissue.

Case presentation

A 19-year-old Japanese female without known medical history was transported to our emergency department because of coma. She complained of fever over 39 °C

* Correspondence: hidetakarina@gmail.com
†Equal contributors
[1]Department of Emergency and Critical Care Medicine, Nara Medical University, Shijo-cho, 840, Kashihara City, Nara, Japan
Full list of author information is available at the end of the article

and severe occipital headache the night before her family found her unconscious. Physical examination revealed that her Glasgow coma scale was 6 (E1V1M4) with blood pressure of 128/72 mmHg, heart rate of 88 beats/min, and respiratory rate of 19 breaths/min. Both pupils were 3.5 mm with a sluggish light reflex. Neurological examination found no motor laterality or pathological reflex, except for nuchal rigidity. A head CT scan revealed no focal region, but diffuse swelling of the brain. Her blood tests showed elevated leukocytes (21,100 cells/μL) and C-reactive protein (20.6 mg/dL). A lumbar tap was performed and turbid yellow spinal fluid was collected. Spinal fluid examination revealed protein 394 mg/dl, glucose 0 mg/dl and a cell count of 10112/mm^3 (96 % polymorphonuclear leukocytes), which confirmed the diagnosis of bacterial meningitis.

She was intubated and admitted to an intensive care unit. Due to poor study of the gram staining, meropenem and vancomycin were administered right after IV dexamethasone. On day 8, *N. meningitides* was cultured from the spinal fluid collected on admission and antibiotic therapy was changed to ampicillin (Fig. 2). Brain MRI study was performed on day 10 (Fig. 1). Postcontrast T1-weighted imaging showed enhanced subarachnoidal space of the cerebellum, typically along the great horizontal fissure (Fig. 1a and b). Additionally, Diffusion-weighted imaging (DWI) found high intensity area and SWI revealed multiple low-intensity spots in subarachoid space along the great horizontal fissure (Fig. 1c and d). Since these spotty low-intensity areas in the cerebellum located nonlinearly and there were no enhanced spots in the axial contrasted T1-weighted imaging, we confirmed that these low-intensity signals were not telangiectasia, but microbleeds. Antibiotic management was successful and her clinical symptoms improved. She was discharged on day 24 without neurological deficits. A follow-up brain MRI was performed on day 42. SWI showed the regions of multiple low-intensity spots in cerebellum persisted, but were disappearing (Fig. 1e). She had no neurological deficits and complained no symptoms on day 42.

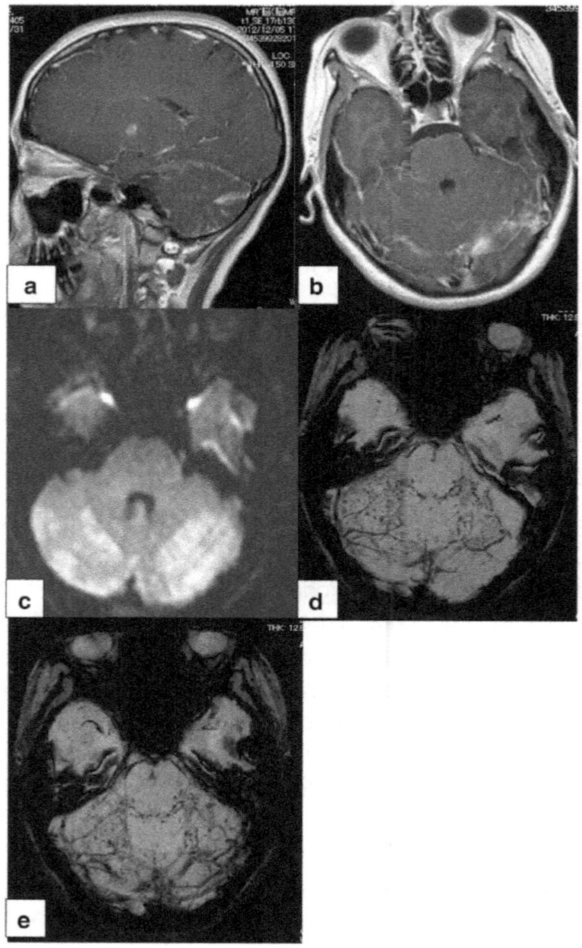

Fig. 1 Brain magnetic resonance imaging of the patient. Postcontrast T1-weighted saggital and axial imaging (**a, b**) showed enhancement in subarachoid space of cerebellum, typically in the great horizontal fissure. Diffusion-weighted imaging (**c**) showed high-intensity area in the great horizontal fissure. Susceptibility-weighted imaging (**d**) showed nonlinear multiple low intensity spots. These multiple spots are not enhanced in axial postcontrast T1-weighted image (**b**). Follow up MRI on day 42 showed that the multiple low-intensity spots persisted, but were disappearing (**e**)

We reported a case of meningitis due to *N. meningitides* in which the patient's SWI findings indicated diffuse microbleeds in the cerebellum. Despite an extensive literature search, we could not find a report of bacterial meningitis with microbleeds in the cerebellum or cerebral cortex identified by SWI.

The most common MRI findings in bacterial meningitis are intraventricular signal alterations, meningeal enhancement, and intraparenchymatous signal changes [7]. In this case, postcontrast T1-weighted imaging revealed enhancement in subarachnoidal space of cerebellum, which is consistent with general MRI findings of bacterial meningitis. Interestingly, DWI showed high intensity areas and SWI revealed multiple low-intensity spots located with veins in subarachnoid space along the great horizontal fissure. On SWI, deoxyhemoglobin, hemorrhagic blood products, and methemoglobin of hemorrhagic lesions can be visualized as low-intensity signals [8]. With the findings of DWI and SWI, we speculated that a collection of purulent exudate in subarachnoid space caused microbleeds on the surface of cerebellum. Animal experiments and a recent autopsy study of bacterial meningitis reported that both macroscopic and microscopic hemorrhages can be observed [4, 6]. In a pneumococcal meningitis mouse model, microscopic hemorrhages can be found in both the subarachnoid space and cortex [4]. An autopsy study of pneumococcal meningitis by Vergouwen et al. [6] also reported that the

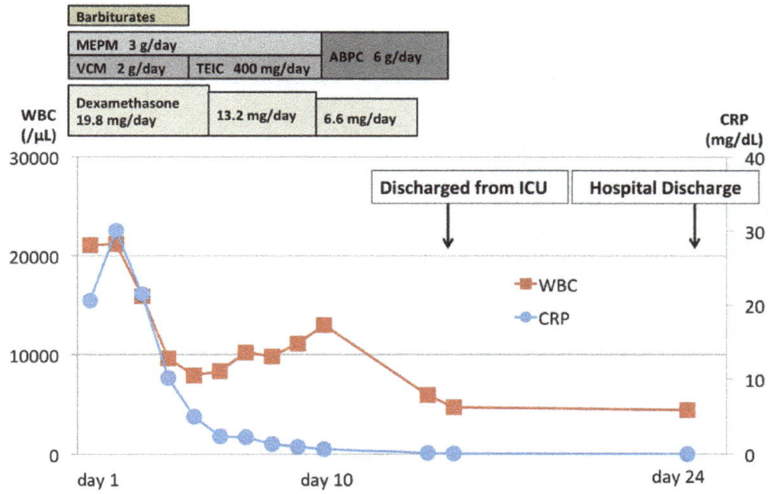

Fig. 2 Clinical course of the case. The patient was managed successfully with antibiotics and dexamethasone and discharged on day 24. MEPM, meropenem; VCM, vancomycin; TEIC, teicoplanin; WBC, white blood cell; ICU, intensive care unit; ABPC, ampicilin

majority of microbleeds were located in the cortex and subcortex with no evidence of infarction. The mechanism of microbleeds is considered as pyogenic vasculitis following vascular wall injury or extravasation of red blood cells from congested small veins caused by severe inflammation [6]. Microbleeds in meningococcal meningitis, however, has not been observed in human studies.

Other pathophysiology which can cause microbleeds detected by SWI are hypertsensive vasculopathy or amyloid angiopathy [9]. This patient, however, had no history indicating these pathophysiologies.

The clinical significance of microbleeds in bacterial meningitis, however, is not well documented. In this current case report, the cerebellar microbleeds did not seem to cause any neurological deterioration. Further studies are needed to investigate the pathogenesis of microbleeds and their clinical significance.

Conclusions

Meningococcal meningitis can cause multiple microbleeds in the cerebellum. In this report, we successfully identified microbleeds by susceptibility-weighed imaging. Using this imaging modality, further investigations will clarify its clinical incidence and significance.

Consent

Written informed consent was obtained from the patient for publication of this case report and any accompanying images. A copy of the written consent is available for review by the Editor of this journal.

Abbreviations

CT: Computed tomography; MRI: Magnetic resonance imaging; DWI: Diffusion-weighted imaging; SWI: Susceptibility-weighted imaging.

Competing interests

The authors have no competing interests to declare.

Authors' contributions

KM – conception, design, and manuscript preparation. HF – manuscript preparation and English translation. YK, TW, and KN – contributed to manuscript preparation. TT – contributed to radiological assessment. KO – substantial contribution to the concept of the manuscript and final correction of the manuscript. All authors have approved the final version of the manuscript.

Authors' information

All authors are medical doctors. TT is currently at Department of radiology, Nagoya University Graduate school of Medicine, Nagoya, Japan.

Acknowledgements

This report received no funding.

Author details

[1]Department of Emergency and Critical Care Medicine, Nara Medical University, Shijo-cho, 840, Kashihara City, Nara, Japan. [2]Department of Neurosurgery, Nara Medical University, Shijo-cho, 840, Kashihara City, Nara, Japan. [3]Department of Neurosurgery, Nara Prefecture General Medical Center, Hiramatsu, 1-30-1, Nara City, Nara, Japan. [4]Department of Radiology, Nara Medical University, Shijo-cho, 840, Kashihara City, Nara, Japan.

References

1. Sigurdardottir B, Bjornsson OM, Jonsdottir KE, Erlendsdottir H, Gudmundsson S. Acute bacterial meningitis in adults. A 20-year overview. Arch Intern Med. 1997;157(4):425–30.
2. Hussein AS, Shafran SD. Acute bacterial meningitis in adults. A 12-year review. Medicine (Baltimore). 2000;79(6):360–8.
3. Bodilsen J, Dalager-Pedersen M, Schonheyder HC, Nielsen H. Stroke in community-acquired bacterial meningitis: a Danish population-based study. Int J Infect Dis. 2014;20:18–22.

4. Mook-Kanamori B, Geldhoff M, Troost D, van der Poll T, van de Beek D. Characterization of a pneumococcal meningitis mouse model. BMC Infect Dis. 2012;12:71.
5. Woehrl B, Brouwer MC, Murr C, Heckenberg SG, Baas F, Pfister HW, et al. Complement component 5 contributes to poor disease outcome in humans and mice with pneumococcal meningitis. J Clin Invest. 2011;121(10):3943–53.
6. Vergouwen MD, Schut ES, Troost D, van de Beek D. Diffuse cerebral intravascular coagulation and cerebral infarction in pneumococcal meningitis. Neurocrit Care. 2010;13(2):217–27.
7. Lummel N, Koch M, Klein M, Pfister HW, Bruckmann H, Linn J. Spectrum and prevalence of pathological intracranial magnetic resonance imaging findings in acute bacterial meningitis. Clin Neuroradiol. 2014. doi:10.1007/s00062-014-0339-x.
8. Haacke EM, Xu Y, Cheng YC, Reichenbach JR. Susceptibility weighted imaging (SWI). Magn Reson Med. 2004;52(3):612–8.
9. Yates PA, Villemagne VL, Ellis KA, Desmond PM, Masters CL, Rowe CC. Cerebral microbleeds: a review of clinical, genetic, and neuroimaging associations. Front Neurol. 2014;4:205.

9

Prospective, randomized comparison of gadopentetate and gadobutrol to assess chronic myocardial infarction applying cardiovascular magnetic resonance

Andre Rudolph[1,2*], Daniel Messroghli[3], Florian von Knobelsdorff-Brenkenhoff[1,2], Julius Traber[1,2], Johannes Schüler[1,2], Ralf Wassmuth[1,2] and Jeanette Schulz-Menger[1,2]

Abstract

Background: We hypothesized that the contrast medium gadobutrol is not inferior compared to Gd-DTPA in identifying and quantifying ischemic late gadolinium enhancement (LGE), even by using a lower dose.

Methods: We prospectively enrolled 30 patients with chronic myocardial infarction as visualized by LGE during clinical routine scan at 1.5 T with 0.20 mmol/kg Gd-DTPA. Participants were randomized to either 0.15 mmol/kg gadobutrol (group A) or 0.10 mmol/kg gadobutrol (group B). CMR protocol was identical in both exams. LGE was quantified using a semiautomatic approach. Signal intensities of scar, remote myocardium, blood and air were measured. Signal to noise (SNR) and contrast to noise ratios (CNR) were calculated.

Results: Signal intensities were not different between Gd-DTPA and gadobutrol in group A, whereas significant differences were detected in group B. SNR of injured myocardium (53.5+/−21.4 vs. 30.1+/−10.4, $p = 0.0001$) and CNR between injured and remote myocardium (50.3+/−20.3 vs. 27.3+/−9.3, $p < 0.0001$) were lower in gadobutrol. Infarct size was lower in both gadobutrol groups compared to Gd-DTPA (group A: 16.8+/−10.2 g vs. 12.8+/−6.8 g, $p = 0.03$; group B: 18.6+/−12.0 g vs. 14.0+/−9.9 g, $p = 0.0016$).

Conclusions: Taking application of 0.2 mmol/kg Gd-DTPA as the reference, the delineation of infarct scar was similar with 0.15 mmol/kg gadobutrol, whereas the use 0.10 mmol/kg gadobutrol led to reduced tissue contrast.

Keywords: Cardiovascular Magnetic Resonance, Contrast media, Gadobutrol, Gd-DTPA, Chronic myocardial infarction, Late gadolinium enhancement

Background

Myocardial infarction is a leading cause of mortality worldwide. Accurate assessment of infarct size and morphology is important for clinical decision making in a lot of clinical settings [1, 2]. Currently, late gadolinium enhancement cardiac magnetic resonance (LGE-CMR) is a well-established and accurate method to assess scar morphology [3] and is widely used in clinical CMR [4, 5]. Until now, Gd-DTPA, a linear ionic gadolinium chelate, is the extracellular contrast agent that is mostly used for detection of myocardial LGE and is commonly administered as double dose (0.2 mmol/kg). After the administration of Gd-DTPA, cases of nephrogenic systemic fibrosis (NSF) in patients with renal failure have been reported, leading to a new risk classification of contrast media [6]. Whereas the detailed mechanism of NSF is not known, it could be shown in animal experiments that the tissue gadolinium distribution is altered in case of renal impairment [7].

* Correspondence: a.rudolph@charite.de
[1]Working Group CMR, Experimental and Clinical Research Center, a joint cooperation between the Charité Medical Faculty and the Max-Delbrück Center for Molecular Medicine, Lindenberger Weg 80, 13125 Berlin, Germany
[2]Dept. of Cardiology and Nephrology, HELIOS-Kliniken Berlin Buch, Schwanebecker Chaussee 50, 13125 Berlin, Germany
Full list of author information is available at the end of the article

Gadobutrol is a macrocyclic nonionic gadolinium chelate with a higher T_1 relaxivity compared to Gd-DTPA (gadobutrol: r1 = 4.7 $mmol^{-1}s^{-1}$; Gd-DTPA: r1 = 3.9 $mmol^{-1}s^{-1}$, at 1.5 Tesla, in human blood plasma, at 37 °C) [8]. The binding profile is known to be more stable, thus through to have a lower risk of NSF. Only three controversially discussed cases of NSF were reported after the use of gadobutrol worldwide until now [9, 10]. Therefore gadobutrol is classified as a low risk contrast-medium. This and the higher relaxivity are driving forces for further evaluations in cardiovascular settings.

Today, there are only limited data available analyzing the influence of contrast agents with different relaxivities on LGE quantification. In this study, we hypothesized that gadobutrol, which is characterized by a higher relaxivity compared to Gd-DTPA, is not inferior to Gd-DTPA in identifying and quantifying ischemic LGE, even when using a lower dose.

Methods

Patients' enrollment

Between September 2010 and December 2011, patients with a history of a chronic myocardial infarction and LGE as assessed during a clinical CMR scan using 0.20 mmol/kg Gd-DTPA were screened and asked for participation in a second study-related CMR scan. All included patients gave written informed consent and were scheduled for a second CMR examination afterwards. The study had been registered under EudraCT number: 2010-020775-22 and was accordingly approved by the ethical board of the city of Berlin (LAGESO).

The sample size of this randomized prospective trial was calculated based on a power calculation. The assumption was, that for a two-sided alpha of 5 % and a power of 80 % based on a delta of 0.15, 15 patients per dose gadobutrol have to be included.

Patients were randomized for either 0.15 mmol/kg (group A) or 0.10 mmol/kg (group B) gadobutrol. All patients were in normofrequent sinus rhythm.

Inclusion criteria

- between 18 and 80 years of age
- chronic myocardial infarction (>3 months old) based on coronary artery disease (CAD), detected by invasive angiography
- successfully performed clinical LGE CMR study within the last 4 weeks
- evidence of single myocardial infarction on LGE CMR with "hyper-enhancement" involving at least two contiguous short-axis slices
- written informed consent

Exclusion criteria

- severe arrhythmia, atrial fibrillation
- history of moderate or severe impairment of renal function (GFR < 60 ml/min)
- additional myocardial infarction or acute coronary syndrome during the last 4 weeks
- general contraindications for CMR

Image acquisition

CMR was performed on a 1.5Tesla cardiac-dedicated clinical MR system (Avanto, Siemens Healthcare, Erlangen, Germany) using a 12-channel coil. Identical CMR protocols were applied for both examinations.

LGE LGE was assessed in all patients starting 13 min after contrast administration in a short axis stack by using a 2D inversion recovery gradient echo sequence (slice thickness 8 mm, no gap, TE 5.0 ms, FA 30°, matrix 256×192, field of view 350×262mm) with an inversion time (TI) adjusted to null signal from normal myocardium. In case of questionable bright signal in the myocardium during the scan, we changed the read out or acquired a perpendicular slice to exclude artefacts. Slice position was identical as for cine imaging using a single slice single breathold approach.

T_1 quantification T_1 quantification was performed with a Modified Look-Locker Inversion-recovery (MOLLI) sequence [11], acquired in a mid-ventricular short-axis slice before and 1, 3, 5, 9, 20 min after contrast administration. Multiple post-contrast measurements were performed to show the optimal time point of image acquisition after contrast administration. Imaging parameters were: non-selective inversion pulse, steady-state free precession single-shot read out in mid-diastole, field of view 223 × 320 mm, matrix 174 × 192, slice thickness 8 mm, TE 1.08 ms, FA 35°, bandwidth 1002Hz/Px, minimum inversion time of 100 ms, maximum inversion time of 3600 ms.

Image analysis

Function For analyzing LV function and volumes, the endocardial and epicardial contours were manually drawn in systole and diastole using dedicated software (CMR^{42}, circle, Calgary, Canada). LV mass was calculated as total myocardial volume multiplied by the specific gravity of the myocardium (1.05 g/ml). LV mass and LV end diastolic volume were indexed to height.

LGE The readers were blinded to the group assignment. For quantification of LGE a semiautomatic gray-scale threshold technique was performed as published previously

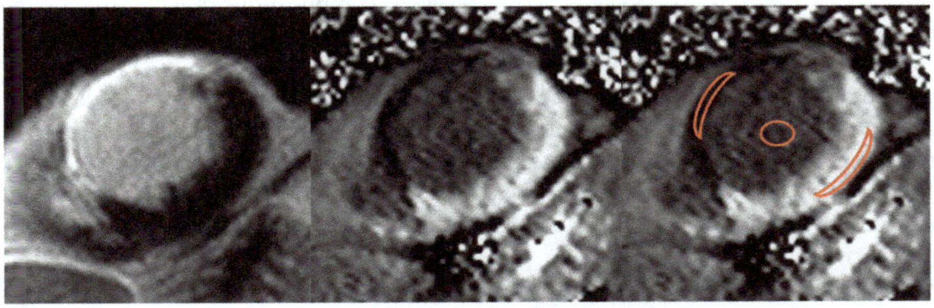

Fig. 1 T_1-Mapping. LGE-image in short axis view (left) with corresponding T_1-map (center and right) show a transmural anteroseptal myocardial infarction. ROIs (infarct region, remote myocardium and blood pool) were drawn on the map (right)

[12]. Areas of LGE were defined as a signal intensity of more than 6 standard deviations (SD) above the mean of remote myocardium.

Signal intensities of scar tissue, remote myocardium, blood and air were measured by drawing free-hand ROIs of approximately 10–20 pixels in each LGE short axis stack. Reproducible locations were achieved by using anatomical landmarks in dedicated software (CMR[42], circle international, Calgary Canada). For signal-to-noise ratio (SNR) and contrast-to-noise ratio (CNR) the following sequations were used [13]:

SNR = mean signal of ROI/standard deviation of background noise. CNR (between tissue A and tissue B) = SNR (A)–SNR (B).

T_1 quantification T_1 maps were constructed offline using MRmap [14, 15] a customized software program written in Interactive Data Language (IDL; RSI International, Boulder, CO, USA). The position of the source images was initially manually adjusted to correct for potential misregistration. A curve fit of the MOLLI source images was then performed, with automatic calculation of T_1 values for each pixel. A T_1 parametric map was subsequently generated and used for further analysis. The parametric maps were evaluated in CMR[42]. Freehand ROI's of approximately 10–20 pixels were placed in scar tissue, remote myocardium and blood for measuring the averaged T_1 time in this tissue. Reference for scar delineation was the LGE image in the same plane (Fig. 1).

Table 1 Patient's characteristics

	Group A	Group B
Male/female	15/0	15/0
Age (years)	70.20 ± 4.70	63.50 ± 10.70
Scar amount (g)	16.77 ± 10.18	18.63 ± 11.98
SNR scar	45.51 ± 22.56	53.45 ± 21.40
CNR between scar tissue and remote myocardium	41.76 ± 21.24	50.27 ± 20.30

Interobserver variability

To test inter-observer variability in LGE quantification, two readers who were blinded to each other's results analyzed all examinations.

Statistical analysis

Statistical analyses were performed using SAS 9.2 (SAS Institute Inc., Cary, NC, USA) and SPSS 21.0 for windows (Chicago, Il, USA). Data are presented as mean ± standard deviation. Statistical tests were performed using non-parametric methods due to the low sample size within each group. Continuous data were compared using the Wilcoxon rank sum tests. Paired data were compared using Wilcoxon signed rank tests. Categorical data were compared using Fisher's exact test. Statistical tests were considered significant with the two-sided $p < 0.05$. Spearman correlation coefficient's were used to determine observer-related variability. Boxplots were generated with SPSS and show median (line in the middle), 1st quartile (bottom of box), 3rd quartile (top of box), lowest case within 1.5 times IQR (bottom whisker), highest case within 1.5 times IQR (top whisker) and outliers.

Table 2 Signal intensities and LGE quantification in group A

	Gd-DTPA (0.2 mmol/kg)	Gadobutrol (0.15 mmol/kg)	p-value
SNR of scar tissue	45.51 ± 22.56	47.04 ± 19.78	>0.9999
CNR between scar tissue and remote myocardium	41.76 ± 21.24	42.83 ± 17.31	>0.9999
SNR of blood	43.97 ± 16.32	44.37 ± 16.20	0.6698
CNR between scar tissue and blood	1.53 ± 17.18	2.65 ± 14.02	0.5153
Amount of LGE (g)	16.77 ± 10.18	12.84 ± 6.79	0.0300

Results

We screened 252 patients and identified 51 who met our criteria. 30 patients agreed to participate in the trial and were prospectively enrolled in the study and randomized to either 0.15 mmol/kg gadobutrol (group A) or 0.10 mmol/kg gadobutrol (group B). 21 patients refused participation due to a lack of motivation or fear of repeated contrast administration. There were no significant differences between groups relating age, scar amount and signal intensities for control agent Gd-DTPA (Table 1). The time duration between both scans was at maximum 30 days. We took the history again to check for clinical events. In none of the patients a clinical event was existing.

No complications related to contrast administration were observed. Infarcts were detectable in all patients.

Comparison of signal intensities and LGE amount

In group A signal intensities showed no differences between Gd-DTPA and gadobutrol (Table 2, Figs. 2 and 3). Amount of LGE was lower in gadobutrol, the absolute difference was small, but reached statistical significance ($p = 0.03$).

In group B signal intensities showed significant differences between Gd-DTPA and gadobutrol. In particular SNR of injured myocardium and CNR between injured and remote myocardium were significantly lower in gadobutrol resulting in a significant smaller

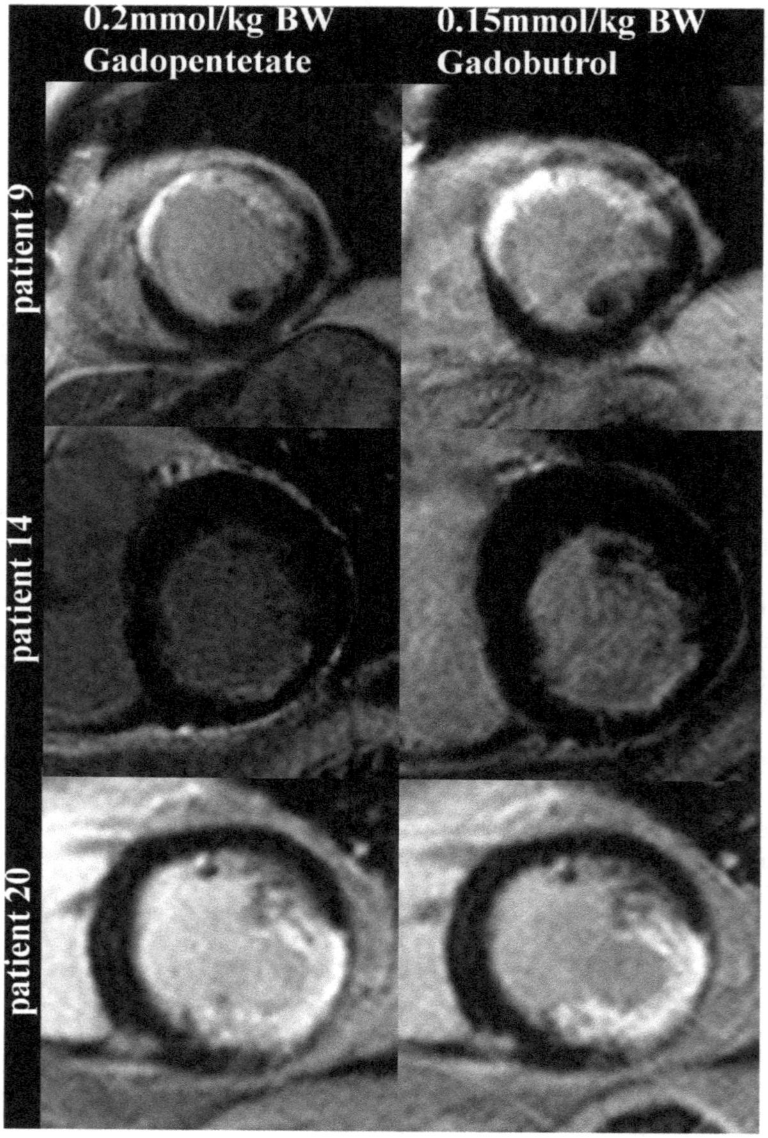

Fig. 2 LGE (short axis view) example images from group A. Left: after 0.2 mmol/kg BW Gd-DTPA. Right: after 0.15 mmol/kg BW gadobutrol

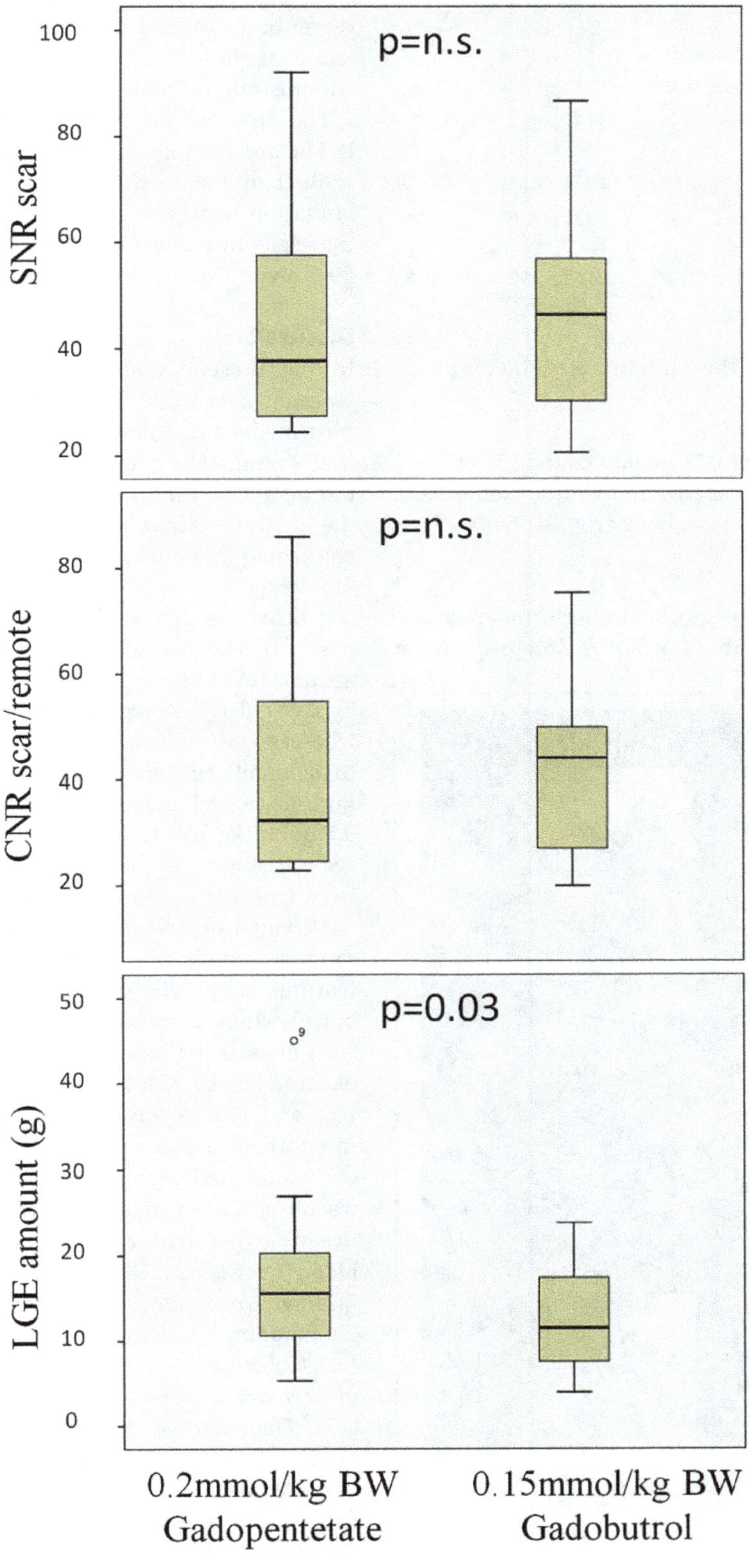

Fig. 3 Boxplots showing SNR-, CNR and LGE amount in group A. Left: after 0.2 mmol/kg BW Gd-DTPA. Right: after 0.15 mmol/kg BW gadobutrol

Table 3 Signal intensities and LGE quantification in group B

	Gd-DTPA (0.2 mmol/kg)	Gadobutrol (0.1 mmol/kg)	p-value
SNR of scar tissue	53.45 ± 21.40	30.11 ± 10.36	0.0001
CNR between scar tissue and remote myocardium	50.27 ± 20.30	27.32 ± 9.28	<0.0001
SNR of blood	48.57 ± 17.69	19.84 ± 6.33	<0.0001
CNR between scar tissue and blood	4.89 ± 12.96	10.29 ± 9.26	0.0554
Amount of LGE (g)	18.63 ± 11.98	14.03 ± 9.92	0.0016

scar size as defined by the amount of LGE (Table 3, Figs. 4 and 5).

Interobserver Variability of LGE quantification

Interobserver variability was low and without differences between the contrast agents in both groups (Table 4).

T_1 mapping

For technical reasons we were able to perform a pairwise analysis in only six patients of group A. Interestingly, in this subgroup we found no significant differences between both contrast media regarding T_1 times of the different tissues at different time- points after contrast administration (Table 5).

The drop-out rate was high due to two main-aspects: I) The applied sequence was a first generation one as described in the method section. II) The most frequent limitation was the registration failure of the raw images especially in regions of wall thinning respectively the infarct area.

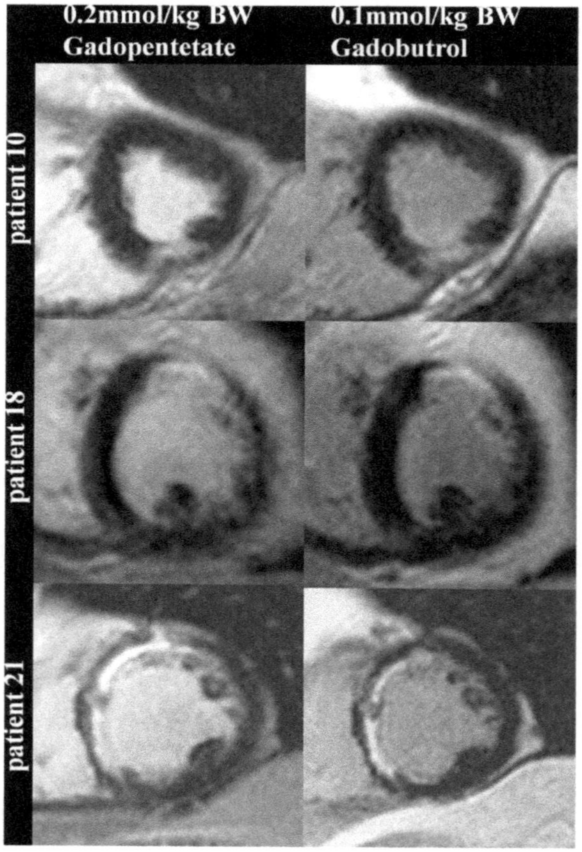

Fig. 4 LGE (short axis view) example images from group B. Left: after 0.2 mmol/kg BW Gd-DTPA. Right: after 0.1 mmol/kg BW gadobutrol

Discussion

In the present study we compared the depiction of chronic myocardial infarction using two different contrast media and different doses in a prospective randomized setting. The null hypothesis of our study was, that the infarct volume with gadobutrol is not equivalent to the infarct volume with the control agent. This was confirmed by our results. The main results are the following:

I) Scar was detectable with each contrast media and dose. II) The use of 0.15 mmol/kg BW (body weight) gadubutrol led to similar results compared to 0.2 mmol/kg BW Gd-DTPA regarding signal intensity and contrast whereas the application of 0.1 mmol/kg gadobutrol led to a significant poorer delineation of scar tissue. III) Both doses gadobutrol led to a smaller infarct size taking 0.2 mmol/kg BW Gd-DTPA as the reference. IV) Observer variability of LGE quantification was independent from type and dose of contrast agent.

Although our sample size was small, but defined in a random setting, we could confirm in part the data by Durmus et al., who compared 0.15 mmol/kg BW gadobutrol with 0.2 mmol/kg BW Gd-DTPA in 20 patients with myocardial infarction [16]. They showed that gadobutrol led to similar infarct size and CNR between scar and remote myocardium compared to Gd-DTPA. In contrast to our results, CNR between scar and blood even increased with gadobutrol in their study, whereas we observed no significant difference in group A between gadubutrol and Gd-DTPA regarding SNR of blood as well as CNR between scar and blood. Our finding are supported by the quantitative parametric T1-mapping results as presented in a subgroup.

DeCobelli et al. compared gadobutrol with Gd-DTPA in patients with positive LGE regardless of its etiology [17]. They showed that 0.1 mmol/kg BW gadobutrol is as effective as 0.2 mmol/kg BW Gd-DTPA regarding signal intensities and quantification of injured tissue. Our data (group B) are different to these results. In our study 0.1 mmol/kg BW gadobutrol led to poorer delineation of infarct scar and reduced amount of LGE as found by both readers. A possible explanation for this discrepancy between both studies could be the different patient

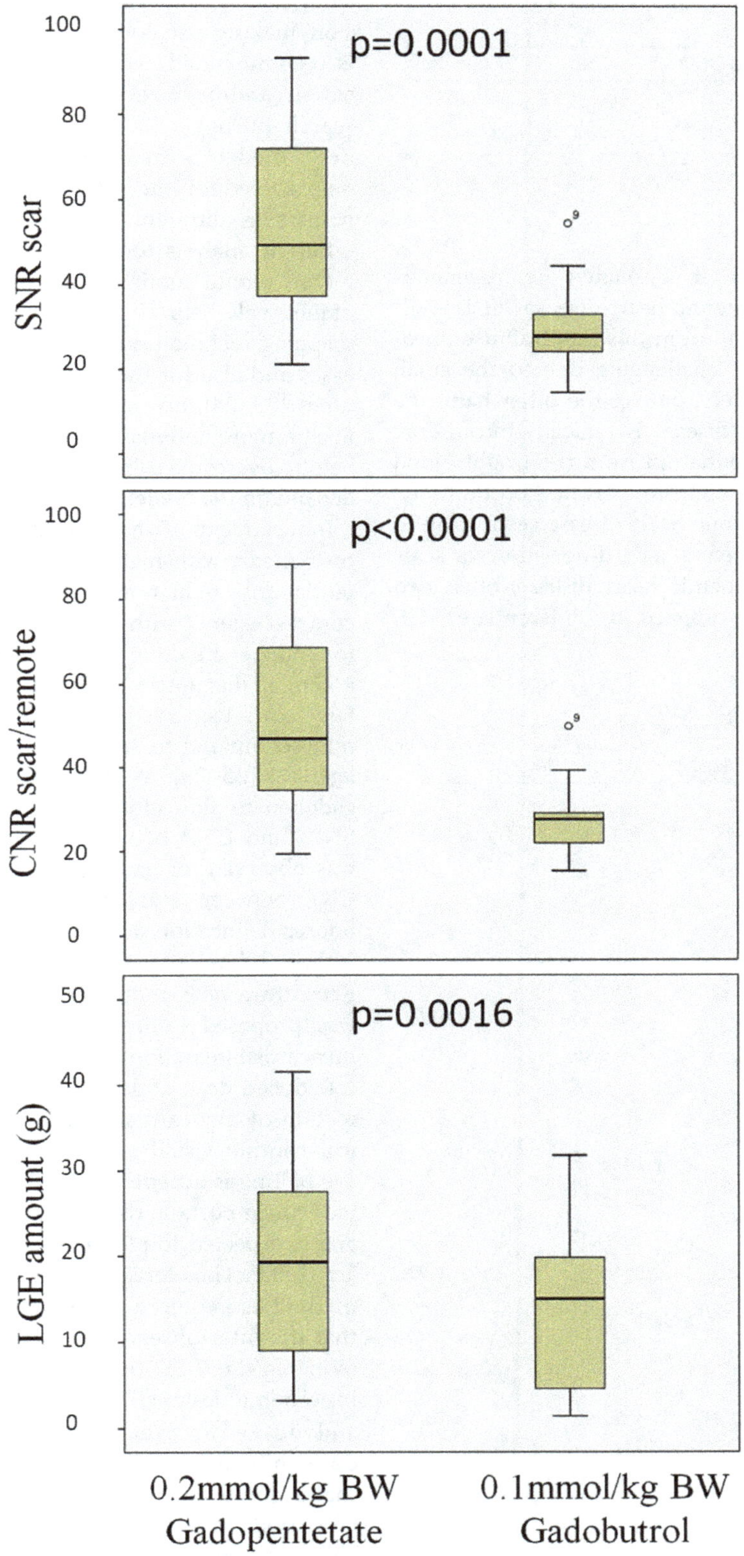

Fig. 5 Boxplots showing SNR-, CNR and LGE amount in group B. Left: after 0.2 mmol/kg BW Gd-DTPA. Right: after 0.1 mmol/kg BW gadobutrol

Table 4 Spearman's correlation coefficients between the two readers

	Gd-DTPA	Gadobutrol
Group A	0.85	0.93
Group B	0.91	0.94

population. DeCobelli et al. evaluated heterogeneous groups including non-ischemic heart-diseases. It is well-known, that the quantification in this more diffuse fibrosis is on one hand more challenging due to the small size and the blurred borders, but on the other hand the location in non-ischemic disease is typically intramural. That facilitates the differentiation from the bright blood pool signal. The different character of the fibrotic tissue in non-ischemic and ischemic heart disease seems to lead to the application of different standard-deviation for scar-sizing. In case of non-ischemic heart disease, often two standard deviations were applied to differentiate LGE from remote myocardium [18, 19]. For clinical decision making usually visual assessment of LGE images is recommended, whereas quantitative analysis of LGE extent and/or "grey-zone" extent is common for research purposes [20]. The integration of pharmacokinetic models with different compartments could also help to reduce the influence of different contrast dynamics in different types of fibrosis [21], as well as different analysis tools [22].

Table 5 T_1 values (ms) in group A ($n = 6$)

Time after contrast administration	Gd-DTPA (0.2 mmol/kgKG)	Gadobutrol (0.15 mmol/kgKG)	p-value
Native			
myocardium	909 ± 199	990 ± 117	0.17
scar	1033 ± 226	978 ± 98	0.92
blood	1407 ± 42	1402 ± 62	0.53
1 min			
myocardium	248 ± 38	250 ± 36	0.92
scar	207 ± 28	210 ± 36	0.75
blood	134 ± 18	144 ± 15	0.35
3 min			
myocardium	305 ± 50	311 ± 23	0.75
scar	227 ± 18	241 ± 36	0.35
blood	181 ± 23	200 ± 17	0.25
5 min			
myocardium	361 ± 57	360 ± 18	0.92
scar	275 ± 31	285 ± 48	0.46
blood	215 ± 21	248 ± 52	0.08
9 min			
myocardium	416 ± 61	405 ± 22	0.6
scar	300 ± 50	308 ± 47	0.35
blood	260 ± 28	265 ± 21	0.6
20 min			
myocardium	472 ± 63	468 ± 35	0.89
scar	351 ± 67	361 ± 64	0.5
blood	330 ± 42	337 ± 26	0.5

One would assume that parametric mapping techniques will help to overcome that problem. Whereas mapping techniques are already applied in different diseases and also for the quantification of extracellular volumes [23, 24], no standardized approach is given today. Furthermore automatic assessment of infarct borders will help to overcome subjective approaches [25], but they also depend on the predefined gold standards.

Independent of the quantification method itself, contrast media with higher relaxivity are warranted for potential dose reduction. The concept of dose reduction in contrast agents with higher relaxivity was also analyzed for gadobenate dimeglumine. Recent studies have shown a similar diagnostic performance and delineation of infarct scars using reduced doses of gadobenate dimeglumine compared to standard dose Gd-DTPA (0.2 mmol/kg BW) [26–28]. When comparing equivalent doses of gadobenate dimeglumine with Gd-DTPA [29], higher SNR- and CNR between scar and remote myocardium was observed for gadobenate dimeglumine, whereas the CNR between scar and blood decreased resulting in poorer delineation of small subendocardial infarcts. New technical developments could help to overcome this limit. Recently, a new multi contrast LGE sequence (MCODE) was proposed to improve detection of subendocardial myocardial infarction [30].

Reduced dose of gadobutrol allows a reproducible detection of myocardial infarction in all patients. In clinical routine visual assessment of scar is accepted and eye balling is accepted [12]. But scar quantification may play an important role in treatment planning in future and is expected to play a crucial role in risk stratification [1, 31, 32]. Therefore, a simple and robust post-processing method is required. The present study demonstrated that the inter-observer variability of LGE quantification by using the 6-SD threshold yielded satisfactory results in ischemic lesions independent from the contrast type and dose. However, we observed that relaxivity and dose influence the absolute results, which underlines that accurate follow-up evaluations need constant CMR conditions in clinical trials. CMR offers the unique capability to bring reliable (semi)quantitative approaches of myocardial tissue differentiation based on contrast- and non-contrast enhanced techniques into clinical routine therefore standardization is of importance.

Limitations

The present study was conducted at a single center with a relatively small sample size. The study only included men to omit the influence of sex on the results. Further studies in women are necessary to extend the conclusions to both sexes.

SNR- and CNR of LGE images are influenced by inversion time. Its adjustment is operator-dependent. T1-mapping was expected to add information on contrast-media timing, but for technical reasons we were only able to complete a pairwise T1 analysis in six patients of group A. Larger studies preferably with mapping techniques are needed to confirm our results.

Conclusions

The use of 0.15 mmol/kg BW gadobutrol led to comparable results as 0.20 mmol/kg BW Gd-DTPA in delineation of myocardial infarction and only to a small, clinically non-relevant deviation in quantification of infarct scar and may be an appropriate alternative under consideration of the lower risk for NSF. In contrast, the dose of 0.10 mmol/kg BW gadobutrol was associated with lower signal intensity and higher discrepancy regarding infarct size. Our results underline that accurate scar evaluation during follow-up depends on type of contrast agent and contrast dose and therefore requires constant study conditions.

Competing interests

The trial was supported by a grant of Bayer HealthCare Medical Care (Bayer Pharma AG, Berlin, Germany) (See: Acknowledgements).

Author' contributions

AR participated in the design of the study, coordinated the scans, evaluated the data and drafted the manuscript, DM conceived of the study, participated in its design and helped to draft parts of the manuscript; FvK in the design of the study, evaluated part of the data, helped to draft the manuscript, JT participated in data postprocessing, partly statistical analysis. JS performed data-analysis. RW participated in the design of the study and performed CMR scans. JSM conceived main parts of the study, participated in the design and helped to draft the manuscript. All authors read and approved the final manuscript."

Acknowledgements

The authors would like to thank our technicians, led by Kerstin Kretschel, for their assistance and great help in acquiring the images.
Furthermore, without the work of our study nurse Annette Köhler this study would not have been possible.
We are thankful for the tremendous help of Edyta Blaszczyk during the revision process.
The trial was supported by a grant of Bayer HealthCare (Bayer Pharma AG, Berlin, Germany). The authors want to thank the HELIOS research center especially Dr. Heinrich and Mr. Welcker for their help in formal work during run the applications. Prof. Petra Thürmann in handling the formal challenges.

Author details

[1]Working Group CMR, Experimental and Clinical Research Center, a joint cooperation between the Charité Medical Faculty and the Max-Delbrück Center for Molecular Medicine, Lindenberger Weg 80, 13125 Berlin, Germany. [2]Dept. of Cardiology and Nephrology, HELIOS-Kliniken Berlin Buch, Schwanebecker Chaussee 50, 13125 Berlin, Germany. [3]Department of Congenital Heart Disease and Pediatric Cardiology, Deutsches Herzzentrum Berlin, Berlin, Germany.

References

1. Boye P, Abdel-Aty H, Zacharzowsky U, Bohl S, Schwenke C, van der Geest RJ, et al. Prediction of life-threatening arrhythmic events in patients with chronic myocardial infarction by contrast-enhanced CMR. JACC Cardiovasc Imaging. 2011;4(8):871–9.
2. de Haan S, Meijers TA, Knaapen P, Beek AM, van Rossum AC, Allaart CP. Scar size and characteristics assessed by CMR predict ventricular arrhythmias in ischaemic cardiomyopathy: comparison of previously validated models. Heart. 2011;97(23):1951–6.
3. Kim RJ, Chen EL, Lima JA, Judd RM. Myocardial Gd-DTPA kinetics determine MRI contrast enhancement and reflect the extent and severity of myocardial injury after acute reperfused infarction. Circulation. 1996;94(12):3318–26.
4. von Knobelsdorff-Brenkenhoff F, Schulz-Menger J. Cardiovascular magnetic resonance imaging in ischemic heart disease. J Magn Reson Imaging. 2012; 36(1):20–38.
5. von Knobelsdorff-Brenkenhoff F, Bublak A, El-Mahmoud S, Wassmuth R, Opitz C, Schulz-Menger J. Single-centre survey of the application of cardiovascular magnetic resonance in clinical routine. Eur Heart J Cardiovasc Imaging. 2013;14(1):62–8.
6. Yang L, Krefting I, Gorovets A, Marzella L, Kaiser J, Boucher R, et al. Nephrogenic systemic fibrosis and class labeling of gadolinium-based contrast agents by the Food and Drug Administration. Radiology. 2012; 265(1):248–53.
7. Wadas TJ, Sherman CD, Miner JH, Duncan JR, Anderson CJ. The biodistribution of [153Gd]Gd-labeled magnetic resonance contrast agents in a transgenic mouse model of renal failure differs greatly from control mice. Magn Reson Med. 2010;64(5):1274–80.
8. Pintaske J, Martirosian P, Graf H, Erb G, Lodemann KP, Claussen CD, et al. Relaxivity of Gadopentetate Dimeglumine (Magnevist), Gadobutrol (Gadovist), and Gadobenate Dimeglumine (MultiHance) in human blood plasma at 0.2, 1.5, and 3 Tesla. Invest Radiol. 2006;41(3):213–21.
9. Wollanka H, Weidenmaier W, Giersig C. NSF after Gadovist exposure: a case report and hypothesis of NSF development. Nephrol Dial Transplant. 2009; 24(12):3882–4.
10. Elmholdt TR, Bettina J, Mette R, Pedersen M, Olesen AB. Two cases of nephrogenic systemic fibrosis after exposure to the macrocyclic compound gadobutrol. NDT Plus. 2010;3:285–7.
11. Messroghli DR, Radjenovic A, Kozerke S, Higgins DM, Sivananthan MU, Ridgway JP. Modified Look-Locker inversion recovery (MOLLI) for high-resolution T1 mapping of the heart. Magn Reson Med. 2004;52(1):141–6.
12. Flett AS, Hasleton J, Cook C, Hausenloy D, Quarta G, Ariti C, et al. Evaluation of techniques for the quantification of myocardial scar of differing etiology using cardiac magnetic resonance. Jacc. 2011;4(2):150–6.
13. Dietrich O, Raya JG, Reeder SB, Reiser MF, Schoenberg SO. Measurement of signal-to-noise ratios in MR images: influence of multichannel coils, parallel imaging, and reconstruction filters. J Magn Reson Imaging. 2007;26(2):375–85.
14. Messroghli DR, Rudolph A, Abdel-Aty H, Wassmuth R, Kuhne T, Dietz R, et al. An open-source software tool for the generation of relaxation time maps in magnetic resonance imaging. BMC Med Imaging. 2010;10:16.
15. Messroghli DR, Walters K, Plein S, Sparrow P, Friedrich MG, Ridgway JP, et al. Myocardial T1 mapping: application to patients with acute and chronic myocardial infarction. Magn Reson Med. 2007;58(1):34–40.
16. Durmus T, Schilling R, Doeblin P, Huppertz A, Hamm B, Taupitz M, et al. Gadobutrol for magnetic resonance imaging of chronic myocardial infarction: intraindividual comparison with gadopentetate dimeglumine. Invest Radiol. 2012;47(3):183–8.
17. De Cobelli F, Esposito A, Perseghin G, Sallemi C, Belloni E, Ravelli S, et al. Intraindividual comparison of gadobutrol and gadopentetate dimeglumine for detection of myocardial late enhancement in cardiac MRI. AJR Am J Roentgenol. 2012;198(4):809–16.
18. Rudolph A, Abdel-Aty H, Bohl S, Boye P, Zagrosek A, Dietz R, et al. Noninvasive detection of fibrosis applying contrast-enhanced cardiac magnetic resonance in different forms of left ventricular hypertrophy relation to remodeling. J Am Coll Cardiol. 2009;53(3):284–91.
19. Assomull RG, Prasad SK, Lyne J, Smith G, Burman ED, Khan M, et al. Cardiovascular magnetic resonance, fibrosis, and prognosis in dilated cardiomyopathy. J Am Coll Cardiol. 2006;48(10):1977–85.

20. Schulz-Menger J, Bluemke DA, Bremerich J, Flamm SD, Fogel MA, Friedrich MG, et al. Standardized image interpretation and post processing in cardiovascular magnetic resonance: Society for Cardiovascular Magnetic Resonance (SCMR) board of trustees task force on standardized post processing. J Cardiovasc Magn Reson. 2013;15:35.
21. Knowles BR, Batchelor PG, Parish V, Ginks M, Plein S, Razavi R, et al. Pharmacokinetic modeling of delayed gadolinium enhancement in the myocardium. Magn Reson Med. 2008;60(6):1524–30.
22. Heiberg E, Sjogren J, Ugander M, Carlsson M, Engblom H, Arheden H. Design and validation of Segment–freely available software for cardiovascular image analysis. BMC Med Imaging. 2010;10:1.
23. Ugander M, Oki AJ, Hsu LY, Kellman P, Greiser A, Aletras AH, et al. Extracellular volume imaging by magnetic resonance imaging provides insights into overt and sub-clinical myocardial pathology. Eur Heart J. 2012; 33(10):1268–78.
24. Mongeon FP, Jerosch-Herold M, Coelho-Filho OR, Blankstein R, Falk RH, Kwong RY. Quantification of extracellular matrix expansion by CMR in infiltrative heart disease. JACC Cardiovasc Imaging. 2012;5(9):897–907.
25. Tao Q, Milles J, Zeppenfeld K, Lamb HJ, Bax JJ, Reiber JH, et al. Automated segmentation of myocardial scar in late enhancement MRI using combined intensity and spatial information. Magn Reson Med. 2010;64(2):586–94.
26. Bauner KU, Reiser MF, Huber AM. Low dose gadobenate dimeglumine for imaging of chronic myocardial infarction in comparison with standard dose gadopentetate dimeglumine. Invest Radiol. 2009;44(2):95–104.
27. Tumkosit M, Puntawangkoon C, Morgan TM, Clark HP, Hamilton CA, Ntim WO, et al. Left ventricular infarct size assessed with 0.1 mmol/kg of gadobenate dimeglumine correlates with that assessed with 0.2 mmol/kg of gadopentetate dimeglumine. J Comput Assist Tomogr. 2009;33(3):328–33.
28. Balci NC, Inan N, Anik Y, Erturk MS, Ural D, Demirci A. Low-dose gadobenate dimeglumine versus standard-dose gadopentate dimeglumine for delayed contrast-enhanced cardiac magnetic resonance imaging. Acad Radiol. 2006; 13(7):833–9.
29. Schlosser T, Hunold P, Herborn CU, Lehmkuhl H, Lind A, Massing S, et al. Myocardial infarct: depiction with contrast-enhanced MR imaging–comparison of gadopentetate and gadobenate. Radiology. 2005;236(3):1041–6.
30. Bandettini WP, Kellman P, Mancini C, Booker OJ, Vasu S, Leung SW, et al. MultiContrast Delayed Enhancement (MCODE) improves detection of subendocardial myocardial infarction by late gadolinium enhancement cardiovascular magnetic resonance: a clinical validation study. J Cardiovasc Magn Reson. 2012;14(1):83.
31. Klem I, Weinsaft JW, Bahnson TD, Hegland D, Kim HW, Hayes B, et al. Assessment of myocardial scarring improves risk stratification in patients evaluated for cardiac defibrillator implantation. J Am Coll Cardiol. 2012;60(5): 408–20.
32. Fluechter S, Kuschyk J, Wolpert C, Doesch C, Veltmann C, Haghi D, et al. Extent of late gadolinium enhancement detected by cardiovascular magnetic resonance correlates with the inducibility of ventricular tachyarrhythmia in hypertrophic cardiomyopathy. J Cardiovasc Magn Reson. 2010;12:30.

10

A semi-automated measuring system of brain diffusion and perfusion magnetic resonance imaging abnormalities in patients with multiple sclerosis based on the integration of coregistration and tissue segmentation procedures

Alfredo Revenaz[1], Massimiliano Ruggeri[2], Marcella Laganà[3], Niels Bergsland[3,4], Elisabetta Groppo[5], Marco Rovaris[6] and Enrico Fainardi[1*]

Abstract

Background: Diffusion-weighted imaging (DWI) and perfusion-weighted imaging (PWI) abnormalities in patients with multiple sclerosis (MS) are currently measured by a complex combination of separate procedures. Therefore, the purpose of this study was to provide a reliable method for reducing analysis complexity and obtaining reproducible results.

Methods: We implemented a semi-automated measuring system in which different well-known software components for magnetic resonance imaging (MRI) analysis are integrated to obtain reliable measurements of DWI and PWI disturbances in MS.

Results: We generated the Diffusion/Perfusion Project (DPP) Suite, in which a series of external software programs are managed and harmonically and hierarchically incorporated by in-house developed Matlab software to perform the following processes: 1) image pre-processing, including imaging data anonymization and conversion from DICOM to Nifti format; 2) co-registration of 2D and 3D non-enhanced and Gd-enhanced T1-weighted images in fluid-attenuated inversion recovery (FLAIR) space; 3) lesion segmentation and classification, in which FLAIR lesions are at first segmented and then categorized according to their presumed evolution; 4) co-registration of segmented FLAIR lesion in T1 space to obtain the FLAIR lesion mask in the T1 space; 5) normal appearing tissue segmentation, in which T1 lesion mask is used to segment basal ganglia/thalami, normal appearing grey matter (NAGM) and normal appearing white matter (NAWM); 6) DWI and PWI map generation; 7) co-registration of basal ganglia/thalami, NAGM, NAWM, DWI and PWI maps in previously segmented FLAIR space; 8) data analysis. All these steps are automatic, except for lesion segmentation and classification.

Conclusion: We developed a promising method to limit misclassifications and user errors, providing clinical researchers with a practical and reproducible tool to measure DWI and PWI changes in MS.

Keywords: DPP Suite, Coregistration, Automatic segmentation, Automatic classification, DWI, PWI

* Correspondence: henryfa@tin.it
[1]Unità Operativa di Neuroradiologia, Dipartimento di Neuroscienze e Riabilitazione, Azienda Ospedaliero-Universitaria of Ferrara, Arcispedale S. Anna, Via Aldo Moro 8, 44124 Cona, Ferrara, Italy
Full list of author information is available at the end of the article

Background

The role of diffusion-weighted imaging (DWI) and perfusion-weighted imaging (PWI) modalities in multiple sclerosis (MS) has recently received increased attention due to the potential of these two advanced magnetic resonance imaging (MRI) techniques in detecting the structural and hemodynamic characteristics of MS-related focal [1–7] and diffuse [8–16] brain abnormalities in gray and white matter, which characterize the well-known heterogeneity of the disease [17]. In fact, although conventional MRI findings are currently considered a valid surrogate marker for MS diagnosis and progression in treated and untreated patients, their diagnostic and prognostic value still remains very limited given the inability of conventional MRI in identifying the specific pathologic substrates of MS lesions [17]. Thus, it could be crucial to understand whether the detection and quantification of focal and diffuse DWI and PWI changes may help in recognizing the different mechanisms implicated in MS damage and, as a consequence, in improving diagnostic accuracy, early outcome prediction and response to treatment monitoring in MS. As DWI and PWI can be easily integrated in the context of MRI examination, this may have a large impact for routine clinical setting and patient quality of life. Therefore, further studies are warranted to clarify the actual significance of DWI and PWI disturbances in MS. However, the evaluation of DWI and PWI alterations in MS is generally restricted to the research field and is currently performed by different software programs, used separately from each other with lack of standardization regarding the overall process [1–16, 18, 19]. This implies several steps including various co-registration and tissue/lesion segmentation tasks which make the analysis rather laborious, time-consuming and prone to inaccuracies due to human intervention. These limitations could explain why the results coming from previous studies were not always concordant. In addition, there are no large-scale studies investigating DWI and PWI abnormalities in MS focal lesions categorized according to different stages of their evolution (acute and chronic) [20]. Thus, a more integrated analysis process incorporating all software packages employed in performing co-registration and tissue/lesion segmentation steps would be beneficial. This approach should be based on the activation of the different software modules according to a logical sequence leading to precise measurements of DWI and PWI values in focal MS lesions, in normal appearing grey matter (NAGM) and in normal appearing white matter (NAWM). For these reasons, the pipeline proposed in this work consists in an implementation of already described algorithms [4, 6, 10, 13, 15] combined according to a hierarchical order in a semi-automated manner. Although many automated methods have recently been developed for MS lesion detection [21–23], we chose semi-automated operations for the identification of focal damage to minimize potential biases due to lesion misclassification [18, 19], which could overcome operator-dependent misinterpretations related to visual inspection. On the other hand, the lack of clear standards renders it difficult to judge the superiority of one approach over other available choices [18, 19, 24]. Accordingly, we included tools commonly used in the MS literature which have been demonstrated to be both efficient and accurate in co-registration and tissue/lesion segmentation procedures. Moreover, the investigators of our group have many combined years of experience using these tools [18, 19, 24–26]. In this way, we sought to provide a promising tool for reducing analysis complexity and obtaining reproducible results.

Methods

Definition and general description of the DPP Suite and modules

The process management system named *Diffusion/ Perfusion Project* (DPP) described in the paper is an in-house developed suite written in Matlab (The MathWorks, Natick, MA, USA) and requiring the Image Processing Toolbox. The DPP is a collection of software modules all related to MRI data management, sharing the same GUI (Graphical User Interface) and exchanging data with each other. DPP Suite integrates commonly used software tools which are able to perform different types of data analysis and management. The primary aim of DPP Suite is to create a uniform environment where it can be possible to assess a considerably larger number of data from MS patients compared to the other current analysis methods, reducing as much as possible analysis complexity, time required and potential human errors. The most relevant procedures manageable through DPP Suite are schematically presented in Fig. 1, where data and operations are shown as a flowchart. In summary, DPP Suite operations include: 1) image pre-processing; 2) registration of T1-weighted images; 3) lesion segmentation and classification; 4) registration of lesion masks; 5) normal appearing tissue segmentation; 6) PWI and DWI map generation; 7) registration of tissue segmentation and quantitative MRI maps; 8) data analysis.

Pre-processing

Image pre-processing starts with the automatic anonymization of MRI sequences for each patient which are exported from a PACS database and copied in a local repository dynamically linked with the DPP Suite. This process aims at protecting patient identity during the whole procedure. Furthermore, demographic data, resulting analysis and patient identity are stored as a protected file controlled by the DPP Suite. The anonymization

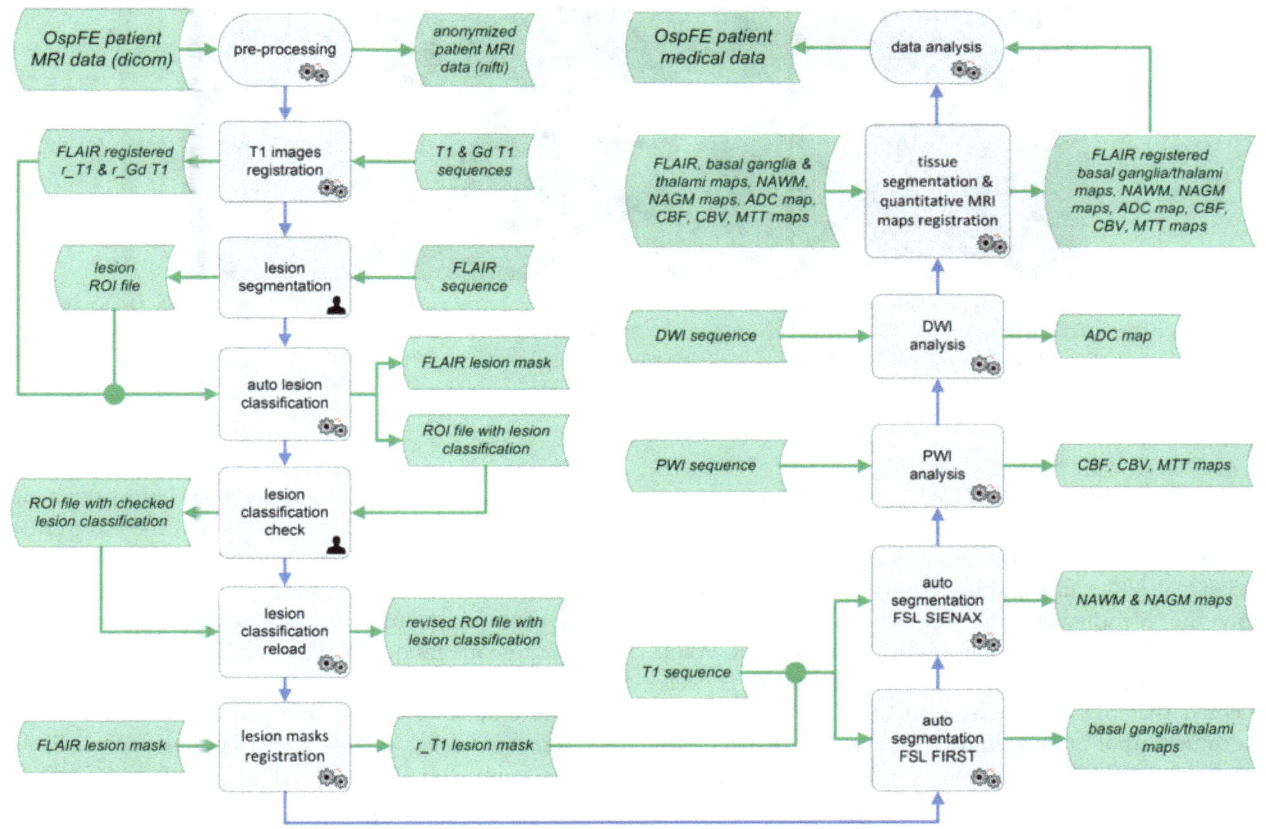

Fig. 1 Flowchart of Diffusion/Perfusion Project (DPP) Suite. The DPP Suite is used for diffusion-weighted imaging (DWI) and perfusion-weighted imaging (PWI) measurements in focal and diffuse abnormalities in multiple sclerosis (MS) patients. OspFE = Ferrara Hospital; MRI = magnetic resonance imaging; FLAIR = axial fluid-attenuated inversion recovery MRI images; T1 = 2D axial non-enhanced T1-weighted spin-Echo or 3D non-enhanced T1-weighted gradient-Echo MRI images; Gd T1 = Gadolinium-enhanced T1-weighted spin-Echo MRI images; r_T1 = registered 2D axial non-enhanced T1-weighted spin-Echo or 3D non-enhanced T1-weighted gradient-Echo MRI images; r_Gd T1 = registered Gadolinium-enhanced T1-weighted spin-Echo MRI images; ROI = regions of interest; NAWM = normal appearing white matter; NAGM = normal appearing grey matter; ADC = apparent diffusion coefficient; CBF = cerebral blood flow; CBV = cerebral blood volume; MTT = mean transit time

procedure is performed by Image Processing Toolbox Matlab function with some adaptations. The original embedded task for data anonymization, called *dicomanon*, was modified generating a function called *dpp_dicomanon* that can strengthen the patient data confidentiality level if needed. After anonymization, DICOM format [27] files are converted in NIFTI format [28] using the Statistical Parametric Mapping (SPM) 8 toolbox (http://www.fil.ion.ucl.ac.uk/spm/) [29] Notably, pre-processing is performed on a limited dataset that includes the following MRI sequences: axial fluid-attenuated inversion recovery (FLAIR); two-dimensional (2D) axial non-enhanced T1-weighted spin-echo or three-dimensional (3D) non-enhanced T1 gradient-echo; axial Gadolinium (Gd)-enhanced T1-weighted spin-echo; axial DWI and axial PWI. Therefore, before data conversion, a DPP function selects patients having all MRI sequences requested for analysis, excluding those with incomplete radiological data. Concurrently, a set of report files containing a checklist of unavailable sequences for each non-conforming patient is generated. In addition, all MRI data are reorganized in a storage structure aimed at making a uniform data format, including sequences names, filenames or data storing and other details, that is independent of that given by different MRI scanners (e.g. Philips, Siemens or GE), without modifications in information content.

Registration of T1-weighted images

In this first step (Fig. 2), both axial 2D non-enhanced T1-weighted spin-echo or 3D non-enhanced T1 gradient-echo and axial Gd-enhanced T1-weighted spin-echo are registered in FLAIR space using an automated process based on the employment of a DPP module invoking one of the two following external software packages: SPM or FMRIB's Linear Image Registration Tool (FLIRT) from FMRIB Software Library (FSL) suite (http://fsl.fmrib.ox.ac.uk/fsl/fslwiki/flirt) [30, 31]. Although T2-weighted images are generally considered the most sensitive in detecting

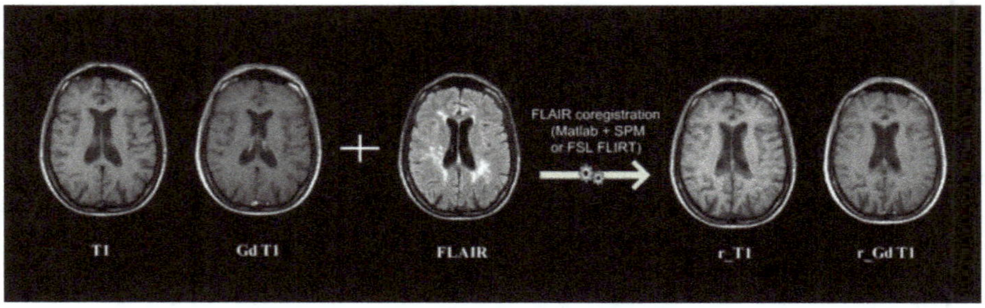

Fig. 2 An illustrative example of registration of T1-weighted images. SPM = Statistical Parametric Mapping; FSL = FMRIB Software Library; FLIRT = FMRIB's Linear Image Registration Tool; FLAIR = axial fluid-attenuated inversion recovery MRI images; T1 = 2D axial non-enhanced T1-weighted spin-Echo or 3D non-enhanced T1-weighted gradient-Echo MRI images; Gd T1 = Gadolinium-enhanced T1-weighted spin-Echo MRI images; r_T1 = registered 2D axial non-enhanced T1-weighted spin-Echo or 3D non-enhanced T1-weighted gradient-Echo MRI images; r_Gd T1 = registered Gadolinium-enhanced T1-weighted spin-Echo MRI images

infratentorial lesions [32], FLAIR images serve for the following lesion segmentation since they improve lesion/brain contrast due to the suppression of cerebrospinal fluid signal [33]. On the other hand, T1-weighted images allow the identification of MS T1 hypointense (black holes) and T1 Gd-enhancing lesions as well as the evaluation of brain atrophy [17]. In this regard, it is well-accepted that 3D are superior to 2D T1 images in the determination of brain volume [34]. However, we chose to process also 2D T1 images since, in clinical practice, not all centers are equipped to routinely perform 3D T1 sequences in MS patients. The choice between SPM and FSL FLIRT is user selectable.

Lesion segmentation and classification

The development of automated techniques for lesion detection is one of the most central challenges in MS research. Therefore, a number of approaches have recently been proposed [21–23]. However, it is generally accepted that there are no automatic lesion segmentation methods with 100 % reliability [18, 19]. This is the reason why a series of semi-automated algorithms were designed and tested in order to support and simplify lesion segmentation and classification. This step is one of the most critical and complex because it involves both human operation and automated processes. In fact, two basic operations are implemented: a) semi-automatic lesion segmentation; b) semi-automatic lesion classification.

Semi-automatic lesion segmentation

As depicted in Fig. 3, this step is performed on FLAIR images using Jim (Jim 6.0, Xinapse Systems, Leicester, UK; http://www.xinapse.com) [34] as an external software package. After visual identification, each lesion is semi-automatically segmented by a local threshold-based technique. In addition, a region of interest (ROI) of the NAWM is manually outlined. The output of this process is an ROI file corresponding to the delineated areas.

Semi-automatic lesion classification

Using the FLAIR-derived lesion ROI file, DDP Suite automatically masks the non-enhanced and Gd-enhanced T1-weighted images (Fig. 4). The DDP Suite then calculates the intensity of each lesion in both non-enhanced

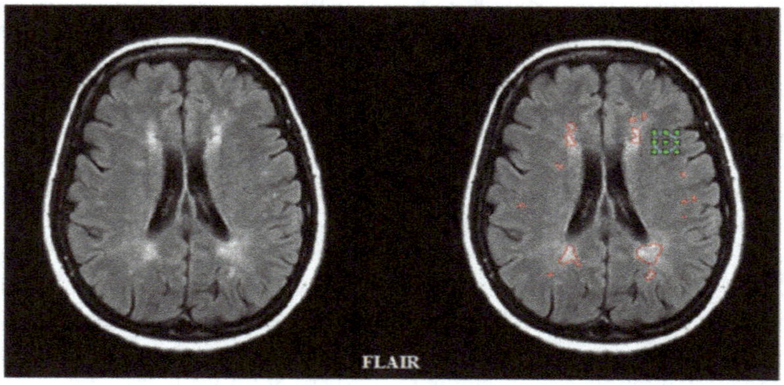

Fig. 3 A descriptive example of semi-automated lesion segmentation process on fluid-attenuated inversion recovery (FLAIR) images. Segmented hyperintense lesions in red; area used for NAWM mean intensity estimation in green

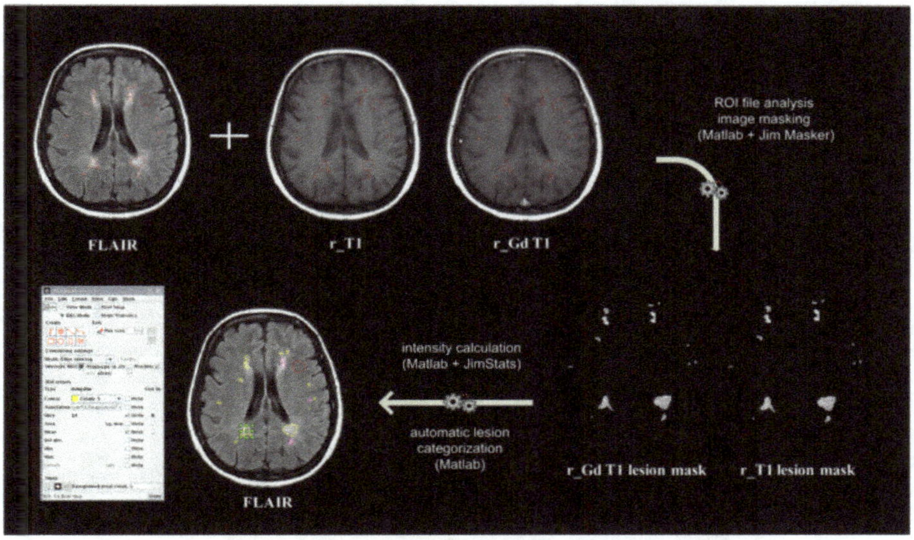

Fig. 4 A demonstrative example showing the automatic lesion classification process. FLAIR = axial fluid-attenuated inversion recovery MRI images; r_T1 = registered 2D axial non-enhanced T1-weighted spin-Echo or 3D non-enhanced T1-weighted gradient-Echo MRI images; r_Gd T1 = registered Gadolinium-enhanced T1-weighted spin-Echo MRI images. ROI = Region Of Interest; area used for NAWM mean intensity estimation in red

and Gd-enhanced T1-weighted sequence. Based on the recently proposed classification [20], the algorithm categorizes each T2-weighted hyperintense lesion, based on its intensity in four classes: 1) Gd-enhancing and T1-weighted isointense (C1); 2) Gd-enhancing and T1-weighted hypointense (C2); 3) non Gd-enhancing and T1-weighted isointense (C3); 4) non Gd-enhancing and T1-weighted hypointense, i.e. black holes (C4). As, in absence of serial MRI examinations, lesion activity is demonstrable only by Gd enhancement [35], C1 and C2 type lesions are considered as acute, whereas C3 and C4 lesions are judged as chronic [36, 37]. The output of the process is a recombined ROI file enriched with classification of each lesion given by a different color code for each lesion type and a descriptive text label where the type and characteristics of the single lesion are briefly reported (Fig. 4). Lesion classification is accomplished using a DPP algorithm based on a lesion intensity comparison to the NAWM ROI intensity level. The thresholds to identify the lesion classes are defined as a configurable multiplier of the standard deviation of the intensity values in the NAWM ROI.

$$Thre_{High} = \bar{I}_{default} + Mf \cdot St\_dev(I_{NAWM}) \quad (1)$$

$$Thre_{Low} = \bar{I}_{default} - Mf \cdot St\_dev(I_{NAWM}) \quad (2)$$

Where $\bar{I}$ is the mean intensity of the NAWM and *Mf* is the multiplier factor and *St_dev* is the standard deviation calculation function. The mean intensity of ach lesion is then calculated and compared with the two thresholds referred to in formulas (1) and (2) that are calculated for both non-enhanced and Gd-enhanced T1-weighted images. The automatic lesion classification algorithm performance is briefly presented in Fig. 5 to document the accuracy of the procedure. The error percentage of automatic classification was less than 1 % for C1 and C2 lesion classes and about 21 % and 23 % for C3 and C4 lesion classes, respectively. It is important to underline that the low error percentage found for C1 and C2 lesion classes could be related to the small number of this type of lesions occurred in the selected patients, as well as in all patients analyzed. Therefore, these results support the need of a visual correction for automatic lesion classification. The output of the automatic lesion classification process is a text file in Jim ROI Analysis Tool format, containing all the ROI definitions and classifications. Automatic lesion classifications are visually checked and revised by the operator. The new checked file is then automatically reloaded and converted by DDP Suite into different revised ROI files, including the lesions categorized as total lesions, lesion classes (C1, C2, C3 and C4) and single lesion, which are then used in the following steps.

Registration of lesion masks

This stage requires the creation of a lesion mask in the T1 space and is performed by SPM or FSL FLIRT external software packages invoked by a DPP module. Briefly, FLAIR images previously segmented are used to automatically produce a lesion mask that is coregistered in the non-enhanced T1-weighted space to obtain a registered lesion mask. When FLIRT is chosen, coregistration is done applying to the lesion mask in the FLAIR space the transformation matrix generated by the registration

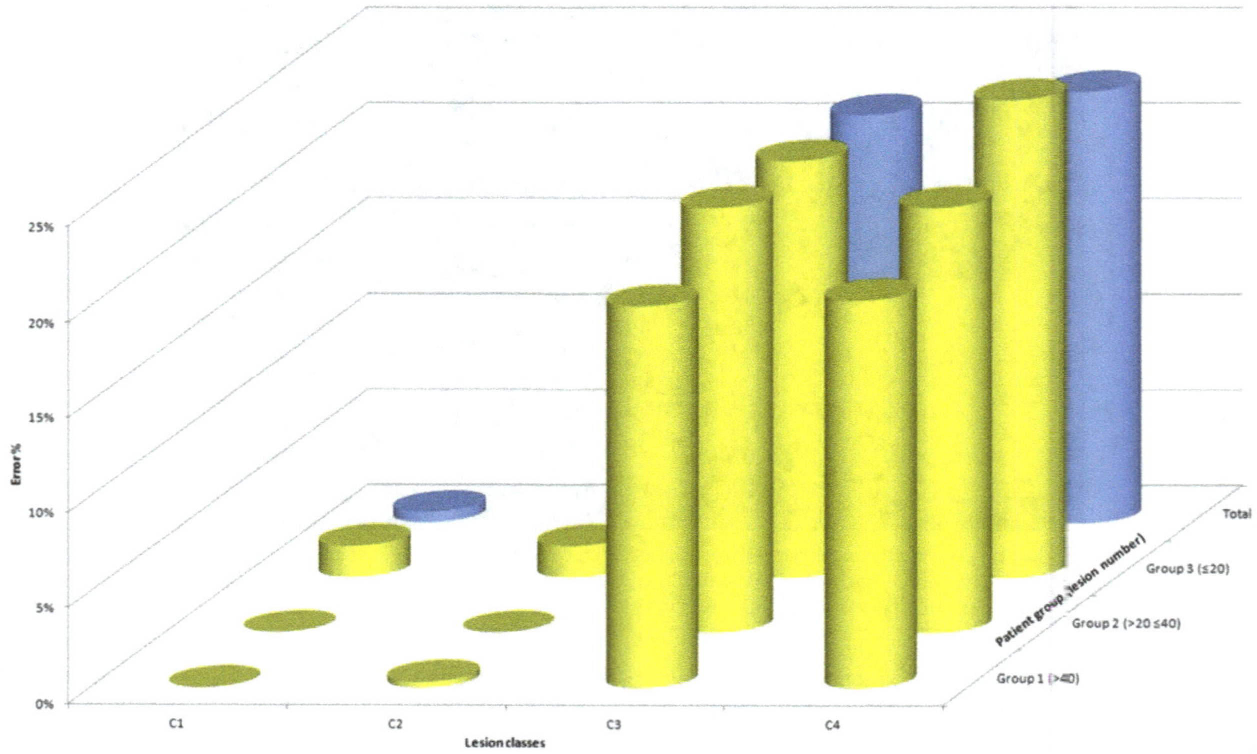

Fig. 5 Automatic lesion classification algorithm performance for a group of 15 randomly selected patients. The automatic classification algorithm is compared with classification of the same lesions performed visually by an expert. Vertical axis shows the error percentage over total number of lesions. Group 1 (>40) = patient group 1 was composed by 5 patients with more than 40 lesions; Group 2 (>20 ≤ 40) = patient group 2 was composed by 5 patients with more than 20 and less than 40 lesions; Group 3 (≤20) = patient group 3 was composed by 5 patients with less than 20 lesions; Total = mean values between group 1, 2 and 3; C1 = lesion class 1; C2 = lesion class 2; C3 = lesion class 3; C4 = lesion class 4

of FLAIR and T1. If SPM is selected, T1 is set as the reference image, FLAIR as source and the lesion mask as other. The result is a black and white lesion mask that is a binarization of the brain lesion area where lesions are white and the remaining brain tissue is black (Fig. 6).

Normal appearing tissue segmentation

As depicted in Fig. 7, DPP Suite invokes automatic segmentation of the basal ganglia and thalami via the external FSL tool FMRIB's Integrated Registration and Segmentation Tool (FIRST) (http://fsl.fmrib.ox.ac.uk/fsl/fslwiki/first)

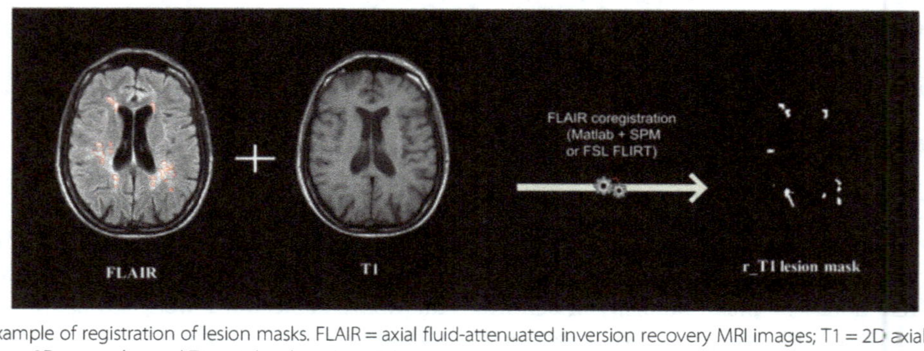

Fig. 6 A graphic example of registration of lesion masks. FLAIR = axial fluid-attenuated inversion recovery MRI images; T1 = 2D axial non-enhanced T1-weighted spin-Echo or 3D non-enhanced T1-weighted gradient-Echo MRI images; SPM = Statistical Parametric Mapping; FSL = FMRIB Software Library; FLIRT = FMRIB's Linear Image Registration Tool; r_T1 = registered 2D axial non-enhanced T1-weighted spin-Echo or 3D non-enhanced T1-weighted

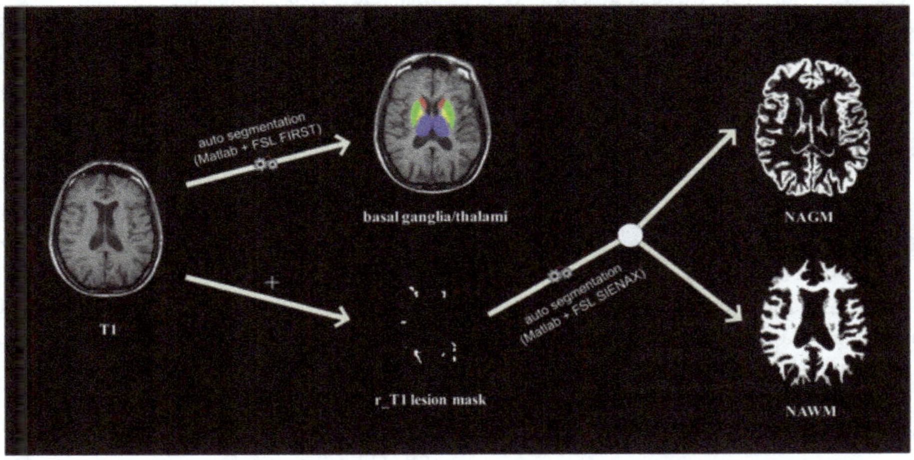

Fig. 7 An illustrative example of normal appearing tissue segmentation. T1 = 2D axial non-enhanced T1-weighted spin-Echo or 3D non-enhanced T1-weighted gradient-Echo MRI images; FSL = FMRIB Software Library; FIRST = FMRIB's Integrated Registration and Segmentation Tool; SIENAX = Structural Image Evaluation using Normalization of Atrophy; r_T1 = registered 2D axial non-enhanced T1-weighted spin-Echo or 3D non-enhanced T1-weighted gradient-Echo MRI images; NAGM = normal appearing grey matter; NAWM = normal appearing white matter

[38]. The input is the non-enhanced T1-weighted sequence. The segmented basal ganglia structures include the right and left caudate, putamen and globus pallidus. The following step is represented by the automatic segmentation of grey and white matter for which DPP Suite invokes FSL SIENAX (Structural Image Evaluation using Normalization of Atrophy) (http://fsl.fmrib.ox.ac.uk/fsl/fslwiki/SIENA) [39]. In this case, the inputs are non-enhanced T1-weighted sequence and registered T1 lesion mask, whereas the output are two files including NAGM and NAWM images obtained after subtracting registered T1 lesion mask from non-enhanced T1-weighted. In addition, FSL SIENAX generates a report file including total brain tissue volume, as a whole and normalized according to skull size, and normalized NAGM and NAWM volumes.

PWI map generation

PWI studies are performed with a dynamic susceptibility contrast (DSC) MRI first-pass bolus-tracking technique using echo-planar gradient-echo T2* sequences. PWI analysis provides relative measurements of brain hemodynamic parameters such as Cerebral Blood Flow (CBF), Cerebral Blood Volume (CBV) and Mean Transit Time (MTT). CBF, CBV and MTT maps are generated by a singular value decomposition (SVD) deconvolution operation based on the measurement of an arterial input function (AIF) [40]. The calculation of PWI maps is automatically performed by Jim Perfusion Analysis tool invoked by DPP Suite. DSC images consist of a time-series of sequences, one volume for each time point, which monitor the concentration of an injected paramagnetic contrast agent transiting from the blood vessels to the brain tissue. Therefore, AIF determination implies the knowledge of the exact volume where the contrast agent is perceptible in the brain (Contrast Arrival Point). For that reason, the DPP Suite implements an algorithm that identifies the contrast arrival volume number using Jim Stats. This algorithm evaluates the mean intensity in volumes, using in subsequent steps the average intensity of the previous analyzed volumes, in order to reduce the noise affecting the images. It detects when the difference of mean intensity between two subsequent volumes is more than an adjustable threshold. The threshold is not an absolute value or an absolute percent, but is a fraction of the difference between maximum and minimum intensity value measured in all volumes of the sequence. Thus, the threshold is less dependent from the volume intensity absolute level.

DWI map generation

DWI studies are often performed with a single-shot echo-planar T2 spin-echo sequence according to the Stejskal-Tanner method [41]. The diffusion gradients are applied in three orthogonal directions (x, y, z) with two b-values (0 and 1000 s/mm^2) to form the isotropic DWI images at b 1000 s/mm^2. DWI analysis takes as input T2 images and extracts from these images apparent Diffusion Coefficient (ADC) maps, related to each Cartesian axis. More precisely, as reported elsewhere [42], ADC maps are generated using T2-weighted images at b 0s/mm^2 and isotropic DWI images at b 1000 s/mm^2 obtained in all three orthogonal directions. All calculations are automatically performed by Jim Image Algebra tool invoked by DPP Suite controlling the entire process. The process output is an average ADC map, obtained calculating the mean of the previously calculated ADC on the three Cartesian axes. After this process, previously generated ADC maps and PWI maps are ready to be registered in the next step (Fig. 8).

Registration of tissue segmentation and quantitative MRI maps

This step is aimed at automatically translating the results of all intermediate processes previously described in the FLAIR space to allow the final data analysis in which DWI and PWI values are measured in every lesion as well as in the basal ganglia and thalami, NAGM and NAWM. DPP Suite invokes SPM or FSL FLIRT external software tools which generate the following registered maps:

From T1 space:

1. Basal ganglia and thalami maps;
2. NAGM map;
3. NAWM map;
   from DWI space:
4. Average ADC map;
   from PWI space:
5. CBV, CBF and MTT maps.

The different maps are registered into the FLAIR space and used in the next data analysis (Fig. 9). The coregistration is performed using a similar method as in registration of lesion masks.

Data analysis

The final step represents the key advance performed by the DPP Suite compared to existing semi-automated methods. Measurements are obtained by the integration of the entire set of images and maps previously generated. This result is obtained using distinct software modules. In this stage, two groups of automatic analysis are developed. In the first one (Fig. 10, panel a), NAGM, NAWM and basal ganglia maps are used to mask ADC and PWI maps owing to Jim Masker invoked by DPP Suite. At this point, DPP Suite activates the Jim Stats tool that is able to calculate ADC, CBF, CBV and MTT values in these brain areas. In addition, the Jim Stats tool also measures NAGM, NAWM and basal ganglia/thalami volumes and voxel number and DPP Suite parses previously saved FSL SIENAX report file including whole and normalized total brain tissue volume and normalized NAGM and NAWM volumes. In the second group of data analysis (Fig. 10, panel b), DPP Suite invokes Jim Masker to mask DWI and PWI maps with FLAIR segmented lesions which DPP Suite has previously saved and stored as total, single class (C1, C2, C3 and C4) and single lesion maps. In this way, it is possible to obtain ADC, CBF, CBV and MTT values in all types of lesions where, in addition, also volume and voxel number are measured. All of these data are stored in a comma separated values (csv) file.

Graphical User Interface

The Graphical user Interface (GUI) is shown in Fig. 11. The GUI keeps hidden all configuration parameters. Thus, the user is unable to modify the system parametrization and has a limited number of operations to perform. The configuration parameters are collected in a text configuration file. However, the configuration can be modified as needed by an expert operator, based on the needs of the study. These parameters are not shown in the GUI to facilitate the use of DPP suite by non-expert operators. The GUI configuration presents two sections: the first area in which all the process steps are singularly selectable and the second area where only three process macro steps can be activated. All these steps are performed automatically by DPP Suite, except

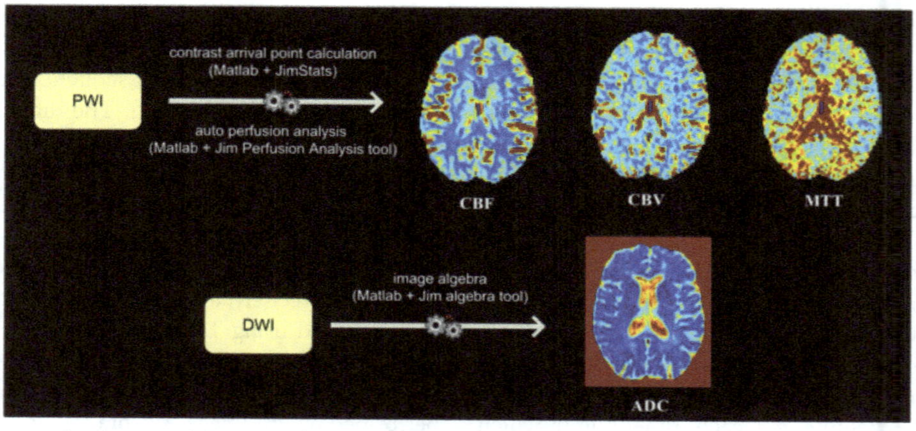

Fig. 8 A descriptive example of generated apparent diffusion coefficient (ADC) and perfusion-weighted imaging (PWI) maps. CBF = Cerebral Blood Flow; CBV = Cerebral Blood Volume; MTT = Mean Transit Time; DWI = Diffusion Weighted Imaging

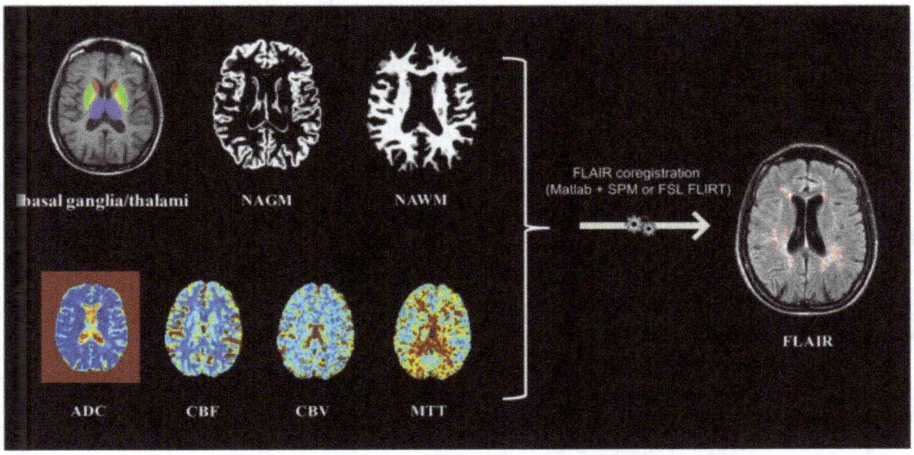

Fig. 9 A graphic example of registration of tissue segmentation and quantitative MRI maps. NAGM = normal appearing grey matter; NAWM = normal appearing white matter; ADC = apparent diffusion coefficient; CBF = cerebral blood flow; CBV = cerebral blood volume; MTT = mean transit time; SPM = Statistical Parametric Mapping; FSL = FMRIB Software Library; FLIRT = FMRIB's Linear Image Registration Tool; FLAIR = axial fluid-attenuated inversion recovery MRI images

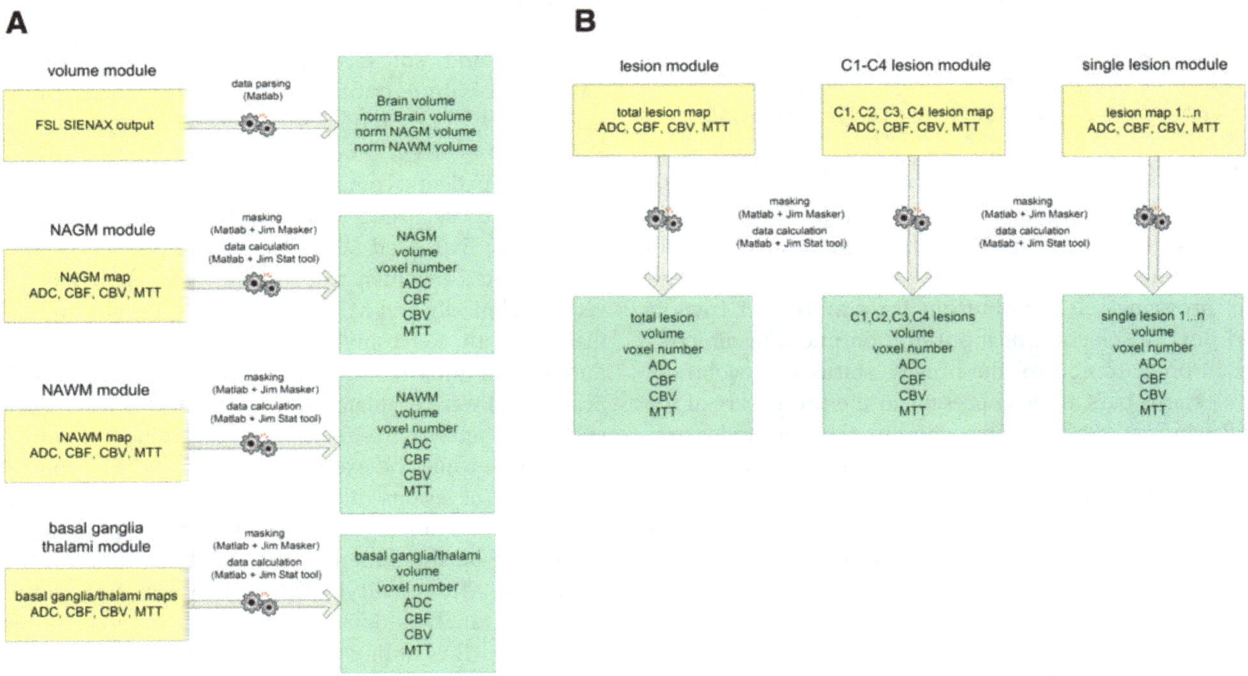

Fig. 10 Two diagrams describing DPP data analysis. Panel **a**: measurements of total, brain normal appearing grey matter (NAGM) and normal appearing white matter (NAWM) volume and voxel number, both as a whole and normalized according to skull size, and measurements of apparent diffusion coefficient (ADC), cerebral blood flow (CBF), cerebral blood volume (CBV) and mean transit time (MTT) in basal ganglia, NAGM and NAWM. Panel **b**: measurements of apparent diffusion coefficient (ADC), cerebral blood flow (CBF), cerebral blood volume (CBV) and mean transit time (MTT) in previously saved and stored FLAIR lesion categorized as total, class C1, C2, C3, C4 and single. norm = normalized; C1 = enhancing T2-weighted hyperintense and T1-weighted isointense; C2 = enhancing T2-weighted hyperintense and T1-weighted ipointense ; C3 = non-enhancing T2-weighted hyperintense and T1-weighted isointense; C4 = non-enhancing T2-weighted hyperintense and T1-weighted ipointense, black holes

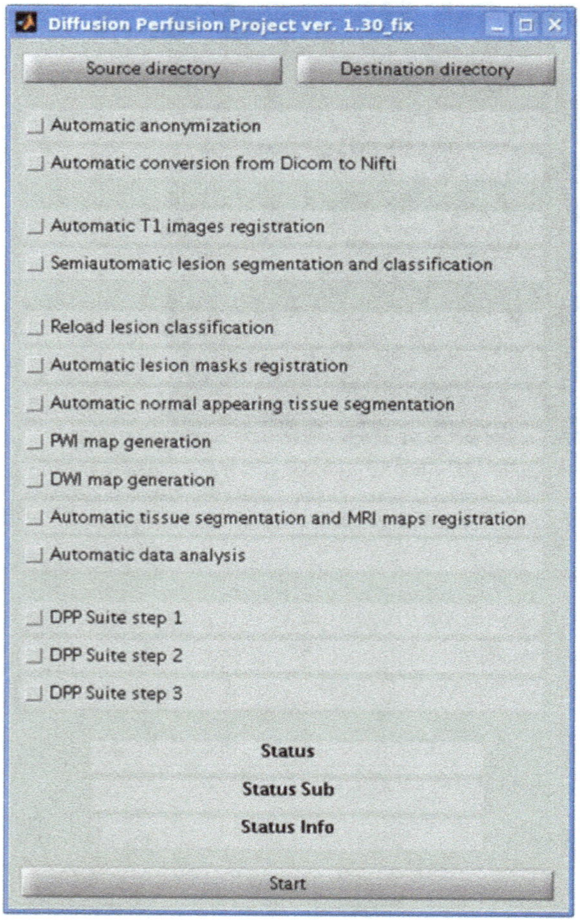

Fig. 11 A picture illustrating the Graphical User Interface (GUI)

lesion segmentation and classification which requires human intervention. The GUI presents also two directory browsing selection buttons for a more user friendly and flexible selection of input and output data directories. In order to control the process status and evolution, three status bars are also present in the lower part of the GUI window: a) a status bar defining the step under execution or the process execution status; b) a status-sub bar describing the sub-module under execution; c) a status-info bar indicating the patient number whose data are under analysis. The lower button is the step/process activation button, which starts the selected operations to be executed in an automated way by the DPP Suite.

Process safety and data security

All process steps, such as utilized parameters, the final results and the intermediate data are logged, saved and stored in the DPP Suite. This ensures complete environment preservation. For example, when an external tool is invoked by the DPP Suite both images and results and the tool's standard output/error data log is read and saved. This approach allows post processing visual verification of e.g. co-registration (SPM or FSL FLIRT), tissue segmentation (SIENAX or FSL FIRST) or automatic detection of AIF-like voxels (Jim Perfusion tool). In Fig. 12 is presented an example of coregistration check performed using the Check Reg tool part of SPM module for functional MRI. Although processing parameters were tuned and optimized for every single step in DPP suite, in case of failure, configuration can be modified to correct processing errors. In this way, a clinician can check the results and make sure that they are accurate. Other security measures are integrated in DPP suite as well. For example, if a set of data represent both an output for the *(n-1)th* step and the input for the *(n)th* step, the entire data are copied before being modified by the *(n)th* step. Moreover, execution times and software version are preserved for every run of the suite (e.g. preprocessing data structure). This approach allows data reconstruction, process verification and software debugging, making it possible to reproduce every single step or the entire process and, thus, future validation of the DPP Suite.

Results

Software metrics

In order to evaluate the DPP Suite performance, the hardware and software configurations are listed in Table 1. It is important to note that the entire suite is carried out by a Linux Virtual Machine running in a Windows based PC. The execution time for all modules in a single patient (woman; 33 year old; clinically and MRI inactive with Relapsing-Remitting MS; disease duration = 84 months; Expanded Disability Status Scale = 2.5) and in five patients (4 women and 1 men; mean age = 46.4 ± 3.7 years; 2 clinically and MRI active and 3 clinically and MRI inactive with Relapsing-Remitting MS; median disease duration = 1 months; median Expanded Disability Status Scale = 1.5) were evaluated to test the DPP Suite performance. This analysis resulted linear regarding the number of patients, while the execution time varied as a function of number of lesions of patients (Fig. 13). Typical execution time for a single patient can vary from 30 to 55 min depending on the patient characteristics (number of lesions and MRI quality). The key information derived from this analysis is that the most time-consuming process is the anonymization with *dpp_dicomanon*. Interestingly, the typical execution time of the entire suite analysis is relatively short (45 min), which seems to be acceptable for a research use. It is important to note that the DPP Suite is able to work with different equipment since it can run on all hardware supporting VMware player (https://www.vmware.com/) or compatible virtualization software.

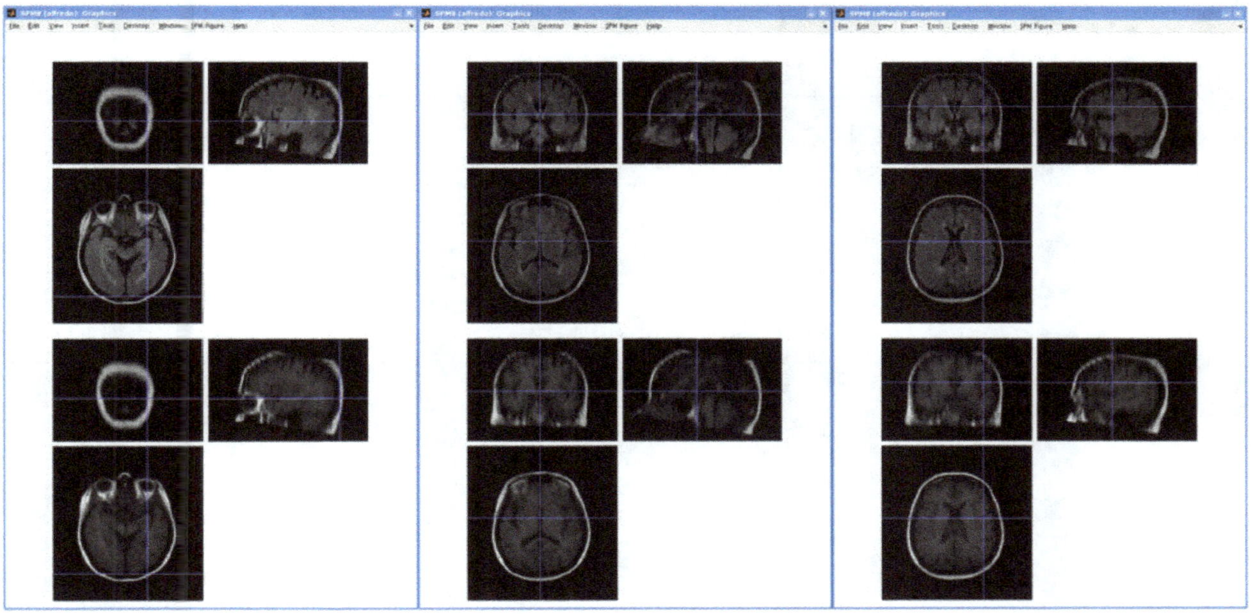

Fig. 12 A visual coregistration check example using Check Reg tool in SPM. Left to right are presented three panels showing the output of Check Reg in case of a T1 (lower images) to FLAIR (higher images) sequences coregistration. Three relevant points were selected in order to check coregistration visually

Reproducibility of results

The repeatability of data coming from DPP Suite was tested with the analysis of lesion number and ADC, CBF, CBV and MTT values obtained from 38 patients with Relapsing-Remitting MS (31 women and 7 men; mean age = 45.8 ± 9.1 years; 8 clinically active and 30 clinically inactive; median disease duration = 9 months; median Expanded Disability Status Scale = 2.0) by two different readers (EG with 2 years of experience; EF with 15 years of experience) who performed a double blinded, independent semi-automatic lesion segmentation and classification of T2-weighted hyperintense lesions. After checking data for normality by using the Kolmogorov-Smirnov test, continuous variables were compared using Mann-Whitney U test or independent-samples t test when appropriate. In addition, kappa inter-observer agreement was calculated. Kappa values were interpreted according to the proposed standards of Landis and Koch: 0–0.20 (slight agreement); 0.21–0.40 (fair agreement); 0.41–0.60 (moderate agreement); 0.61–0.80 (substantial agreement); 0.81–1.00 (almost perfect agreement) [43]. Tables 2 and 3 show that there were not statistically significant differences between the two readers in the evaluation of lesion number and ADC, CBF, CBV and MTT values detected in the four classes of T2-weighted hyperintense lesions. Inter-observer agreement between the two readers was substantial for lesion number and ADC, CBF, CBV and MTT values in C1 lesion class and for lesion number and ADC and MTT values in C2 lesion class, almost perfect for all parameters assessed in C3 and C4 lesion classes, and only moderate for CBF and CBV values in C2 lesion class. These findings argue for a good reproducibility of results provided by DPP Suite. On the other hand, the discrepancies observed between the two readers could be mainly attributable to differences in how the users have outlined and categorized the lesions, even if the selection of co-registration (FSL FLIRT versus SPM) and decision of whether an automated analysis passes quality control or not could represent other potential explanations. The modest inter-observer agreement between the two readers found for CBF and CBV values in C2 lesion class could be also affected by the current limitations in discriminating between acute active and chronic active Gd-enhancing and T1-weighted hypointense T2-weighted hyperintense lesions [44]. In any case, such differences can be minimized based on having some type of training between the

Table 1 Test Bench Hardware and Software

Hardware Host PC	
CPU	Intel Core i7-4770
Ram	8 Gb
Hard Disk	SSD + Raid 1 disk
Software Host PC	
Operating System	Windows 7 professional
Virtualization	VMware player 6.0.3
Software Guest PC	
Operating System	Scientific Linux 5.5

CPU Central Processing Unit, *SSD* Solid State Drive, *Raid* Redundant array of independent disks

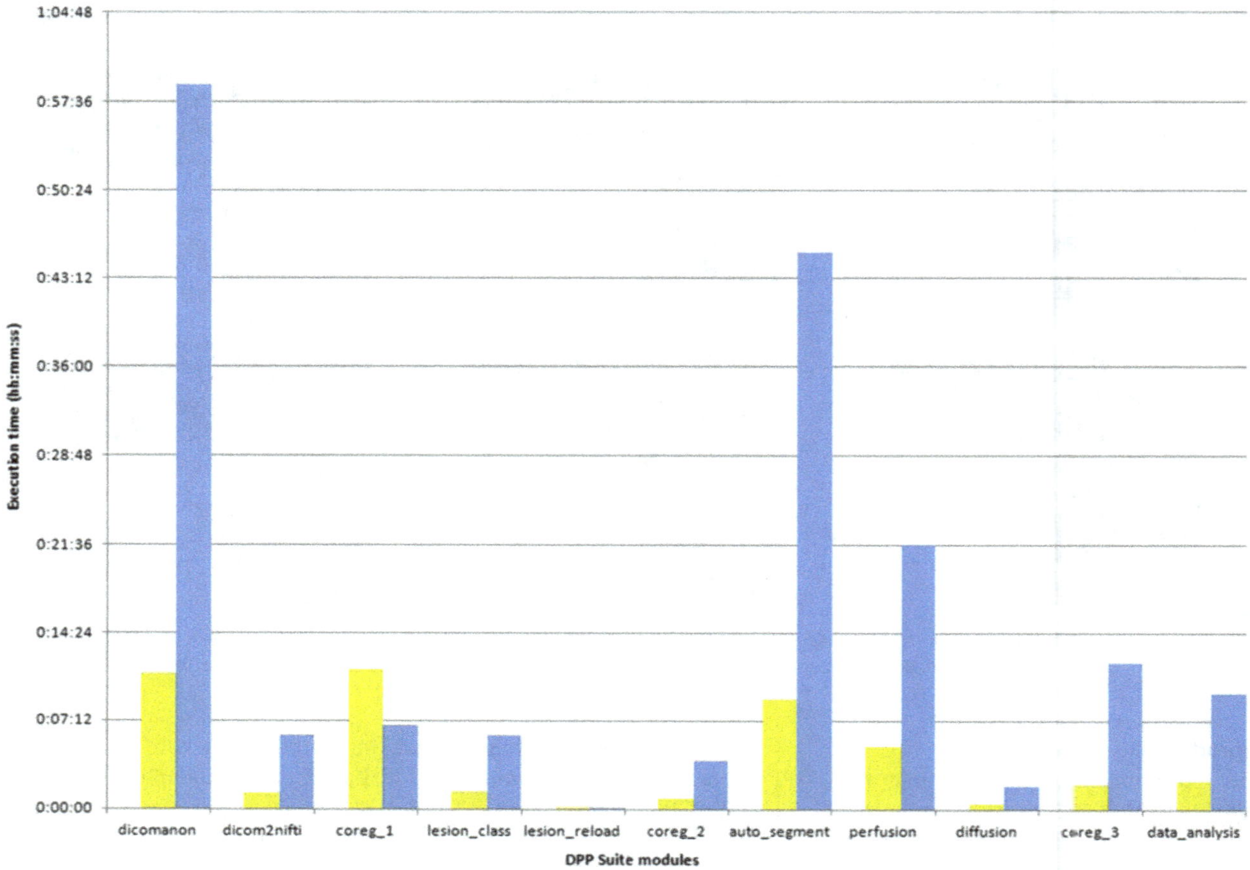

Fig. 13 Execution time benchmark in a single patient (yellow/left) and 5 patients (blue/right). Vertical axis shows the execution times in the *hours:minutes:seconds* format. Matlab R2010a, Xinapse Jim 6.0, FMRIB Software library (FSL) 4.1.9 and Statistical Parametric Mapping (SPM) 8 were the software systems employed. coreg_1 = registration of T1-weighted images; lesion_class = lesion classification; coreg_2 = registration of lesion masks; auto_segment = normal appearing tissue segmentation; coreg_3 = registration of tissue segmentation and quantitative MRI maps

users (i.e. which option should be selected and how to assess the quality of the analysis).

Written informed consent was given by all patients before inclusion and the study design was approved by the Research Ethics Board of Azienda Ospedaliero-Universitaria di Ferrara (Italy) that is our Local Committee for Medical Ethics in Research

Discussion and conclusions

In this work we implemented an alternative system to analyze DWI and PWI abnormalities in various classes of lesions and in normal appearing brain tissues from patients with MS. The novelty of our approach is represented by a semi-automated integration of several previously validated software packages which are sequentially activated instead of separately utilized. This has the effect of significantly reducing human intervention that can be a source of bias and improper tissue and/or lesion classification. This approach makes the analysis quicker, simpler and provides reliable results. In fact, except for two checkpoints represented by lesion segmentation and classification, DPP Suite procedures offer a highly automatic elaboration of a large amount of MRI data in which the different algorithms are harmonically and hierarchically incorporated. The main objective of the development of our DPP Suite is to provide clinical researchers with a practical and reproducible tool to clarify the actual significance of DWI and PWI disturbances in MS. On the other hand, the coherent integration process obtained with the DPP Suite offers an intuitive time improvement compared to manually performing the individual steps. Finally, the DPP Suite provides a "best of breed" approach for the external tool choice and usage for each specific operation, a software modularity leading to a better management of method complexity and reusability in the setting of process safety. However, the evaluation of the DPP Suite in terms of usability, sustainability and maintainability by using different target users remains to be addressed.

Table 2 Number of focal lesions and ADC, CBF, CBV and MTT values in C1 and C2

	C1 lesions				C2 lesions			
	First reader	Second reader	*p* value*	Kappa value	First reader	Second reader	*p* value*	Kappa value
Lesion number (sum, median, IQR, mean ± SD, range)	4, 0, 0-0, 0.1 ± 0.3, 0-1	7, 0, 0-0, 0.2 ± 0.5, 0-2	$p = 0.242$	0.692	9, 0, 0-0, 0.3 ± 0.6, 0-2	12, 0, 0-0, 0.2 ± 0.7, 0-3	$p = 0.148$	0.614
ADC x 10-3 s/mm2 (median, IQR, mean ± SD, range)	0, 0-0, 0.1 ± 0.3, 0-0.9	0, 0-0, 0.1 ± 0.3, 0-0.9	$p = 0.256$	0.792	0, 0-0, 0.2 ± 0.4, 0-1.1	0, 0-0, 0.1 ± 0.3, 0-1.2	$p = 0.146$	0.721
CBF ml/100g/min (median, IQR, mean ± SD, range)	0, 0-0, 15.8 ± 50.2, 0-244.9	0, 0-0, 24 ± 59.3, 0-244.9	$p = 0.2400$	0.686	0, 0-0, 35.3 ± 76.2, 0-342.2	0, 0-0, 14.5 ± 39, 0-136.6	$p = 0.108$	0.450
CBV 100g/min (median, IQR, mean ± SD, range)	0, 0-0, 0 ± 0, 0-0.2	0, 0-0, 0 ± 0.1, 0-0.2	$p = 0.248$	0.742	0, 0-0, 0 ± 0.1, 0-0.4	0, 0-0, 0 ± 0.1, 0-0.3	$p = 0.114$	0.464
MTT seconds (median, IQR, mean ± SD, range)	0, 0-0, 0.8 ± 2.8, 0-15.3	0, 0-0, 1.1 ± 2.7, 0-11.2	$p = 0.251$	0.719	0, 0-0, 2 ± 3.8, 0-13.5	0, 0-0, 1.2 ± 3.3, 0-13.5	$p = 0.136$	0.673

Values obtained by two different readers in Gd-enhancing and T1-weighted isointense (C1) and Gd-enhancing and T1-weighted hypointense (C2) T2-weighted hyperintense lesions from 38 patients with Relapsing-Remitting Multiple Sclerosis. *ADC* Apparent Diffusion Coefficient, *CBF* Cerebral Blood Flow, *CBV* Cerebral Blood Volume, *MTT* Mean Transit Time, *First reader* EG, *Second reader* EF, *SD* Standard deviation, *IQR* Interquartile range, *Mann-Whitney

Table 3 Number of focal lesions and ADC, CBF, CBV and MTT values in C3 and C4

	C3 lesions				C4 lesions			
	First reader	Second reader	*p* value	Kappa value	First reader	Second reader	*p* value	Kappa value
Lesion number (sum, median, IQR, mean ± SD, range)	1075, 18, 5.5-33.8, 28.3 ± 30.8, 0-129	1138, 19, 5.5-38.8, 29.9 ± 32.6, 0-132	$p = 0.446$*	0.921	689, 11, 3-21.5, 18.1 ± 22.8, 0-99	623, 8, 2-20, 16.4 ± 20.3, 0-87	$p = 0.420$*	0.904
ADC x 10-3 s/mm2 (median, IQR, mean ± SD, range)	0.9, 0.9-1, 0.9 ± 0.2, 0-1.2	0.9, 0.9-1, 0.9 ± 0.2, 0-1.2	$p = 0.350$*	0.872	1, 0.9-1.1, 1 ± 0.2, 0-1.2	1, 0.9-1.1, 1 ± 0.2, 0-1.3	$p = 0.448$*	0.812
CBF ml/100g/min (median, IQR, mean ± SD, range)	131.6, 88.6-183.8, 137.5 ± 60.2, 0-295.9	139.3, 99.9-191.1, 141.8 ± 58.8, 0-295.9	$p = 0.376$**	0.844	124.3, 84.8-165.9, 124.6 ± 58.5, 0-263	105.5, 76.5-150, 115.1 ± 59.6, 0-270.8	$p = 0.243$**	0.848
CBV 100g/min (median, IQR, mean ± SD, range)	0.1, 0.1-0.2, 0.1 ± 0, 0-0.3	0.1, 0.1-0.2, 0.1 ± 0, 0-0.3	$p = 0.500$**	0.824	0.1, 0.1-0.2, 0.1 ± 0.1, 0-0.3	0.1, 0.1-0.1, 0.1 ± 0.1, 0-0.3	$p = 0.181$**	0.769
MTT seconds (median, IQR, mean ± SD, range)	8.3, 6.9-9, 8 ± 2.2, 0-12.1	8.1, 6.6-8.6, 7.8 ± 2.2, 0-12.1	$p = 0.384$**	0.836	8.4, 6.8-9.7, 8.2 ± 2.6, 0-15	8.4, 6.8-9.7, 81. ± 2.9, 0-15	$p = 0.463$**	0.828

Values obtained by two different readers in non Gd-enhancing and T1-weighted isointense (C3) and non Gd-enhancing and T1-weighted hypointense (C4) T2-weighted hyperintense lesions from 38 patients with Relapsing-Remitting Multiple Sclerosis. *ADC* Apparent Diffusion Coefficient, *CBF* Cerebral Blood Flow, *CBV* Cerebral Blood Volume, *MTT* Mean Transit Time, *First reader* EG, *Second reader* EF; *SD* Standard deviation, *IQR* Interquartile range, *Mann-Whitney; **t-test

Competing interests
The author(s) declare that they have no competing interests.

Authors' contributions
AR designed and implemented the algorithm, participated in the study concept and design, in data acquisition and interpretation and in manuscript preparation, editing and review. MRuggeri participated in manuscript preparation and editing. ML participated in the study design, in data analysis and in manuscript editing and review. NB participated in the study design, in data analysis and in manuscript editing and review. EG contributed to data acquisition and interpretation. MRovaris contributed to the study design, in data analysis and in manuscript editing and review. EF conceived the study, participated in the study design, performed the statistical analysis, contributed to data acquisition and interpretation and in manuscript preparation, editing and review. All authors read and approved the final manuscript.

Author details
[1]Unità Operativa di Neuroradiologia, Dipartimento di Neuroscienze e Riabilitazione, Azienda Ospedaliero-Universitaria of Ferrara, Arcispedale S. Anna, Via Aldo Moro 8, 44124 Cona, Ferrara, Italy. [2]Consiglio Nazionale delle Ricerche, 44124 Ferrara, Italy. [3]MR Research Laboratory, IRCCS Don Gnocchi Foundation ONLUS, Milan, Italy. [4]Buffalo Neuroimaging Analysis Center, Department of Neurology, University at Buffalo SUNY, Buffalo, NY, USA. [5]Sezione di Neurologia, Dipartimento di Scienze Biomediche e Chirurgiche Specialistiche, Università di Ferrara, Ferrara, Italy. [6]Unità Operativa di Sclerosi Multipla, Fondazione Don Gnocchi ONLUS, IRCCS S. Maria Nascente, 20148 Milano, Italy.

References
1. Balashov KE, Lindzen E. Acute demyelinating lesions with restricted diffusion in multiple sclerosis. Mult Scler. 2012;18:1745–53.
2. Zeid NA, Pirko I, Erickson B, Weigand SD, Thomsen KM, Scheithauer B, et al. Diffusion-weighted imaging characteristics of biopsy-proven demyelinating brain lesions. Neurology. 2012;78:1655–62.
3. Eisele P, Szabo K, Griebe M, Rossmanith C, Förster A, Hennerici M, et al. Reduced diffusion in a subset of acute MS lesions: a serial multiparametric MRI study. AJNR Am J Neuroradiol. 2012;33:1369–73.
4. Wuerfel J, Bellmann-Strobl J, Brunecker P, Aktas O, McFarland H, Villringer A, et al. Changes in cerebral perfusion precede plaque formation in multiple sclerosis: a longitudinal perfusion MRI study. Brain. 2004;127:111–9.
5. Ge Y, Law M, Johnson G, Herbert J, Babb JS, Mannon LJ, et al. Dynamic susceptibility contrast perfusion MR imaging of multiple sclerosis lesions: characterizing hemodynamic impairment and inflammatory activity. AJNR Am J Neuroradiol. 2005;26:1539–47.
6. Peruzzo D, Castellaro M, Calabrese M, Veronese E, Rinaldi F, Bernardi V, et al. Heterogeneity of cortical lesions in multiple sclerosis: an MRI perfusion study. J Cereb Blood Flow Metab. 2013;33:457–63.
7. Narayana PA, Zhou Y, Hasan KM, Datta S, Sun X, Wolinsky JS. Hypoperfusion and T1-hypointense lesions in white matter in multiple sclerosis. Mult Scler. 2014;20:365–73.
8. Werring DJ, Brassat D, Droogan AG, Clark CA, Symms MR, Barker GJ, et al. The pathogenesis of lesions and normal-appearing white matter changes in multiple sclerosis: a serial diffusion MRI study. Brain. 2000;123:1667–76.
9. Filippi M, Iannucci G, Cercignani M, Rocca MA, Pratesi A, Comi G. A quantitative study of water diffusion in multiple sclerosis lesions and normal-appearing white matter using echo-planar imaging. Arch Neurol. 2000;57:1017–21.
10. Tavazzi E, Dwyer MG, Weinstock-Guttman B, Lema J, Bastianello S, Bergamaschi R, et al. Quantitative diffusion weighted imaging measures in patients with multiple sclerosis. Neuroimage. 2007;36:746–54.
11. Garaci FG, Colangelo V, Ludovici A, Gaudiello F, Marziali S, Centonze D, et al. A diffusion longitudinal MR imaging study in normal-appearing white matter in untreated relapsing-remitting multiple sclerosis. AJNR Am J Neuroradiol. 2007;28:475–8.
12. Law M, Saindane AM, Ge Y, Babb JS, Johnson G, Mannon LJ, et al. Microvascular abnormality in relapsing remitting multiple sclerosis: perfusion MR imaging findings in normal-appearing white matter. Radiology. 2004;231:645–52.
13. Adhya S, Johnson G, Herbert J, Jaggi H, Babb JS, Grossman RI, et al. Pattern of hemodynamic impairment in multiple sclerosis: dynamic susceptibility contrast perfusion MR imaging at 3.0 T. Neuroimage. 2006;33:1029–35.
14. Inglese M, Park S-J, Johnson G, Babb JS, Miles L, Jaggi H, et al. Deep gray matter perfusion in multiple sclerosis: dynamic susceptibility contrast perfusion magnetic resonance imaging at 3.0 T. Arch Neurol. 2007;64:196–202.
15. Zamboni P, Menegatti E, Weinstock-Guttman B, Dwyer MG, Schirda CV, Malagoni AM, et al. Hypoperfusion of brain parenchyma is associated with the severity of chronic cerebrospinal venous insufficiency in patients with multiple sclerosis: a cross-sectional preliminary report. BMC Med. 2011;9:22.
16. Paling D, Thade Petersen E, Tozer DJ, Altmann DR, Wheeler-Kingshott CA, Kapoor R, et al. Cerebral arterial bolus arrival time is prolonged in multiple sclerosis and associated with disability. J Cereb Blood Flow Metab. 2014;34:34–42.
17. Filippi M, Rocca MA. MR imaging of multiple sclerosis. Radiology. 2011;259: 659–81.
18. Mortazavi D, Kouzani AZ, Soltanian-Zadeh H. Segmentation of multiple sclerosis lesions in MR images: a review. Neuroradiology. 2012;54:299–320.
19. Lladó X, Ganiler O, Oliver A, Martí R, Freixenet J, Valls L, et al. Automated detection of multiple sclerosis lesions in serial brain MRI. Neuroradiology. 2012;54:787–807.
20. Zivadinov R, Stosic M, Cox JL, Ramasamy DP, Dwyer MG. The place of conventional MRI and newly emerging MRI techniques in monitoring different aspects of treatment outcome. J Neurol. 2008;255:61–74.
21. Datta S, Sajja BR, He R, Wolinsky JS, Gupta RK, Narayana PA. Segmentation and quantification of black holes in multiple sclerosis. Neuroimage. 2006;29: 467–74.
22. Datta S, Sajja BR, He R, Gupta RK, Wolinsky JS, Narayana PA. Segmentation of gadolinium-enhanced lesions on MRI in multiple sclerosis. J Magn Reson Imaging. 2007;25:932–7.
23. Schmidt P, Gaser C, Arsic M, Buck D, Förschler A, Berthele A, et al. An automated tool for detection of FLAIR-hyperintense white-matter lesions in multiple sclerosis. Neuroimage. 2012;59:3774–83.
24. Vrenken H, Jenkinson M, Horsfield MA, Battaglini M, van Schijndel RA, Rostrup E, et al. Recommendations to improve imaging and analysis of brain lesion load and atrophy in longitudinal studies of multiple sclerosis. J Neurol. 2013;260:2458–71.
25. Tavazzi E, Laganà MM, Bergsland N, Tortorella P, Pinardi G, Lunetta C, et al. Grey matter damage in progressive multiple sclerosis versus amyotrophic lateral sclerosis: a voxel-based morphometry MRI study. Neurol Sci. 2015;36: 371–7.
26. Bergsland N, Laganà MM, Tavazzi E, Caffini M, Tortorella P, Baglio F, et al. Corticospinal tract integrity is related to primary motor cortex thinning in relapsing-remitting multiple sclerosis. Mult Scler. 2015. [Epub ahead of print].
27. Lim J, Zein R. The digital imaging and communications in medicine (DICOM): description, structure and applications. In: Kamrani AK, Nasr EA, editors. Rapid Prototyping: Theory and practice. New York: Springer; 2006. p. 63–86.
28. Larobina M, Murino L. Medical image file formats. J Digit Imaging. 2014;27:200–6.
29. Ashburner J, Andersson JLR, Friston KJ. Image registration using a symmetric prior-in three-dimensions. Hum Brain Mapping. 2000;9:212–25.
30. Jenkinson M, Smith S. A global optimisation method for robust affine registration of brain images. Med Image Anal. 2001;5:143–56.
31. Jenkinson M, Beckmann CF, Behrens TEJ, Woolrich MW, Smith SM. FSL. Neuroimage. 2012;62:782–90.
32. Gawne-Cain ML, O'Riordan JI, Thompson AJ, Moseley IF, Miller DH. Multiple sclerosis lesion detection in the brain: a comparison of fast fluid-attenuated inversion recovery and conventional T2-weighted dual spin echo. Neurology. 1997;49:364–70.
33. Hennig J, Nauerth A, Friedburg H. RARE imaging: a fast imaging method for clinical MR. Magn Reson Med. 1986;3:823–33.
34. Bermel RA, Sharma J, Tjoa CW, Puli SR, Bakshi R. A semiautomated measure of whole-brain atrophy in multiple sclerosis. J Neurol Sci. 2003;208:57–65.
35. Lublin FD, Reingold SC, Cohen JA, Cutter GR, Sørensen PS, Thompson AJ, et al. Defining the clinical course of multiple sclerosis: the 2013 revisions. Neurology. 2014;83:278–86.
36. Ge Y. Multiple Sclerosis: The Role of MR Imaging. AJNR Am J Neuroradiol. 2006;27:1165–76.
37. Zivadinov R, Bergsland N, Stosic M, Sharma J, Nussenbaum F, Durfee J, et al. Use of perfusion- and diffusion-weighted imaging in differential diagnosis of acute and chronic ischemic stroke and multiple sclerosis. Neurol Res. 2008;30:816–26.

38. Patenaude B, Smith SM, Kennedy DN, Jenkinson M. A Bayesian model of shape and appearance for subcortical brain segmentation. Neuroimage. 2011;56:907–22.
39. Smith SM, Zhang Y, Jenkinson M, Chen J, Matthews PM, Federico A, et al. Accurate, robust, and automated longitudinal and cross-sectional brain change analysis. Neuroimage. 2002;17:479–89.
40. Østergaard L, Weisskoff RM, Chesler DA, Gyldensted C, Rosen BR. High resolution measurement of cerebral blood flow using intravascular tracer bolus passages. Part I. Mathematical approach andstatistical analysis. Magn Reson Med. 1996;36:715–25.
41. Stejskal EO, Tanner JE. Spin diffusion measurements: spin echoes in the presence of a time dependent field gradient. J Chem Phys. 1965;42:288.
42. Le Bihan D, Breton E, Lallemand D, Grenier P, Cabanis E, Laval-Jeantet M. MR imaging of intravoxel incoherent motions: application to diffusion and perfusion in neurologic disorders. Radiology. 1986;161:401–7.
43. Landis JR, Koch GG. The measurement of observer agreement for categorical data. Biometrics. 1977;33:159–74.
44. Campbell Z, Sahm D, Donohue K, Jamison J, Davis M, Pellicano C, et al. Characterizing contrast-enhancing and re-enhancing lesions in multiple sclerosis. Neurology. 2012;78:1493–9.

11

Are two readers more reliable than one? A study of upper neck ligament scoring on magnetic resonance images

Ansgar Espeland[1,2*], Nils Vetti[1,2] and Jostein Kråkenes[1,2]

Abstract

Background: Magnetic resonance imaging (MRI) studies typically employ either a single expert or multiple readers in collaboration to evaluate (read) the image results. However, no study has examined whether evaluations from multiple readers provide more reliable results than a single reader. We examined whether consistency in image interpretation by a single expert might be equal to the consistency of combined readings, defined as independent interpretations by two readers, where cases of disagreement were reconciled by consensus.

Methods: One expert neuroradiologist and one trained radiology resident independently evaluated 102 MRIs of the upper neck. The signal intensities of the alar and transverse ligaments were scored 0, 1, 2, or 3. Disagreements were resolved by consensus. They repeated the grading process after 3–8 months (second evaluation). We used kappa statistics and intraclass correlation coefficients (ICCs) to assess agreement between the initial and second evaluations for each radiologist and for combined determinations. Disagreements on score prevalence were evaluated with McNemar's test.

Results: Higher consistency between the initial and second evaluations was obtained with the combined readings than with individual readings for signal intensity scores of ligaments on both the right and left sides of the spine. The weighted kappa ranges were 0.65-0.71 vs. 0.48-0.62 for combined vs. individual scoring, respectively. The combined scores also showed better agreement between evaluations than individual scores for the presence of grade 2–3 signal intensities on any side in a given subject (unweighted kappa 0.69-0.74 vs. 0.52-0.63, respectively). Disagreement between the initial and second evaluations on the prevalence of grades 2–3 was less marked for combined scores than for individual scores ($P \geq 0.039$ vs. $P \leq 0.004$, respectively). ICCs indicated a more reliable sum score per patient for combined scores (0.74) and both readers' average scores (0.78) than for individual scores (0.55-0.69).

Conclusions: This study was the first to provide empirical support for the principle that an additional reader can improve the reproducibility of MRI interpretations compared to one expert alone. Furthermore, even a moderately experienced second reader improved the reliability compared to a single expert reader. The implications of this for clinical work require further study.

* Correspondence: ansgar.espeland@helse-bergen.no
[1]Department of Radiology, Haukeland University Hospital, Jonas Liesvei 65, 5021, Bergen, Norway
[2]Department of Surgical Sciences, University of Bergen, Bergen, Norway

Background

A key feature of any imaging test is its reliability [1]. A conclusive image reading should be reliable, regardless of the number of readers involved. Higher reliability might be expected when multiple readers interpret the images and their readings are combined than when only one reader interprets the images. However, we have found no empirical data to support or refute this assumption. A majority or consensus view is not necessarily more reliable than the view of one expert alone. Two readers combined could, in theory, be less consistent than one reader (as exemplified by the hypothetical data shown in Additional file 1). Double, or repeated readings can also affect validity; this approach can prevent errors [2,3], but it can also increase false positive rates [4].

Radiologists provide a large number of expert opinions in their daily work. This work could be significantly impacted by data that showed a single expert opinion was insufficient or that a second opinion provided additional benefit. In research settings, it is more feasible for a single expert to study large numbers of images, rather than multiple readers. Indeed, many studies have reported conclusive image findings based on the determination of only one expert reader [5-7]. In other studies, multiple readers were used to determine the final image results [8-11]. We compared these two approaches for scoring the signal intensities of the alar and transverse ligaments on upper neck magnetic resonance images (MRIs). Consistent image readings are required in research to assess the presence and clinical relevance of high intensity signals [11-13]. Our aim was to determine whether consistency in image interpretation by a single expert might be equal to the consistency of combined readings, defined as independent interpretations by two readers, where cases of disagreement were reconciled by consensus.

Methods

This study included 102 prospectively recruited subjects (49 men and 53 women; mean age 47.2 years) that comprised 68 healthy volunteers, 18 patients with rheumatoid arthritis, and 16 patients with chronic neck pain. These subjects represented random subsamples of participants included in a larger project on MRIs of upper neck ligaments. Based on a computer generated list of random numbers, the present study included the same relative numbers of healthy individuals, patients with arthritis, and patients with neck pain as were included in the larger project. All subjects gave written informed consent to participate. The study was in compliance with the Helsinki Declaration and was approved by The Regional Committee for Medical Research Ethics, Western-Norway.

All subjects were imaged with their head and neck in a neutral position in a standard, one-channel, circular, polarized, receive-only, head coil, with a 1.5 Tesla scanner (Symphony Mastroclass, Siemens Medical System, Erlangen, Germany). We used an established protocol for MRI of upper neck ligaments [14]. This protocol included proton-density-weighted fast-spin echo sequences of the upper neck in the axial, coronal, and sagittal planes with the following parameters: repetition time: 2150–2660 ms, echo time: 15 ms, slice thickness: 1.5 mm, interslice gap: 0.0 mm or 0.3 mm (sagittal), field of view: 175 mm × 200 mm or 200 mm × 200 mm (coronal), voxel size: 0.6-0.7 × 0.4 × 1.5 mm^3, and echo train length: 13.

The alar and transverse ligaments were scored on a scale of 0, 1, 2, or 3 based on the ratio of the largest cross-sectional area of a high intensity signal (observed in at least two imaging planes) to the total cross-sectional area of the ligament [15,16]. A high intensity signal in 1/3 or less of the total cross sectional area was scored 1; a high intensity signal in 1/3 to 2/3 of the total cross sectional area was scored 2; and a high intensity signal in 2/3 or more of the total cross sectional area was scored 3. Homogenous grey ligaments were scored 2. Ligaments with no high intensity signal were scored 0. The right and left sides of the spine were scored separately; alar ligaments were scored on sagittal sections, and transverse ligaments were scored on sagittal or coronal sections, depending on ligament orientation.

One neuroradiologist (reader A) with 26 years experience and one radiology resident (reader B) with 6 years experience independently scored the signal intensities of the ligaments. Then, all disagreements were resolved by consensus. This process resulted in individual scores for each reader and combined scores for both readers (based on independent readings followed by consensus reading in cases of disagreement). Prior to this study, both readers were trained in the scoring system used and had discussed scores in joint meetings. Reader A had previously scored several thousand ligaments and reader B had scored about one thousand ligaments.

The images were de-identified, presented in a random order (according to a computer generated list of random numbers), and interspersed among similar images that were not used in this study. After 3–8 months, the same images were presented in a new random order (according to a new list of random numbers), and again, interspersed among similar images. The readers were not told that they had assessed the images previously. Readers A and B independently re-scored the signal intensities of the ligaments and resolved any disagreements by consensus. Thus, they repeated the entire process followed in the first evaluations.

Agreements between the initial and second evaluations were analyzed for each reader and for the combined determinations. We analyzed evaluations of each of the four ligament parts separately (left and right alar ligaments, left and right parts of the transverse ligament) and all the ligament parts combined. We calculated linearly weighted kappa values to assess agreement on scores 0–3 for each side. We used unweighted kappa values to assess agreement on scores 2–3 vs. scores 0–1 per subject on any side (right and/or left). Kappa values are expressed with 95% confidence intervals (CIs) based on SEs (non-zero) and were interpreted as follows: k ≤ 0.20, poor; 0.21-0.40, fair; 0.41-0.60, moderate; 0.61-0.80, good; and 0.81-1.00, very good agreement beyond chance [17]. Disagreements on the prevalence of scores 2–3 were assessed with McNemar's test. $P < 0.05$ was taken to indicate statistical significance.

We compared the sum of the scores for all four ligament parts (MRI sum score, 0–12) between reader A vs. reader B vs. their combined scoring vs. their average scoring regarding a) intra-reader reliability using intraclass correlation coefficients (ICCs, two-way model, assuming normality), b) smallest detectable change (SDC), and c) difference between the second and first evaluation using Bland Altman plots with 95% limits of agreement. ICC ≥ 0.70 suggested adequate reliability [18]. SDC was defined as 1.96×√2SEM (standard error of measurement) and indicated the smallest change in MRI sum score that, with $P < 0.05$, could be interpreted as a "real change" above measurement error in one individual [18]. Data were analyzed using WINPEPI 10.0 (http://www.brixtonhealth.com/pepi4windows.html).

A statistical power assessment indicated that, with a true, unweighted kappa of 0.70 and a prevalence of 30% for the relevant MRI finding (e.g., intensity signal scores of 2–3), 85 paired observations would provide 80% power to give a significant result at the 5% level in a two-sided test of k = 0.40 [19]. With a true, unweighted kappa of 0.60 and a prevalence of 30%, 191 paired observations would provide 80% power to give a significant result. This study included 102 paired observations, or 408 paired observations, including all ligament parts.

Results

Better agreement between the initial and second evaluations of alar and transverse ligament signal intensities was obtained with the combined readings than with the individual readings (Table 1, Figure 1). This applied to either ligament side (weighted kappa range was 0.65-0.71 for combined readings vs. 0.48-0.62 for individual readings) and to the presence of grade 2–3 signal intensities on any ligament side in a given subject (unweighted kappa range was 0.69-0.74 for combined readings vs. 0.52-0.63 for individual readings) (Table 1). For all ligament parts combined (n = 408), the weighted kappas for agreement between the initial and the second evaluations were 0.56 (95% CI: 0.50, 0.62) for reader A, 0.55 (95% CI: 0.48, 0.62) for reader B, and 0.68 (95% CI: 0.63, 0.74) for the combined reading.

A higher prevalence of signal intensity scores of 2–3 per subject was reported in the second evaluations compared to the initial evaluations (Table 2). The P values for the difference between evaluations were smaller for individual reader scoring than for combined scoring ($P \leq 0.004$ vs. $P \geq 0.039$ for individual vs. combined differences, respectively) (Table 2).

In the initial evaluation, the combined scores agreed with reader A's scores in 86.0% of cases and with reader B's scores in 80.1% of cases. In the second evaluation, the combined scores agreed with reader A's scores in 83.3% of cases and with reader B's scores in 77.7% of cases. Weighted kappa values for agreement between A and B was 0.49 (95% CI: 0.41, 0.57) in the initial evaluation and 0.56 (95% CI: 0.49, 0.62) in the second evaluation (all ligament parts combined, n = 408).

The MRI sum score for all ligament parts had higher intra-reader reliability with combined scoring (ICC 0.74, 95% CI: 0.64, 0.82) and both readers' average scoring (ICC 0.78, 95% CI: 0.68, 0.84) than with individual reader scoring (A: ICC 0.55, 95% CI: 0.40, 0.67; B: ICC 0.69, 95% CI: 0.58, 0.78). SDC in MRI sum score was lowest for average scoring (2.9) followed by combined (3.3) and individual scoring (A: 4.2, B: 4.4). Similarly, MRI sum score differed less between the two evaluations when average scoring or combined scoring was used (Figure 2).

Discussion

In this study on the reliability of two readers compared to one, the combined reading was more reproducible than a single expert's reading. Therefore, research designs should preferentially use a combined reading for conclusive results.

Table 1 Kappa values for agreement between initial and second evaluations

	Alar ligament scores 0-3			Transverse ligament scores 0-3		
Scored by	**Right side**	**Left side**	**Any side, scores 2-3**	**Right side**	**Left side**	**Any side, scores 2-3**
Reader A	0.59 (0.47, 0.70)	0.62 (0.51, 0.73)	0.63 (0.48, 0.78)	0.50 (0.35, 0.64)	0.51 (0.38, 0.64)	0.59 (0.43, 0.75)
Reader B	0.51 (0.39, 0.63)	0.57 (0.44, 0.70)	0.52 (0.35, 0.68)	0.48 (0.32, 0.64)	0.58 (0.45, 0.72)	0.53 (0.38, 0.68)
A and B combined	0.68 (0.56, 0.79)	0.71 (0.61, 0.81)	0.74 (0.61, 0.88)	0.66 (0.53, 0.79)	0.65 (0.54, 0.77)	0.69 (0.54, 0.84)

Values represent linearly weighted kappa values for scores 0, 1, 2, or 3 on each side of the spine, and unweighted kappa values for scores 2–3 vs. scores 0–1 per subject on any side (right and/or left), with 95% confidence intervals in parenthesis, based on magnetic resonance imaging in 102 subjects.

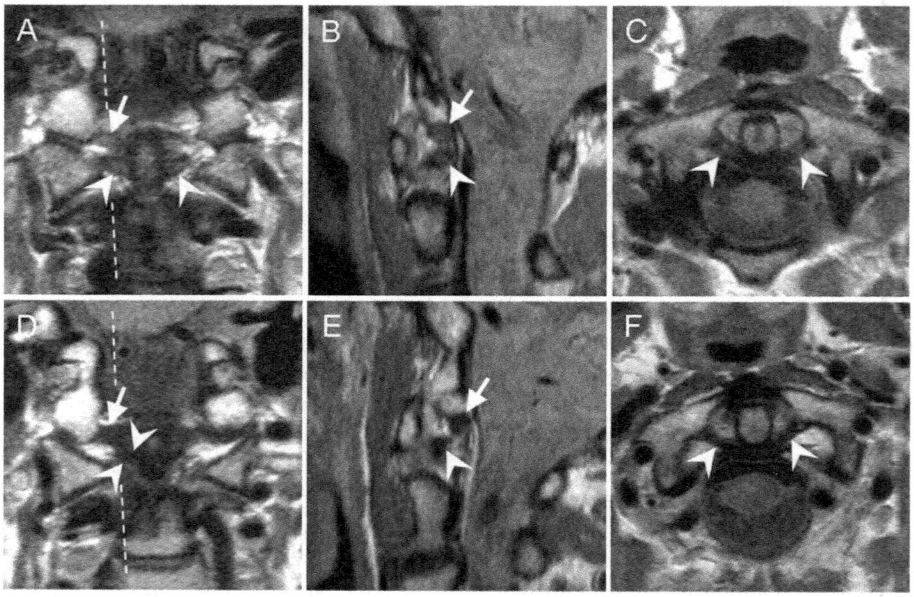

Figure 1 Scoring high signal intensities of alar and transverse ligaments on upper neck MRIs. Proton-density-weighted, fast-spin echo, 1.5 Tesla MRI sections were performed in **(A, D)** coronal, **(B, E)** sagittal, and **(C, F)** axial directions. MRIs were from two healthy women, aged **(A-C)** 44 years old, and **(D-F)** 60 years old. Broken lines mark the sagittal plane. **(A-C)** The transverse ligament is indicated with arrow heads. The high intensity signal was scored 2 by reader A, 1 by reader B, and 2 by consensus; in the second evaluation, the same signal was scored 2 by both readers independently. The alar ligament is indicated with arrows. **(A, B)** The high intensity signal was graded 2 by both readers independently; in the second evaluation, the same signal was scored 2 by reader A, 3 by reader B, and 2 by consensus. **(D-F)** The transverse ligament (arrow heads) and alar ligament (arrows) were scored 0 by both readers independently in both evaluations.

When reporting a sum score for several MRI findings, two readers' average score can be used. Importantly, the two readers in our study first interpreted all images independently; then, they solved all disagreements in consensus. They did not perform a consensus reading without prior separate readings. This approach makes it impossible to assess observer variation, and it is not advised in research settings [20].

Three other points should be noted. First, the combined reading improved the reliability of results, despite the fact that the expert alone achieved moderate to good reliability. Because this level of reliability is common in diagnostic imaging [21-23], our findings may be generalized to many types of imaging examinations. Second, the additional reader had moderate experience. A second expert might have provided even more improvement in the reliability. Third, the consensus reading in cases of agreement may be useful, because consensus discussions can improve agreement between readers [2,24].

The prevalence of a high signal intensity score increased from the first to the second reading (Table 2). This was probably due to uncertainty in interpretation or due to a response bias (i.e., the readers' tendency to prefer scoring high or low, particularly when in doubt, independently of the signal characteristics [25]). Interestingly, the prevalence of a high signal intensity score increased between evaluations less when based on both readers' combined reading, probably because ambiguous cases were more likely to be discussed in consensus and scored consistently. In a prior study [16], each of two readers evaluated

Table 2 Prevalence of scores 2–3 on initial and second evaluations

	Alar ligament scores 2-3*			Transverse ligament scores 2-3*		
Scored by	**Initial %**	**Second %**	***P* value§**	**Initial %**	**Second %**	***P* value§**
Reader A	29.4	43.1	0.001	27.5	40.2	0.004
Reader B	22.5	40.2	<0.001	25.5	46.1	<0.001
A and B combined	31.4	39.2	0.039	28.4	36.3	0.057

The data are based on magnetic resonance imaging in 102 subjects.
* Highest assigned score when different intensities were noted on the right and left sides of the spine.
§ *P* value for difference in prevalence (%), based on McNemar's test.

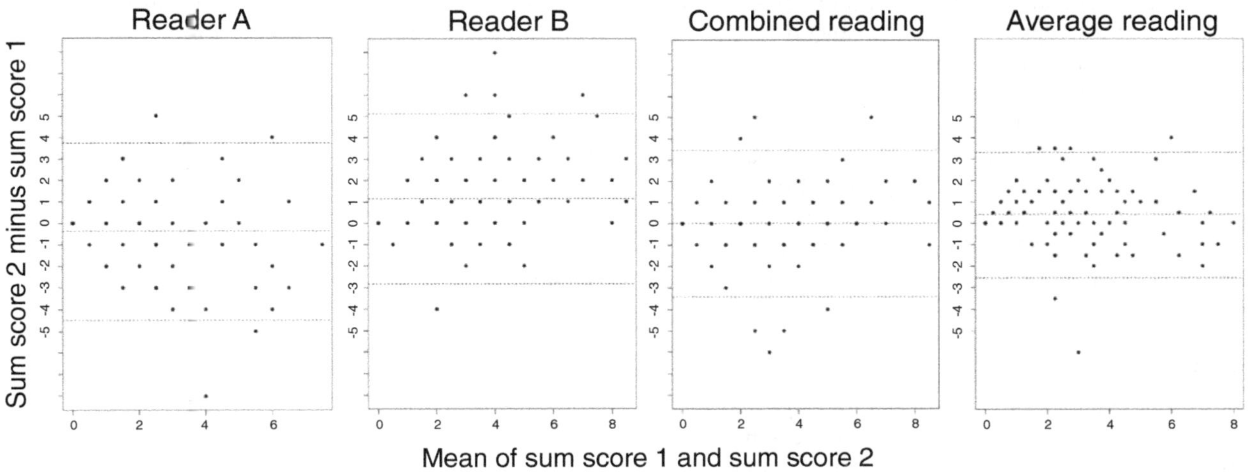

Figure 2 Bland Altman plots of difference in MRI sum score between second and first evaluations. On 102 upper neck MRIs, two readers A and B independently graded the signal intensities of the alar and transverse ligaments on both sides of the spine (i.e. four ligament parts) on a scale of 0, 1, 2 or 3 and then resolved disagreements by consensus (combined reading). They also repeated the grading process (second evaluation). The sum of the scores for all ligament parts (MRI sum score, possible values 0–12) was calculated. In each plot, the difference between sum score 2 (second evaluation) and sum score 1 (first evaluation) is plotted against the mean of the two sum scores. Dotted lines represent mean difference and 95% limits of agreement. The plots show generally smaller differences for both readers' combined reading and for the average of both readers' scores (average reading) than for individual reader scores. Mean difference in sum score (with 95% limits of agreement) was for reader A −0.4 (−4.4, 3.7), reader B 1.2 (−2.7, 5.1), combined reading 0.0 (−3.4, 3.4) and average reading 0.4 (−2.5, 3.3).

the signal intensity of the alar ligament, and assigned lower scores in the second reading than in the first.

In some previous MRI studies of the alar and transverse ligaments, conclusive ligament interpretations were based on one reader's evaluation [26,27], two readers' consensus evaluation (without prior separate readings) [28], or two readers' combined reading (i.e., separate readings followed by consensus reading in cases of disagreement) [13,29,30]. Many factors affected the quality of these studies in addition to the reliability of the conclusive ligament interpretation. Nevertheless, our data indicated that the conclusive interpretation was more reproducible when based on the combined reading, compared to a single expert reading.

Combined readings were performed in our larger studies on high signal intensities of alar and transverse ligaments. In those studies, the same two readers that were used in the present study independently scored all ligaments, solved all disagreements in consensus, and reported a conclusive combined score [11,12,31,32]. Based on that conclusive score, the high intensity signal differed little between healthy volunteers and patients with rheumatoid arthritis, chronic neck pain, or acute whiplash; furthermore, the conclusive score did not affect outcome after acute whiplash [11,12,31,32]. The process of conclusive image reading had been optimized to improve the reliability, which is essential before assessing validity [1]. Neglecting this optimization might lead to underestimations of the finding's potential relationship to clinical features, outcome, or treatment effects [33,34].

Our findings support the use of two or more readers for determining conclusive image readings in research, particularly for images with some ambiguity. In cases where a reliable result was previously documented, one expert's reading might be sufficient for a conclusive reading. The use of two readers must be weighted against the additional effort required to solve disagreements in consensus or to employ additional readers. MRIs of upper neck ligaments yield limited clinical information, and they are not recommended for routine clinical use [12,13,31,32,35,36]. It has been speculated that the ligament high signal intensities may represent normal morphological ligament variants with loose connective tissue and/or fat [13,27,31]. Nevertheless, the present study suggested that more than one reader would provide benefit, e.g., on MRI findings in a whiplash patient. Further studies of clinically important image findings are required to confirm the higher reliability of two readers compared to one.

An important unresolved question is whether a "two readers approach" provides better agreement with a clinical "gold" standard than readout with one single expert, or has better predictive utility. No "gold" standard exists and no predictive utility has been documented for the MRI findings evaluated in this study. It is also not clear whether a "multiple readers approach" with use of more than two independent readers' majority score may be more reliable, accurate or clinically useful, or whether an assessment of discrepant reads *per se* may provide clinically more relevant information than consensus reading in cases of disagreement.

A major strength of this study was that the readers were blinded to the study design. The study had a moderate sample size and power. However, all differences in kappa values, in *P* values for disagreement on prevalence, in ICCs, in SDC, and on Bland Altman plots were in the same direction; this indicated higher reliability with two readers than with one. The kappa for all ligament parts together indicated significantly higher reliability based on non-overlapping CIs. These CIs assumed independent scoring of the four ligament parts; however, all four parts were visible on the same image. Thus, some dependency in the scoring probably existed and may have narrowed the CIs. The kappa value is affected by the prevalence of the evaluated finding, and it is difficult to compare between groups that differ in prevalence [19]. However, this effect on kappa is largest for prevalence below 10% and above 90% and smaller for the prevalence reported in our study (22.5% - 46.1%, Table 2). Normality plots suggested only small deviations from the assumed normal distribution and the ICCs were also higher with two readers than with one based on log transformed data. Our study included more healthy subjects than patients. Images from a sample with a higher proportion of patients would be likely to show a similar prevalence of high signal intensities in the ligaments (based on findings in our main project). However, those images might have been more difficult to interpret, which might have led to lower reliability, and ultimately, a larger improvement in reliability with the inclusion of a second reader. Therefore, this limitation tends to strengthen our findings.

Conclusions

To our knowledge, this study was the first to provide empirical data on the reliability of two readers compared to one. For scoring the signal intensities of ligaments on upper neck MRIs, image reading by a single expert was less consistent than combined reading by the same expert in collaboration with a second reader. The latter approach implied independent readings followed by consensus reading in cases of disagreement. This approach was used to determine conclusive interpretations of high intensity signals in neck ligament studies that have previously shown that high signal intensities had limited clinical relevance [11-13,31,32,36]. Two or more readers may be needed to provide reliable conclusive image reading results in research. In this study, a moderately experienced second reader improved the reliability compared to a single expert reader. The implications of this for clinical work should be assessed in further studies of more clinically relevant imaging findings.

Competing interests

The authors declare that they have no competing interests.

Authors' contributions

AE conceived, designed, and coordinated the study, performed statistical analyses, and drafted the manuscript. NV interpreted the MRI examinations, performed statistical analyses, and helped draft the manuscript. JK interpreted the MRI examinations, participated in the data analysis, and reviewed the manuscript. All authors read and approved the final manuscript.

Acknowledgements

This study received funding from the Grieg Foundation and the Norwegian ExtraFoundation for Health and Rehabilitation. We thank Øivind Salvesen for help with Bland Altman plots.

References

1. Thornbury JR: **Eugene W. Caldwell Lecture. Clinical efficacy of diagnostic imaging: love it or leave it.** *AJR Am J Roentgenol* 1994, **162:**1–8.
2. D'agostino MA, Aegerter P, Jousse-Joulin S, Chary-Valckenaere I, Lecoq B, Gaudin P, Brault I, Scmitz J, Dehaut F, Le Parc J, Breban M, Landais P: **How to evaluate and improve the reliability of power Doppler ultrasonography for assessing enthesitis in spondylarthritis.** *Arthritis Rheum* 2009, **61:**61–69.
3. Yoon LS, Haims AH, Brink JA, Rabinovici R, Forman HP: **Evaluation of an emergency radiology quality assurance program at a level I trauma center: abdominal and pelvic CT studies.** *Radiology* 2002, **224:**42–46.
4. Canon CL, Smith JK, Morgan DE, Jones BC, Fell SC, Kenney PJ, Ferrante D, Lockhart ME, Westfall AO, Koehler RE: **Double reading of barium enemas: is it necessary?** *AJR Am J Roentgenol* 2003, **181:**1607–1610.
5. Cheung KM, Samartzis D, Karppinen J, Mok FP, Ho DW, Fong DY, Luk KD: **Intervertebral disc degeneration: new insights based on "skipped" level disc pathology.** *Arthritis Rheum* 2010, **62:**2392–2400.
6. Kjaer P, Leboeuf-Yde C, Korsholm L, Sorensen JS, Bendix T: **Magnetic resonance imaging and low back pain in adults: a diagnostic imaging study of 40-year-old men and women.** *Spine (Phila Pa 1976)* 2005, **30:**1173–1180.
7. Esposito L, Saam T, Heider P, Bockelbrink A, Pelisek J, Sepp D, Feurer R, Winkler C, Liebig T, Holzer K, Pauly O, Sadikovic S, Hemmer B, Poppert H: **MRI plaque imaging reveals high-risk carotid plaques especially in diabetic patients irrespective of the degree of stenosis.** *BMC Med Imaging* 2010, **10:**27.
8. Jagadeesan BD, Gado Almandoz JE, Moran CJ, Benzinger TL: **Accuracy of susceptibility-weighted imaging for the detection of arteriovenous shunting in vascular malformations of the brain.** *Stroke* 2011, **42:**87–92.
9. Jensch S, de Vries AH, Peringa J, Bipat S, Dekker E, Baak LC, Bartelsman JF, Heutinck A, Montauban van Swijndregt AD, Stoker J: **CT colonography with limited bowel preparation: performance characteristics in an increased-risk population.** *Radiology* 2008, **247:**122–132.
10. Peterson CK, Saupe N, Buck F, Pfirrmann CW, Zanetti M, Hodler J: **CT-guided sternoclavicular joint injections: description of the procedure, reliability of imaging diagnosis, and short-term patient responses.** *AJR Am J Roentgenol* 2010, **195:**W435–W439.
11. Vetti N, Krakenes J, Damsgaard E, Rorvik J, Gilhus NE, Espeland A: **MRI of the alar and transverse ligaments in acute whiplash-associated disorders 1–2 - a cross-sectional controlled study.** *Spine (Phila Pa 1976)* 2011, **36:**E434–E440.

12. Vetti N, Alsing R, Krakenes J, Rorvik J, Gilhus NE, Brun JG, Espeland A: **MRI of the transverse and alar ligaments in rheumatoid arthritis: feasibility and relations to atlantoaxial subluxation and disease activity.** *Neuroradiology* 2010, **52**:215–223.

13. Myran R, Kvistad KA, Nygaard OP, Andresen H, Folvik M, Zwart JA: **Magnetic resonance imaging assessment of the alar ligaments in whiplash injuries: a case-control study.** *Spine (Phila Pa 1976)* 2008, **33**:2012–2016.

14. Vetti N, Krakenes J, Eide GE, Rorvik J, Gilhus NE, Espeland A: **MRI of the alar and transverse ligaments in whiplash-associated disorders (WAD) grades 1–2: high-signal changes by age, gender, event and time since trauma.** *Neuroradiology* 2009, **51**:227–235.

15. Krakenes J, Kaale BR: **Magnetic resonance imaging assessment of craniovertebral ligaments and membranes after whiplash trauma.** *Spine (Phila Pa 1976)* 2006, **31**:2820–2826.

16. Krakenes J, Kaale BR, Moen G, Nordli H, Gilhus NE, Rorvik J: **MRI assessment of the alar ligaments in the late stage of whiplash injury–a study of structural abnormalities and observer agreement.** *Neuroradiology* 2002, **44**:617–624.

17. Altman DG: *Practical statistics for medical research.* 1st edition. London: Chapman & Hall; 1991.

18. Terwee CB, Bot SDM, de Boer MR, van der Windt DAWM, Knol DL, Dekker J, Bouter LM, de Vet HCW: **Quality criteria were proposed for measurement properties of health status questionnaires.** *J Clin Epidemiol* 2007, **60**:34–42.

19. Sim J, Wright CC: **The kappa statistic in reliability studies: use, interpretation, and sample size requirements.** *Phys Ther* 2005, **85**:257–268.

20. Bankier AA, Levine D, Halpern EF, Kressel HY: **Consensus interpretation in imaging research: is there a better way?** *Radiology* 2010, **257**:14–17.

21. Umans H, Wimpfheimer O, Haramati N, Applbaum YH, Adler M, Bosco J: **Diagnosis of partial tears of the anterior cruciate ligament of the knee: value of MR imaging.** *AJR Am J Roentgenol* 1995, **165**:893–897.

22. van Rijn JC, Klemetso N, Reitsma JB, Majoie CB, Hulsmans FJ, Peul WC, Stam J, Bossuyt PM, den Heeten GJ: **Observer variation in MRI evaluation of patients suspected of lumbar disk herniation.** *AJR Am J Roentgenol* 2005, **184**:299–303.

23. Johnson J, Kline JA: **Intraobserver and interobserver agreement of the interpretation of pediatric chest radiographs.** *Emerg Radiol* 2010, **17**:285–290.

24. Pirisi M, Leutner M, Pinato DJ, Avellini C, Carsana L, Toniutto P, Fabris C, Boldorini R: **Reliability and reproducibility of the edmondson grading of hepatocellular carcinoma using paired core biopsy and surgical resection specimens.** *Arch Pathol Lab Med* 2010, **134**:1818–1822.

25. Ker M: **Issues in the use of kappa.** *Invest Radiol* 1991, **26**:78–83.

26. Kaale BR, Krakenes J, Albrektsen G, Wester K: **Whiplash-associated disorders impairment rating: neck disability index score according to severity of MRI findings of ligaments and membranes in the upper cervical spine.** *J Neurotrauma* 2005, **22**:466–475.

27. Dullerud R, Gjertsen O, Server A: **Magnetic resonance imaging of ligaments and membranes in the craniocervical junction in whiplash-associated injury and in healthy control subjects.** *Acta Radiol* 2010, **51**:207–212.

28. Kim HJ, Jun BY, Kim WH, Cho YK, Lim MK, Suh CH: **MR imaging of the alar ligament: morphologic changes during axial rotation of the head in asymptomatic young adults.** *Skeletal Radiol* 2002, **31**:637–642.

29. Roy S, Hol PK, Laerum LT, Tillung T: **Pitfalls of magnetic resonance imaging of alar ligament.** *Neuroradiology* 2004, **46**:392–398.

30. Pfirrmann CW, Binkert CA, Zanetti M, Boos N, Hodler J: **MR morphology of alar ligaments and occipitoatlantoaxial joints: study in 50 asymptomatic subjects.** *Radiology* 2001, **218**:133–137.

31. Vetti N, Krakenes J, Eide GE, Rorvik J, Gilhus NE, Espeland A: **Are MRI high-signal changes of alar and transverse ligaments in acute whiplash injury related to outcome?** *BMC Musculoskelet Disord* 2010, **11**:260.

32. Vetti N, Krakenes J, Ask T, Erdal KA, Torkildsen MD, Rorvik J, Gilhus NE, Espeland A: **Follow-Up MR Imaging of the Alar and Transverse Ligaments after Whiplash Injury: A Prospective Controlled Study.** *AJNR Am J Neuroradiol*, in press.

33. Jarvik JG, Deyo RA: **Moderate versus mediocre: the reliability of spine MR data interpretations.** *Radiology* 2009, **250**:15–17.

34. Feinstein AR: **An additional basic science for clinical medicine: IV. The development of clinimetrics.** *Ann Intern Med* 1983, **99**:843–848.

35. Lummel N, Zeif C, Kloetzer A, Linn J, Bruckmann H, Bitterling H: **Variability of morphology and signal intensity of alar ligaments in healthy volunteers using MR imaging.** *AJNR Am J Neuroradiol* 2011, **32**:125–130.

36. Myran R, Zwart JA, Kvistad KA, Folvik M, Lydersen S, Ro M, Woodhouse A, Nygaard OP: **Clinical characteristics, pain, and disability in relation to alar ligament MRI findings.** *Spine (Phila Pa 1976)* 2011, **36**:E862–E867.

12

Counter-clockwise vortical blood flow in the main pulmonary artery in a patient with patent ductus arteriosus with pulmonary arterial hypertension

Gert Reiter[1], Ursula Reiter[2*], Gabor Kovacs[3], Gabriel Adelsmayr[2], Andreas Greiser[4], Aurelien F. Stalder[4], Horst Olschewski[3] and Michael Fuchsjäger[2]

Abstract

Background: In patients with pulmonary hypertension (PH), duration of vortical blood flow along the main pulmonary artery enables estimation of the mean pulmonary arterial pressure (mPAP) non-invasively. It remains to date not known, if this method is applicable in patients with pulmonary arterial hypertension (PAH) and abnormal aortic-to-pulmonary shunting.

Case presentation: The present case analyzes the effect of a patent ductus arteriosus (PDA) on pulmonary artery flow patterns in PAH (mPAP from right heart catheterization, 75 mmHg). PH-associated vortical blood flow, which is typically observed rotating in a clockwise direction when viewed in right ventricular outflow tract orientation, was found nested in PDA left-to-right shunting. Even though rotating counter-clockwise, duration of vortical flow translated into correct non-invasive mPAP estimate.

Conclusions: This case indicates that PH-associated vortex rotation is not restricted to clockwise direction, and that vortex-based estimation of elevated mPAP might also be feasible in patients with PAH and PDA.

Keywords: Pulmonary arterial hypertension, 4D blood flow, Patent ductus arteriosus, Cardiac magnetic resonance imaging

Background

In patients with pulmonary hypertension (PH) without abnormal aortic-to-pulmonary shunting, PH is associated with vortical blood flow along the main pulmonary artery, whose duration is linearly related to elevated mean pulmonary arterial pressure (mPAP) [1, 2]. Typically, vortex formation takes place at the posterior wall of the main pulmonary artery, and the vortex rotates in a clockwise direction when viewed in the right ventricular outflow tract (RVOT) orientation [1, 3–5].

Pulmonary arterial hypertension (PAH) is a complication in patients with patent ductus arteriosus (PDA), and the retrograde blood flow in the main pulmonary artery caused by left-to-right shunting via the PDA might modify flow patterns typically observed in PH [6]. Potentially, it might affect the presence of a vortex per se, the vortex location, the rotational direction, and also the relationship between vortex duration and mPAP. To approach these issues, pulmonary arterial blood flow patterns were analyzed in a patient with PDA and PAH.

Case presentation

A 21-year-old male patient (Table 1) with PDA and PAH (mPAP, 75 mmHg; systolic/diastolic pulmonary arterial pressures, 102/58 mmHg; systolic/diastolic systemic

* Correspondence: ursula.reiter@medunigraz.at
[2]Division of General Radiology, Department of Radiology, Medical University of Graz, Auenbruggerplatz 9/P, A-8036 Graz, Austria
Full list of author information is available at the end of the article

Table 1 Timeline

1993:	Preterm birth (35th week of pregnancy); bronchopulmonary dysplasia; severe obstructive pulmonary disease
1994:	Echocardiography: enlarged RV and RA; normal LV and LA; small PDA with left-to-right shunt
2006:	Aortic angiography: PDA diameter, 3.5 mm
	Right heart catheterization and PDA trial occlusion: mPAP, 70 mmHg; RV pressures did not significantly decrease after trial occlusion
	Echocardiography: RV/LV/PV diameter, 24/55/34 mm; maximal pressure gradient across PDA, 16 mmHg
2006 – 2014:	Bosentan therapy and close meshed therapy monitoring
2008:	Echocardiography: RV/LV/PV diameter, 28/54/35 mm; maximal pressure gradient across PDA, 16 mmHg
	Right heart catheterization and PDA trial occlusion: PAP, 94/53/70 mmHg; RAP, 4 mmHg. RV pressures did not significantly decrease after trial occlusion
2013:	Echocardiography: RV/LV/PV diameter, 24/59/39 mm
2014:	Right heart catheterization: see case presentation. Clinical classification: PAH associated with congenital heart disease (PDA) according to positive treatment effect of Bosentan
	Cardiac MR: see case presentation
since 2014:	Macitentan therapy

PDA, patent ductus arteriosus. *RV* right ventricle, *LV* left ventricle, *PV* pulmonary valve, *RVP* systolic/diastolic/mean, right ventricular pressure, *PAP* systolic/diastolic/mean, pulmonary arterial pressure, *RAP* right atrial pressure, *PAH* pulmonary arterial hypertension

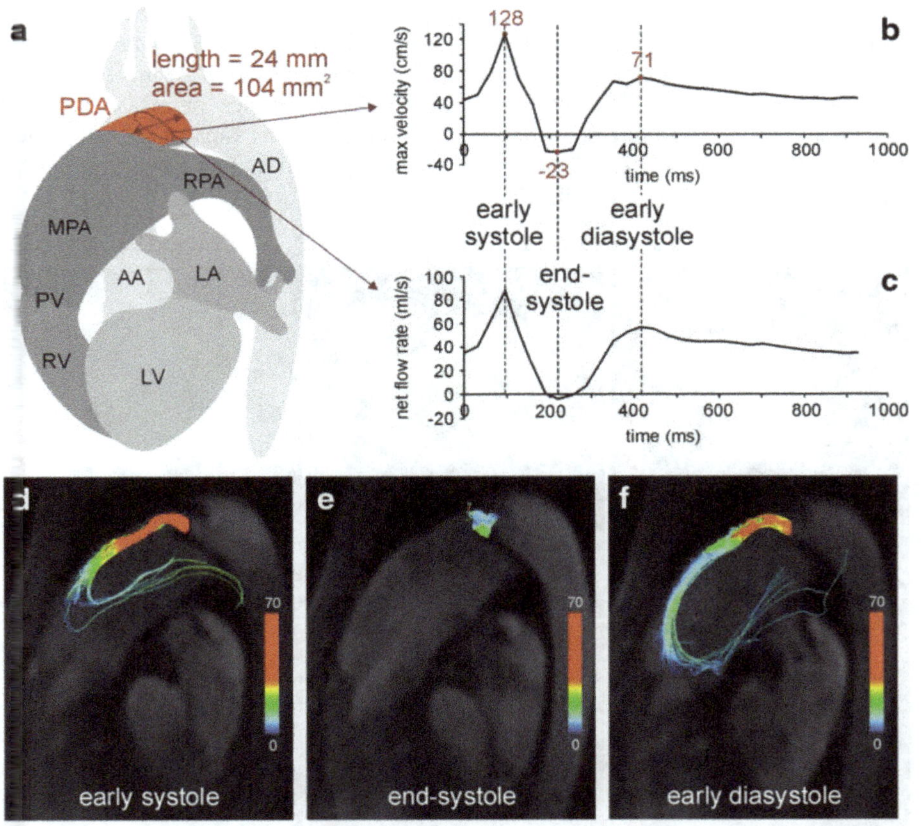

Fig. 1 4D flow evaluation of the PDA. Schematic 3D anatomy (**a**) of the PDA and surrounding cardiovascular structures based on 3D reconstruction of the anatomical phase contrast images. PDA length and time-averaged cross-sectional area at the center of the PDA were evaluated by multi-planar reformation. Time courses of maximal velocity (**b**) and net flow rate (**c**) across the central cross-section of the PDA demonstrate an early systolic and an early diastolic left-to-right peak and small right-to-left flow at end-systole. Velocity-color-encoded streamlines originating from PDA at early systole (**d**), end-systole (**e**) and early diastole (**f**) projected onto multi-planar reformatted anatomical images reflect these bi-phasic PDA flow characteristics. In early systole (**d**) and diastole (**f**) there is fast left-to-right flow through the PDA that reverses direction in the main pulmonary artery. In end-systole (**e**) blood spirals from right-to-left but no streamlines (and particles in Additional file 1: in the online-only Data Supplement) enter the aorta. PDA = patent ductus arteriosus; MPA = main pulmonary artery; RPA = right pulmonary artery; PV = pulmonary valve; AD = aorta descendens; AA = aorta ascendens, LV = left ventricle, RV = right ventricle, LA = left atrium

arterial pressures, 112/67 mmHg; pulmonary arterial wedge pressure, 9 mmHg; right atrial pressure, 7 mmHg; cardiac index, 3.4 L/min/m^2, pulmonary vascular resistance, 11.5 Wood units) was referred for 3 T cardiac magnetic resonance (MR) function and 4D flow imaging (Magnetom Trio, Siemens Healthcare, Erlangen, Germany) after right heart catheterization (RHC) within a prospective study approved by the local ethical review board (ClinicalTrials.gov Identifier NCT01725763). Cardiac function was assessed by cine steady-state free precession real-time imaging during free breathing. Volumetric evaluation revealed enlarged left (LV) and right (RV) ventricular volumes (end-diastolic volume, LV: 126 mL/m^2, RV: 121 mL/m^2; end-systolic volume, LV: 55 mL/m^2, RV: 70 mL/m^2; ejection fraction, LV: 56 %, RV: 42 %), normal left (65 g/m^2) and increased right ventricular mass (61 g/m^2). Left (LA) and right (RA) atrial volumes (maximum volume, LA: 39 mL/m^2, RA: 65 mL/m^2; minimum volume, LA: 19 mL/m^2, RA: 30 mL/m^2) were within normal ranges [7].

MR 4D flow data were acquired in free breathing, covering the heart, pulmonary artery and aorta with gapless slices of a retrospectively ECG-gated, segmented, two-dimensional spoiled gradient-echo-based cine phase-contrast sequence with three-directional velocity encoding in RVOT orientation. Velocity fields were calculated, visualized and analyzed by dedicated prototype software (4D Flow V2.4, Siemens Healthcare, Erlangen, Germany) [8].

Multi-planar reformatted anatomical phase contrast images demonstrated a dilatated main pulmonary artery (cross-sectional area, 15.8 cm^2), and a tubular ductus arteriosus 24 mm in length and 104 mm^2 in cross-sectional area connecting the proximal descending aorta to the left pulmonary artery near its origin (Fig. 1). Time-course of PDA maximal velocity (Fig. 1b) and net blood flow rate (Fig. 1c) during the cardiac cycle, as well as streamlines (Fig. 1d, e, f) and particle traces (see Additional file 1) originating from the PDA, demonstrated biphasic left-to-right shunting without Eisenmenger's syndrome. The systolic/diastolic pressure gradients between aorta and pulmonary artery of 7/2 mmHg, calculated from systolic/diastolic peak velocities across the PDA (Fig. 1b) via the Bernoulli equation (pressure gradient in mmHg = $4 \cdot v^2$, with v being the PDA peak velocity in m/s), matched the difference between systemic and pulmonary systolic/diastolic pressures. Shunt volume across the PDA was 33 mL, which was in agreement with the difference of measured net forward volumes in the ascending aorta (120 mL) and main pulmonary artery (81 mL). The resulting pulmonary-to-systemic flow ratio was 0.7.

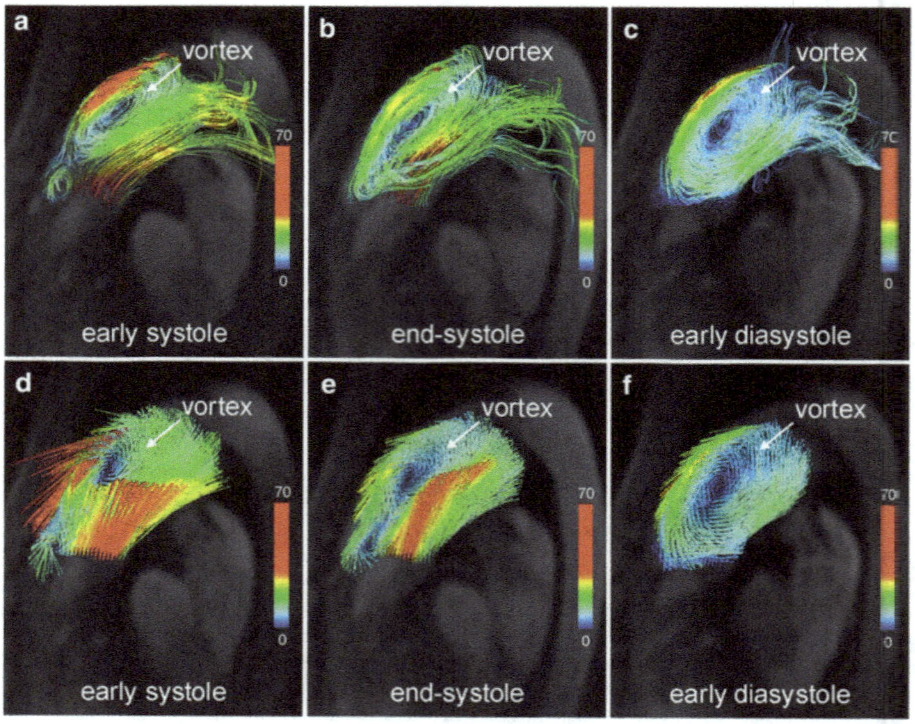

Fig. 2 Vortical blood flow in the main pulmonary artery. Velocity-color-encoded streamlines (**a**, **b**, **c**) and 3D velocity vectors (**d**, **e**, **f**) projected onto multi-planar reformatted anatomical images demonstrate counter-clockwise rotating vortical blood flow nested in bi-directional pulmonary flow caused by PDA. This structure is present throughout the entire cardiac cycle (Additional file 2: in the online-only Data Supplement)

Streamlines (Figs. 2a, b, c) and particle traces (see Additional file 2) originating from the main pulmonary artery, as well as 3D velocity vector fields (Figs. 2d, e, f), demonstrated that left-to-right ductal shunting caused retrograde blood flow along the anterior wall of the main pulmonary artery, reversing direction from retrograde to anterograde above the pulmonary valve. This anterograde flow adhered to the forward flow through the pulmonary valve during systole.

The typical flow pattern in patients with PAH (Fig. 3) - i.e., vortex formation at the posterior wall of the main pulmonary artery - was not seen. Instead there was a vortex at the anterior wall of the main pulmonary artery nested between retrograde and anterograde PDA-caused blood flow and rotating counter-clockwise (i.e., opposite the typical clockwise direction) (Fig. 2). The duration of this vortical blood flow was the complete cardiac interval (t_{vortex} = 100 %), which translated into mPAP of 79 mmHg (according to the formula mPAP in mmHg = 16 + 0.63 · t_{vortex}) [2] and was very close to the value measured during RHC.

Discussion

Irrespectively of the underlying etiology of PH, vortical blood flow along the main pulmonary artery has been identified as a marker of elevated mPAP [1–3]. The formation of this vortical flow has been attributed to the appearance of a thickened boundary layer in the main pulmonary artery caused by increased pulmonary vascular resistance, reduced compliance and altered pulse wave reflection [1, 3]. Owing to the curvature of the vessel this thickened boundary layer is located at the posterior wall of the main pulmonary, which leads to the formation of a clockwise rotating vortex.

In the present case of PDA and PAH, vortex formation is observed at the anterior wall of the main pulmonary artery and its rotational direction is counter-clockwise. This flow topology has not been described neither in PH in general, nor in PAH in particular [1–5, 9]. It could be speculated that the PDA jet which is pressing the pulmonary arterial forward flow against the posterior vessel wall impedes vortex formation in this region. Jet stream

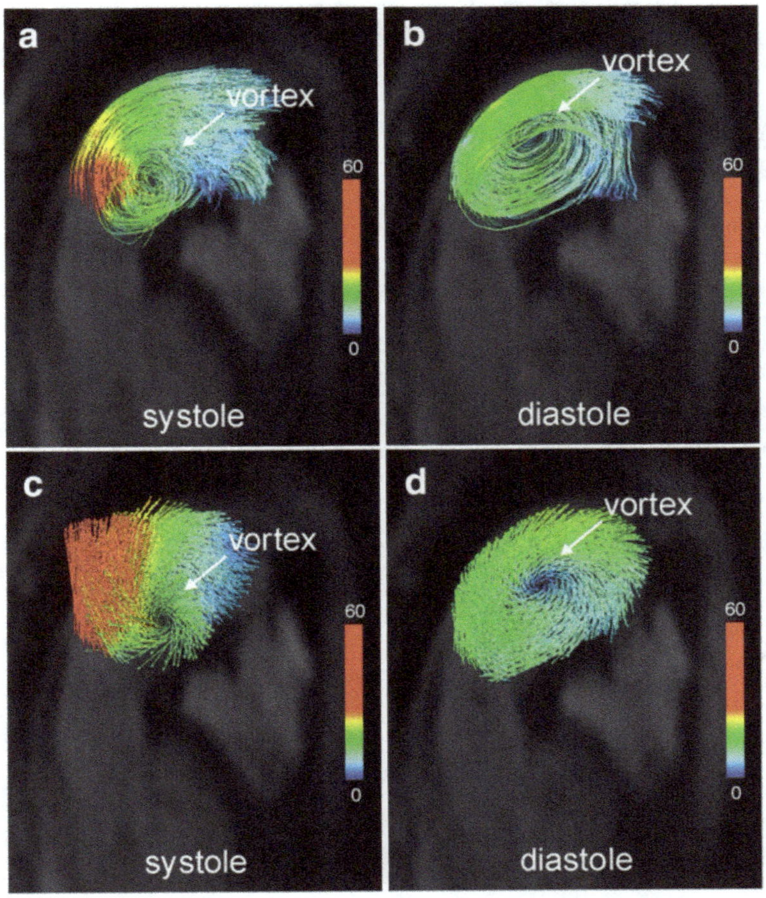

Fig. 3 Typical vortical blood flow in the main pulmonary artery in a patient with pulmonary arterial hypertension (mPAP = 82 mmHg) without PDA. Velocity-color-encoded streamlines (**a**, **b**) and 3D velocity vectors (**c**, **d**) projected onto multi-planar reformatted anatomical images demonstrate clockwise rotating vortical blood flow and forward flow along the posterior wall of the main pulmonary artery

boundaries on the other hand give generally rise to zones of turbulent mixing [10]; PDA jet could therefore favor vortex formation at the anterior wall of the main pulmonary artery.

In PH patients without PDA, duration of vortical blood flow in the main pulmonary artery was found to be closely related to mPAP [2]. Notably, mPAP calculated from the duration of vortical blood flow in the present case revealed good agreement with the mPAP measured by RHC. It could therefore be conjectured that the observed counter-clockwise rotating vortex is similarly related to inadequate release of blood from the main pulmonary artery into the pulmonary vasculature as the clockwise rotating vortex in patients with elevated mPAP without PDA. This would mean that the vortex – irrespectively of its rotational direction – represents a mechanism of "kinetic energy storage", counteracting the increased vascular resistance and the reduced compliance in PH. Clinical studies including patients with PDA with/without PAH and with/without Eisenmenger's syndrome are needed to gain better insights into the complex hemodynamics of PDA with PAH.

Conclusions

The current case indicates that vortex-based estimation of elevated mPAP might be feasible in patients with PDA. However, this case also shows that in a patient with PDA, the location and direction of vortical blood flow may differ from those typically seen in patients with PH without PDA.

Abbreviations

mPAP, mean pulmonary arterial pressure; MR, magnetic resonance; PAH, pulmonary arterial hypertension; PDA, patent ductus arteriosus; PH, pulmonary hypertension; RHC, right heart catheterization; RVOT, right ventricular outflow tract; t_{vortex}, period of existence of vortical blood flow

Acknowledgements

The authors thank Ada Muellner, MSc for reviewing the manuscript.

Funding

The study has received funding from the Styrian government, Department 8 for Science and Research (grant number A3-16.R-8/2012-8). G.A. was supported by the Oesterreichische Nationalbank, Anniversary Fund (grant number 141223).

Authors' contributions

UR and GR drafted the manuscript and acquired and analyzed 4D flow data. GA and MF performed and reported the cardiac MRT investigation; GK and HO performed and evaluated RHC. AG and AFS provided 4D Flow software for image analysis and visualization. All authors read and approved the final manuscript.

Competing interests

G.R., A.G., and A.F.S. are employed by Siemens Healthcare. All authors declare that they have no conflicts of interest relevant to this manuscript.

Author details

[1]Siemens Healthcare, Graz, Austria. [2]Division of General Radiology, Department of Radiology, Medical University of Graz, Auenbruggerplatz 9/P, A-8036 Graz, Austria. [3]Division of Pulmology, Department of Internal Medicine, Medical University of Graz, & LBI for Lung Vascular Research Graz, Graz, Austria. [4]Siemens Healthcare, Erlangen, Germany.

References

1. Reiter G, Reiter U, Kovacs G, Kainz B, Schmidt K, Maier R, Olschewski H, Rienmueller R. Magnetic resonance-derived 3-dimensional blood flow patterns in the main pulmonary artery as a marker of pulmonary hypertension and a measure of elevated mean pulmonary arterial pressure. Circ Cardiovasc Imaging. 2008;1(1):23–30.
2. Reiter G, Reiter U, Kovacs G, Olschewski H, Fuchsjager M. Blood flow vortices along the main pulmonary artery measured with MR imaging for diagnosis of pulmonary hypertension. Radiology. 2015;275(1):71–9.
3. Helderman F, Mauritz GJ, Andringa KE, Vonk-Noordegraaf A, Marcus JT. Early onset of retrograde flow in the main pulmonary artery is a characteristic of pulmonary arterial hypertension. J Magn Reson Imaging. 2011;33(6):1362–8.
4. Odagiri K, Inui N, Miyakawa S, Hakamata A, Wei J, Takehara Y, Sakahara H, Sugiyama M, Alley MT, Tran QK, Watanabe H. Abnormal hemodynamics in the pulmonary artery seen on time-resolved 3-dimensional phase-contrast magnetic resonance imaging (4D-flow) in a young patient with idiopathic pulmonary arterial hypertension. Circ J. 2014;78(7):1770–2.
5. Ota H, Sugimura K, Miura M, Shimokawa H. Four-dimensional flow magnetic resonance imaging visualizes drastic change in vortex flow in the main pulmonary artery after percutaneous transluminal pulmonary angioplasty in a patient with chronic thromboembolic pulmonary hypertension. Eur Heart J. 2015;36(25):1630.
6. Schneider DJ, Moore JW. Patent ductus arteriosus. Circulation. 2006; 114(17):1873–82.
7. Kawel-Boehm N, Maceira A, Valsangiacomo-Buechel ER, Vogel-Claussen J, Turkbey EB, Williams R, Plein S, Tee M, Eng J, Bluemke DA. Normal values for cardiovascular magnetic resonance in adults and children. J Cardiovasc Magn Reson. 2015;17:29.
8. Reiter U, Reiter G, Kovacs G, Stalder AF, Gulsun MA, Greiser A, Olschewski H, Fuchsjager M. Evaluation of elevated mean pulmonary arterial pressure based on magnetic resonance 4D velocity mapping: comparison of visualization techniques. PLoS One. 2013;8(12):e82212.
9. Frydrychowicz A, Bley TA, Dittrich S, Hennig J, Langer M, Markl M. Visualization of vascular hemodynamics in a case of a large patent ductus arteriosus using flow sensitive 3D CMR at 3 T. J Cardiovasc Magn Reson. 2007;9(3):585–7.
10. Oertel H. Prandtl's essentials of fluid mechanics. 2nd ed. New York: Springer; 2004.

Age-related normal structural and functional ventricular values in cardiac function assessed by magnetic resonance

Michael Fiechter[1,3†], Tobias A Fuchs[1†], Catherine Gebhard[1], Julia Stehli[1], Bernd Klaeser[1], Barbara E Stähli[2], Robert Manka[1,2], Costantina Manes[2], Felix C Tanner[2,3], Oliver Gaemperli[1,2] and Philipp A Kaufmann[1,3*]

Abstract

Background: The heart is subject to structural and functional changes with advancing age. However, the magnitude of cardiac age-dependent transformation has not been conclusively elucidated.

Methods: This retrospective cardiac magnetic resonance (CMR) study included 183 subjects with normal structural and functional ventricular values. End systolic volume (ESV), end diastolic volume (EDV), and ejection fraction (EF) were obtained from the left and the right ventricle in breath-hold cine CMR. Patients were classified into four age groups (20–29, 30–49, 50–69, and ≥70 years) and cardiac measurements were compared using Pearson's rank correlation over the four different groups.

Results: With advanced age a slight but significant decrease in ESV (r=−0.41 for both ventricles, P<0.001) and EDV (r=−0.39 for left ventricle, r=−0.35 for right ventricle, P<0.001) were observed associated with a significant increase in left (r=0.28, P<0.001) and right (r=0.27, P<0.01) ventricular EF reaching a maximal increase in EF of +8.4% (P<0.001) for the left and +6.1% (P<0.01) for the right ventricle in the oldest compared to the youngest patient group. Left ventricular myocardial mass significantly decreased over the four different age groups (P<0.05).

Conclusions: The aging process is associated with significant changes in left and right ventricular EF, ESV and EDV in subjects with no cardiac functional and structural abnormalities. These findings underline the importance of using age adapted values as standard of reference when evaluating CMR studies.

Keywords: CMR, Age, LV-EF, RV-EF, Normal values

Background

Cardiac structural and functional ventricular values are important prognostic parameters for predicting patient outcome and are therefore commonly assessed with various methods [1,2] whereby cardiac magnetic resonance (CMR) imaging has emerged as a new gold standard. With an aging Western population, the impact of age on these cardiac parameters is critical for identification of pathology. The ventricular systolic phase represents a synergistic interplay of multiple kinetic components, each of which confers added prognostic information such as short and long-axis shortening and twisting around the ventricular long axis [3]. From the second to seventh decade a substantial decrease in longitudinal shortening (−20%) but an increase in short-axis diameter shortening (+18%) [4] is associated with a prolonged isovolumetric contraction phase [5].

However, the precise impact of aging on the ventricular function has remained controversial. Several studies involving different methods concluded that aging does not have any impact on LV function [6,7], whereas others found a slightly decreased [8-10] LV ejection fraction (LV-EF) in healthy subjects. A recent study assessing cardiac function using echocardiography in a large patient population revealed an increase in LV-EF with a decrease in end-diastolic volume (EDV) and end-systolic

* Correspondence: pak@usz.ch
†Equal contributors
[1]Department of Radiology, Cardiac Imaging, University Hospital Zurich, Zurich, Switzerland
[3]Zurich Center for Integrative Human Physiology (ZIHP), University of Zurich, Zurich, Switzerland
Full list of author information is available at the end of the article

volume (ESV) in older compared to younger individuals [11]. A small study using CMR imaging observed an age-dependent increase in LV-EF [12].

However, the impact of age on both LV and in particular right ventricular (RV) function as assessed by CMR has not been investigated in large study populations. The aim of the present study was to compare LV and RV dimensions and EF over consecutive age decades.

Methods

Study population

This retrospective study enrolled patients who underwent CMR for assessment of myocardial function including those individuals who had normal function and no cardiac pathology. In addition, the following exclusion criteria were applied: history of any cardiac disease, LV-EF <50% and/or RV-EF <45%, and EDV >235 ml (males) and >174 ml (females) as assessed by CMR [13]. As a result 1016 patients were excluded and 183 patients were included into the final analysis. Study patients were classified into four age groups (20–29, 30–49, 50–69, and ≥70 years). Need to obtain written informed consent was waived by the institutional review board due to the nature of the study with sole clinical data collection.

Image acquisition and analysis

Supine cardiac magnetic resonance imaging was performed using a 1.5 Tesla magnetic resonance (MR) scanner (Philips Achieva, Best, NL) using electrocardiogram (ECG) triggered breath-hold fast field echo acquisition imaging covering the heart from the valve plane to the apex with a slice thickness of 8 mm with no gap. The field of view was 450 × 400 × 96 mm. Sequence parameters included plane pixel size of 2.1 × 1.8 mm, acquisition time of 25 heart beats, flip angle of 60°, and repetition time/echo time of 3.4/1.7 ms. A cardiac synergy coil was used for signal acquisition and cardiac synchronization was performed with a vector ECG. Standard projections (short axis, two-, three-, and four-chamber view) were obtained for functional and structural assessment. Quantification of left and right ventricular values was performed using a dedicated software and workstation (Extended Work Space, Philips Medical Systems, NL) by two independent CMR observers. In brief, LV and RV endocardial border were delineated in end-systolic and end-diastolic phases in all planes and EDV/ESV were calculated. LV mass was determined from the end-diastolic frames.

Statistical analysis

Quantitative variables were expressed as mean ± standard deviation (SD) and categorical variables as frequencies or percentages. SPSS 20 (SPSS, Chicago, IL) was used for all statistical analysis. The Pearson's correlation analysis was used to determine a correlation between the parameters of interest. P-values of less than 0.05 were considered statistically significant.

Results

This study included 183 subjects with functional and structural assessment of LV parameters. The quantitative RV parameters were available in 111 patients and the LV mass in 147 patients. The mean age of the study population was 52±14.7 years. The mean LV-EF was 64±7.0% while the mean RV-EF was 59±6.6% (Table 1). The most relevant and statistically significant change in LV and RV parameters was observed between the age group 30–49 years and 50–69 years as well as between 50–69 years and ≥70 years.

There was a modest but significant correlation of the LV-EF with increasing age (n=183 r=0.28, P<0.001) whereas LV-ESV (n=183, r=–0.41, P<0.001), LV-EDV (n=183, r=–0.39, P<0.001), and LV myocardial mass (n=147, r=–0.21, P<0.05) decreased significantly at advanced age (Figure 1).

Table 1 Patient baseline characteristics (n=183)

Age (yrs)	52±14.7
Male, n (%)	117 (64)
Mean LV values	
EF (%)	64±7.0
ESV (ml)	50±17.9
EDV (ml)	137±34.2
Mass (g/m^2)	57±16.7
Mean RV values	
EF (%)	59±6.6
ESV (ml)	52±18
EDV (ml)	126±34.2
Cardiovascular risk factors, n (%)	
Smoking	31 (17)
Hypertension	46 (25)
Diabetes	13 (7)
Dyslipidemia	32 (17)
Positive family history	39 (21)
Medications, n (%)	
Aspirin	50 (27)
Beta-blocker	41 (41)
ACE/angiotensin II inhibitor	43 (23)
Statin	37 (20)
Calcium channel blocker	5 (3)
Nitrate	2 (1)

LV left ventricle; *EF* ejection fraction; *ESV* end systolic volume; *EDV* end diastolic volume; *RV* right ventricle; *ACE* Angiotensin converting enzyme.

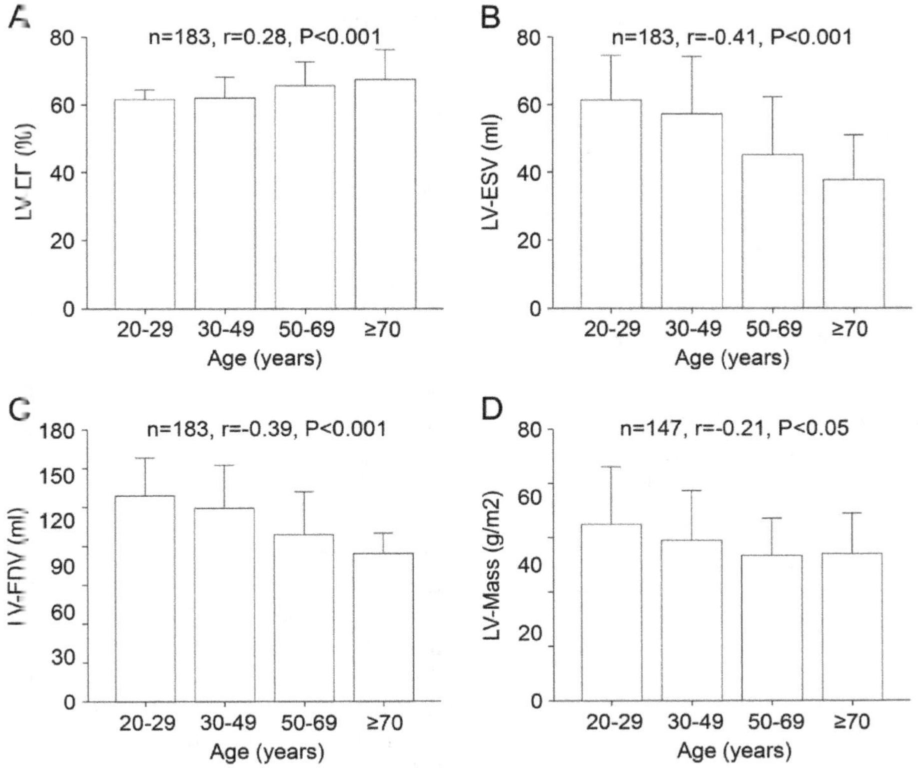

Figure 1 Age-dependent change of LV values by CMR. LV-EF (panel **A**) significantly increased over the four age categories whereas LV-ESV (panel **B**), LV-EDV (panel **C**), and LV myocardial mass (panel **D**) significantly decreased with the aging process.

This was paralleled by a significant increase of RV-EF (n=111, r=0.27, P<0.01) whereas RV-ESV (n=111, r=−0.41, P<0.001) and RV-EDV (n=111, r=−0.35, P<0.001) significantly decreased with increasing age (Figure 2).

The results in the different age groups are summarized in Table 2.

Discussion

The present CMR study documents that increasing age is associated with a significant decrease in LV and RV volumes but an increase in EF. Furthermore, LV myocardial mass significantly decreased over the four age groups. There is increasing awareness on the fact that changes in cardiac ventricular structure and function attributable to the aging process may play an important role in modulating the cardiovascular response to disease [7]. The knowledge of age-dependent normal structural and functional cardiac values is critical for identification of pathology and prediction of patient outcome. The rapid growth of the elderly population renders definition of normal values in advanced age even more important and may particularly help to reduce expensive and unnecessary follow-up examinations while there is a broad consensus on the decline in diastolic function with age. Controversial findings exist for age-related structural and functional cardiac values ranging from increase over no correlation to a decrease in LV-EF with advancing age [7,8,11,14], mainly obtained from echocardiographic studies. In fact, despite several limitations echocardiography has been the modality applied in most of these reports, reflecting the multi-purpose use of this widely available non-invasive tool. Comparable data as assessed from CMR are limited and particularly scarce for the RV. This is particularly important in view of the fact that in the past decade CMR has emerged as a new gold standard of non-invasive LV and RV assessment which is now increasingly available while the evaluation of mechanistic insights in metabolic and pathophysiological mechanisms remains a privilege of highly sophisticated CMR techniques such as tagging and spectroscopy [15].

Differences in myocyte loss on the one hand and trophic effects on the other hand may eventually shift the tip of the balance towards changes in EF in the aging process. The observed decline in ventricular dimensions seems to favourably counterbalance the decrease in LV muscle mass resulting in an increase in EF. This is supported by the observation that twisting and torsion of the left ventricle are more pronounced in the elderly population [16] and it may help explaining recent

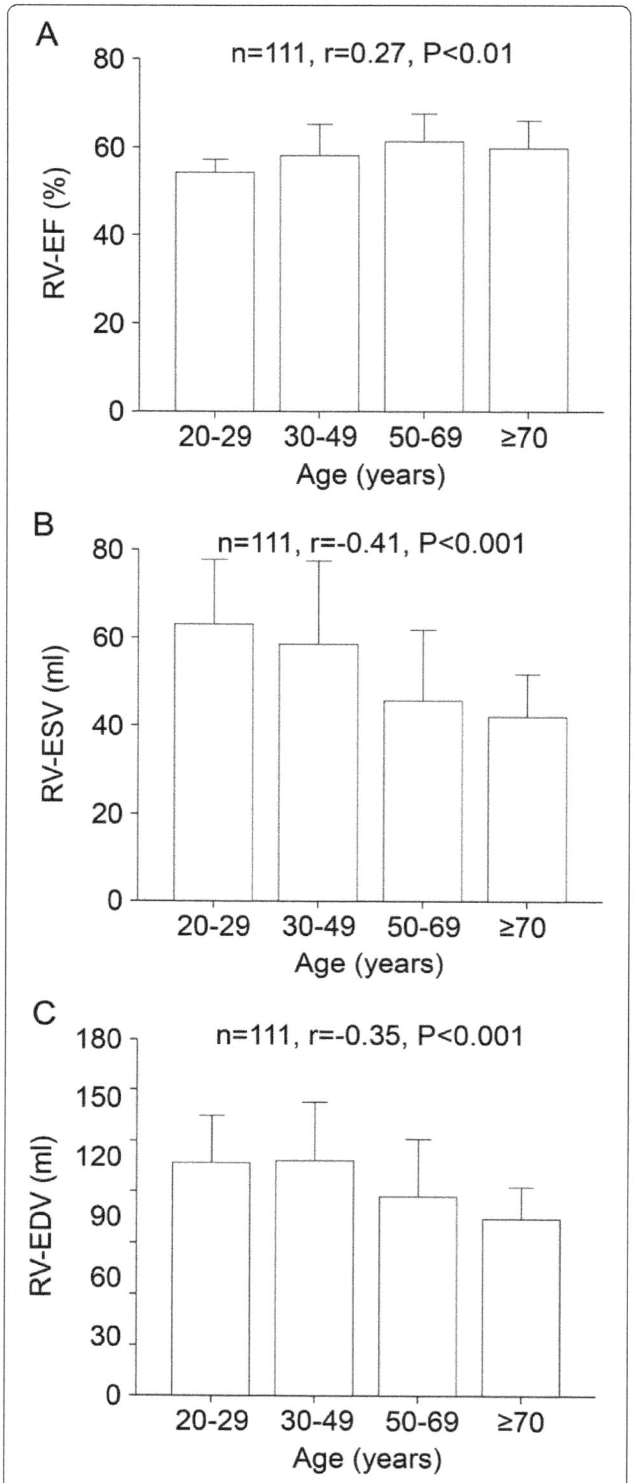

Figure 2 Age-dependent change of RV values in CMR. RV-EF (panel **A**) significantly increased over the four age categories whereas RV-ESV (panel **B**), and RV-EDV (panel **C**) significantly decreased with advancing age.

Table 2 LV and RV measurements in increasing age categories

	20-29 years	30-49 years	50-69 years	≥70 years	P-value
LV	(n = 17)	(n = 61)	(n = 86)	(n = 19)	
EF (%)	60.9±3.2	60.8±5.7	65.2±7.0	69.3±8.7	<0.001
ESV (ml)	63.2±15.2	59.0±17.1	45.1±16.0	35.2±10.4	<0.001
EDV (ml)	161.3±34.6	149.8±33.9	127.6±30.7	114.4±7.6	<0.001
Mass (g/m^2, n)	62.6±19.9 (16)	56.3±16.2 (52)	50.0±1[illegible].2 (63)	52.9±13.9 (16)	<0.05
RV	(n = 12)	(n = 43)	(n = 41)	(n = 15)	
EF (%)	54.1±3.1	57.6±6.8	60.9±6.4	60.2±6.3	<0.01
ESV (ml)	62.4±15.2	59.5±18.7	45.5±16.0	41.4±10.4	<0.001
EDV (ml)	135.0±28.5	139.4±34.7	115.3±31.4	103.6±19.4	<0.001

LV left ventricle; *EF* ejection fraction; *ESV* end systolic volume; *EDV* end diastolic volume; *RV* right ventricle.

observations describing that normal EF can be present despite impaired myocardial contractility [17]. While our results on a decrease in LV volume are in line with the majority of echocardiography and CMR studies, the findings with regard to LV mass seem more controversial. In some studies, LV mass was unchanged during aging [12] while in other studies an increase was found [14,18,19]. Interestingly, there was no association between age and LV mass in the Framingham study detectable by echocardiography [20], while findings were described in a recent CMR analysis of the Framingham study [21] showing a decrease over age. As the latter revealed LV mass as an important predictor of morbidity and mortality [18], a decrease in LV mass could also reflect a survival selection bias. Due to its cross-sectional design our study avoids such bias and provides data from a real live cohort. However, for adequate interpretation it is crucial to review the techniques used, as the results may not necessarily be interchangeable [22]. As mentioned above, most previous studies have assessed LV mass by M-mode echocardiography based on models which take into account LV wall thickness and short-axis dimensions neglecting the real LV shape. In addition, this method is dependent on operator skills. A recent study using latest advancements in echocardiography, i.e. real time 3-dimensional echocardiography, found the lowest values for LV mass and volumes in the eldest patients (seventh decade of life) largely in line with our results. This was further supported by other observations using CMR [23,24].

We acknowledge the following potential study limitations: First, in line with the data mentioned above we present a cross-sectional study of individuals at various ages, whereas patients would need to be followed in time to be more conclusive about age-related changes in cardiac parameters. Second, we did not verify our data with values obtained from another imaging modality and thus are not able to exclude potential modality bias. However, CMR is a well-accepted gold standard itself for such measurements [12]. Third, despite the fact that this is the largest study analysing structural and functional cardiac values in CMR a potential bias towards supernormals as well as a survival selection bias cannot be excluded with final certainty. Furthermore, the limited sample size within subgroups of age does not allow gender-specific analysis. Fourth, we did not standardize loading conditions which may potentially have affected our measurements. However, in healthy individuals the impact of variations in loading conditions appears limited within a broad range of physiologic conditions. In addition, measurements without active interaction by the observer may prevent distortion of the findings closely reflecting real life conditions. Finally, we did not correct the chamber volumes for body size although an association between an increase in body surface area and an increase in chamber dimensions has been reported. However, the aim of the present study was to evaluate the structural and functional changes of the ventricles. As the aging process is per se associated with a decrease in body size normalization of the volumes would have at least in part masked the changes in ventricular volumes observed with aging. This would render meaningful comparison with changes in EF difficult, as for the calculation of EF the normalization cancels out resulting in an uncorrected value [25,26].

Conclusions

In conclusion, the aging process has significant impact on ventricular EF, ESV and EDV in healthy CMR patients with normal functional and structural cardiac values. These findings underline the importance of using age adapted values as standard of reference in CMR studies.

Competing interests

The authors have no competing interests to declare.

Authors' contribution

MF, TAF and PAK were substantially involved in conceptual design of the study, statistical analysis of the data and drafting of the manuscript. CG, JS, BK, and BS were involved in critical review of data integrity, and gave their intellectual input concerning manuscript drafting. RM, CM, TAF and MF were substantially involved in acquisition of imaging data in daily clinical routine. Further, RM and CM gave substantial technical input regarding cardiac magnetic resonance imaging. FT, OG, and PAK critically reviewed the manuscript and gave important intellectual input. All authors have critically reviewed and approved the final version of the manuscript.

Acknowledgments

The study was supported by a grant from the Swiss National Science Foundation to PAK. Furthermore, we thank Ennio Mueller for his excellent technical support.

Author details

[1]Department of Radiology, Cardiac Imaging, University Hospital Zurich, Zurich, Switzerland. [2]Department of Cardiology, Cardiovascular Center, University Hospital Zurich, Zurich, Switzerland. [3]Zurich Center for Integrative Human Physiology (ZIHP), University of Zurich, Zurich, Switzerland.

References

1. White HD, Norris RM, Brown MA, Brandt PW, Whitlock RM, Wild CJ: **Left ventricular end-systolic volume as the major determinant of survival after recovery from myocardial infarction.** *Circulation* 1987, **76**(1):44–51.
2. Wong M, Johnson G, Shabetai R, Hughes V, Bhat G, Lopez B, Cohn JN: **Echocardiographic variables as prognostic indicators and therapeutic monitors in chronic congestive heart failure. Veterans Affairs cooperative studies V-HeFT I and II. V-HeFT VA Cooperative Studies Group.** *Circulation* 1993, **87**(6 Suppl):VI65–VI70.
3. Matter C, Mandinov L, Kaufmann P, Nagel E, Boesiger P, Hess OM: **Function of the residual myocardium after infarct and prognostic significance.** *Z Kardiol* 1997, **86**(9):684–690.
4. Wandt B, Bojo L, Hatle L, Wranne B: **Left ventricular contraction pattern changes with age in normal adults.** *J Am Soc Echocardiogr* 1998, **11**(9):857–863.
5. Harrison TR, Dixon K, Russell RO Jr, Bidwai PS, Coleman HN: **The Relation of Age to the Duration of Contraction, Ejection, and Relaxation of the Normal Human Heart.** *Am Heart J* 1964, **67:**189–199.
6. Kaku K, Takeuchi M, Otani K, Sugeng L, Nakai H, Haruki N, Yoshitani H, Watanabe N, Yoshida K, Otsuji Y, *et al*: **Age- and gender-dependency of left ventricular geometry assessed with real-time three-dimensional transthoracic echocardiography.** *J Am Soc Echocardiogr* 2011, **24**(5):541–547.
7. Ruan Q, Nagueh SF: **Effect of age on left ventricular systolic function in humans: a study of systolic isovolumic acceleration rate.** *Exp Physiol* 2005, **90**(4):527–534.
8. Pfisterer ME, Battler A, Zaret BL: **Range of normal values for left and right ventricular ejection fraction at rest and during exercise assessed by radionuclide angiocardiography.** *Eur Heart J* 1985, **6**(8):647–655.
9. Port S, Cobb FR, Coleman RE, Jones RH: **Effect of age on the response of the left ventricular ejection fraction to exercise.** *N Engl J Med* 1980, **303**(20):1133–1137.
10. Salmasi AM, Alimo A, Jepson E, Dancy M: **Age-associated changes in left ventricular diastolic function are related to increasing left ventricular mass.** *Am J Hypertens* 2003, **16**(6):473–477.
11. Gebhard C, Stähli BE, Gebhard CE RJ, Tanner FC: **Effect of age on left ventricular ejection fraction assessed by echocardiography.** *Cardiovasc Med* 2012, **15**(Suppl 21).
12. Nikitin NP, Loh PH, de Silva R, Witte KK, Lukaschuk EI, Parker A, Farnsworth TA, Alamgir FM, Clark AL, Cleland JG: **Left ventricular morphology, global and longitudinal function in normal older individuals: a cardiac magnetic resonance study.** *Int J Cardiol* 2006, **108**(1):76–83.
13. Plein S, Greenwood JP, Ridgway JP: *Cardiovascular MR Manual.* 1st edition. London: Springer; 2011.
14. Gerstenblith G, Frederiksen J, Yin FC, Fortuin NJ, Lakatta EG, Weisfeldt ML: **Echocardiographic assessment of a normal adult aging population.** *Circulation* 1977, **56**(2):273–278.
15. Hollingsworth KG, Blamire AM, Keavney BD, Macgowan GA: **Left ventricular torsion, energetics, and diastolic function in normal human aging.** *Am J Physiol Heart Circ Physiol* 2012, **302**(4):H885–892.
16. van Dalen BM, Soliman OI, Vletter WB, ten Cate FJ, Geleijnse ML: **Age-related changes in the biomechanics of left ventricular twist measured by speckle tracking echocardiography.** *Am J Physiol Heart Circ Physiol* 2008, **295**(4):H1705–1711.
17. Yu CM, Lin H, Yang H, Kong SL, Zhang Q, Lee SW: **Progression of systolic abnormalities in patients with "isolated" diastolic heart failure and diastolic dysfunction.** *Circulation* 2002, **105**(10):1195–1201.
18. Anversa P, Palackal T, Sonnenblick EH, Olivetti G, Meggs LG, Capasso JM: **Myocyte cell loss and myocyte cellular hyperplasia in the hypertrophied aging rat heart.** *Circ Res* 1990, **67**(4):871–885.
19. Shub C, Klein AL, Zachariah PK, Bailey KR, Tajik AJ: **Determination of left ventricular mass by echocardiography in a normal population: effect of age and sex in addition to body size.** *Mayo Clin Proc* 1994, **69**(3):205–211.

20. Dannenberg AL, Levy D, Garrison RJ: **Impact of age on echocardiographic left ventricular mass in a healthy population (the Framingham Study).** *Am J Cardiol* 1989, **64**(16):1066–1068.
21. Cheng S, Fernandes VR, Bluemke DA, McClelland RL, Kronmal RA, Lima JA: **Age-related left ventricular remodeling and associated risk for cardiovascular outcomes: the Multi-Ethnic Study of Atherosclerosis.** *Circ Cardiovasc Imaging* 2009, **2**(3):191–198.
22. Schepis T, Gaemperli O, Koepfli P, Valenta I, Strobel K, Brunner A, Leschka S, Desbiolles L, Husmann L, Alkadhi H, *et al*: **Comparison of 64-slice CT with gated SPECT for evaluation of left ventricular function.** *J Nucl Med* 2006, **47**(8):1288–1294.
23. Germans T, Gotte MJ, Nijveldt R, Spreeuwenberg MD, Beek AM, Bronzwaer JG, Visser CA, Paulus WJ, van Rossum AC: **Effects of aging on left atrioventricular coupling and left ventricular filling assessed using cardiac magnetic resonance imaging in healthy subjects.** *Am J Cardiol* 2007, **100**(1):122–127.
24. Sandstede J, Lipke C, Beer M, Hofmann S, Pabst T, Kenn W, Neubauer S, Hahn D: **Age- and gender-specific differences in left and right ventricular cardiac function and mass determined by cine magnetic resonance imaging.** *Eur Radiol* 2000, **10**(3):438–442.
25. Maceira AM, Prasad SK, Khan M, Pennell DJ: **Normalized left ventricular systolic and diastolic function by steady state free precession cardiovascular magnetic resonance.** *J Cardiovasc Magn Reson* 2006, **8**(3):417–426.
26. Maceira AM, Prasad SK, Khan M, Pennell DJ: **Reference right ventricular systolic and diastolic function normalized to age, gender and body surface area from steady-state free precession cardiovascular magnetic resonance.** *Eur Heart J* 2006, **27**(23):2879–2888.

Improved operator agreement and efficiency using the minimum area contour change method for delineation of hyperintense multiple sclerosis lesions on FLAIR MRI

David S Wack[1,2*], Michael G Dwyer[1], Niels Bergsland[1], Deepa Ramasamy[1], Carol Di Perri[3], Laura Ranza[3], Sara Hussein[1], Christopher Magnano[1], Kevin Seals[5] and Robert Zivadinov[1,4]

Abstract

Background: Activity of disease in patients with multiple sclerosis (MS) is monitored by detecting and delineating hyper-intense lesions on MRI scans. The Minimum Area Contour Change (MACC) algorithm has been created with two main goals: a) to improve inter-operator agreement on outlining regions of interest (ROIs) and b) to automatically propagate longitudinal ROIs from the baseline scan to a follow-up scan.

Methods: The MACC algorithm first identifies an outer bound for the solution path, forms a high number of iso-contour curves based on equally spaced contour values, and then selects the best contour value to outline the lesion. The MACC software was tested on a set of 17 FLAIR MRI images evaluated by a pair of human experts and a longitudinal dataset of 12 pairs of T2-weighted Fluid Attenuated Inversion Recovery (FLAIR) images that had lesion analysis ROIs drawn by a single expert operator.

Results: In the tests where two human experts evaluated the same MRI images, the MACC program demonstrated that it could markedly reduce inter-operator outline error. In the longitudinal part of the study, the MACC program created ROIs on follow-up scans that were in close agreement to the original expert's ROIs. Finally, in a post-hoc analysis of 424 follow-up scans 91% of propagated MACC were accepted by an expert and only 9% of the final accepted ROIS had to be created or edited by the expert.

Conclusion: When used with an expert operator's verification of automatically created ROIs, MACC can be used to improve inter- operator agreement and decrease analysis time, which should improve data collected and analyzed in multicenter clinical trials.

Keywords: Multiple sclerosis, Detection error, Outline error, Rater agreement, Operator agreement, Metric, Jaccard index, Similarity index, Kappa, Lesion, Assessment, Minimum area contour change

* Correspondence: dswack@buffalo.edu
[1]Buffalo Neuroimaging Analysis Center, Department of Neurology, School of Medicine and Biomedical Sciences, University at Buffalo, State University of New York at Buffalo, Buffalo, NY, USA
[2]Department of Nuclear Medicine, University at Buffalo, State University of New York at Buffalo, Buffalo, NY, USA
Full list of author information is available at the end of the article

Background

Large agreement differences often exist between operators drawing regions of interest (ROIs) of hyperintense lesions on Fluid Attenuated Inversion Recovery (FLAIR) MRI brain scans of patients with multiple sclerosis (MS) despite training and standards designed to minimize inter-operator variability [1-4]. These differences can be broken down into two categories: a) lesion outline disagreement and b) lesion detection disagreement. Differences in how operators outline a lesion account for the majority of difference (measured by volume) between operators. The size of this outline error (OE) between human experts increases with the level of lesion burden revealed in the patient's scan. Detection error (DE), the total area of ROIs chosen by one operator that do not match with another operator's ROIs, remains comparatively compensated with increasing lesion burden of the underlying scan. For MRI scans revealing high lesion burden, OE between raters' ROIs can be much greater than DE [5]. ROIs can be visually very similar, yet have large area differences. As an example, if a 10x10 pixel ROI increased by a half pixel in each direction, the new area would be 21% larger.

Operators often analyze a sequential set of scans that were collected over the course of months or years. Finding a lesion at a given location on a baseline scan is a good indication that a lesion can be found (detected) at the same location on a follow-up scan, though the size and shape (outline) may vary. For this reason, each image must be analyzed and have ROIs drawn for each time point. Despite the similarities between the placements of ROIs between scans of the same individual, there is not a significant time saving in a subsequent lesion analysis compared to the baseline.

A commonly used tool for outlining lesions in MS is the Java Image Manipulation (JIM) software package (version 4.0, Xynapse System, Leichester, UK), which allows an operator to delineate a lesion by clicking near the edge of the lesion. JIM calculates a contour value by choosing the image intensity value associated with the steepest gradient value in a small surrounding neighborhood of the cursor. Using the determined contour value, the program outlines the lesion with an iso-contour curve. This application works well and is an indication that a large percentage of lesion delineations can be represented by a single contour value. There have been many other applications designed to aid operator efficiency and precision in ROI creation such as live wire, active contours, and snakes [6-8]. Lesion growth methods [9,10] have been previously applied to images to delineate MS lesions in order to reduce inter-rater variability. Furthermore, curve evolution has been applied post lesion detection [11]. Re-contouring methods have been applied to auto-propagate an ROI from one phase of a 4D CT image to another [12,13]. The intended application of these tools is to increase operator productivity and reduce inter-operator variability.

Against this background, the Minimum Area Contour Change (MACC) algorithm has been created with two main goals: a) to improve inter-operator agreement on outlining ROIs and b) to automatically propagate longitudinal ROIs from a baseline scan to a follow-up scan (i.e. by "propagate" we mean MACC is run using the baseline ROI set and a follow-up image, to produce ROIs for the follow-up image that have been re-contoured to account for changes in a lesion's size and shape). For each lesion that has a previously drawn ROI, the MACC software selects a unique/best contour value, and uses the iso-contour curve as the lesion outline. The use of MACC virtually assures an improvement in inter-operator agreement because MACC will settle on a unique ROI from a large range of input ROIs. What is less clear is whether the MACC ROIs are an acceptable replacement for the original ROIs. Therefore, in the present study we test whether MACC meets the following four requirements:

1) Differences between ROIs drawn by MACC and the operators' original ROIs should be similar to (or smaller than) the differences found between two operators;
2) ROIs outlined by two operators and reanalyzed by MACC should be significantly closer to each other than the comparison between the operators' original hand-drawn ROIs;
3) If MACC is used to propagate (which includes re-contouring) ROIs to a follow-up image (from the ROIs of the previous scan), differences between ROIs drawn by MACC and the operator's hand-drawn ROIs (of the current scan) should be similar to differences found between two operators;
4) MACC should process a set of ROIs fast enough to be routinely used by an operator.

Methods

MACC algorithm

The MACC algorithm uses an image and an input set of ROIs to create an output set of ROIs, in the same locations as the input ROIs, but outlined according to the rules of the algorithm. For a given ROI (each individual 2d outline of a single lesion, from a single rater), Figure 1, the algorithm restricts the analysis to a rectangular region around the ROI, Figure 2. Then a large set of iso-contours is created for the restricted image, Figure 3. The program searches for the best contour to be the new outline of the lesion, and applies restrictions to candidate contours. For instance, a contour curve cannot be chosen as the final ROI if it: 1) meets the edge of the bounding box, 2) increases or decreases the ROI size from the original by more than a user specified ratio, or 3) does not intersect

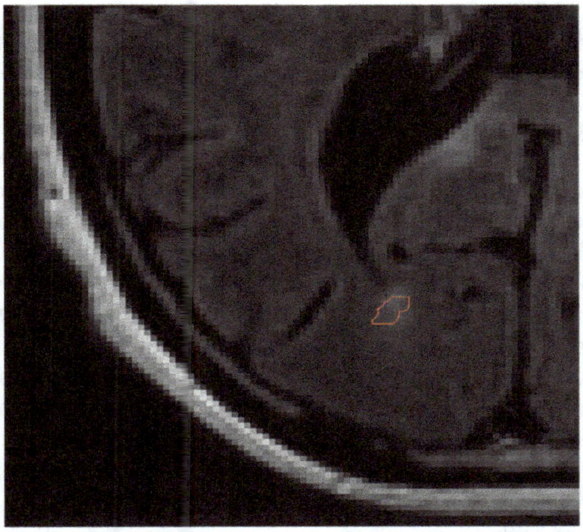

Figure 1 Flair MRI, with a hand-drawn ROI of a lesion shown in lower left.

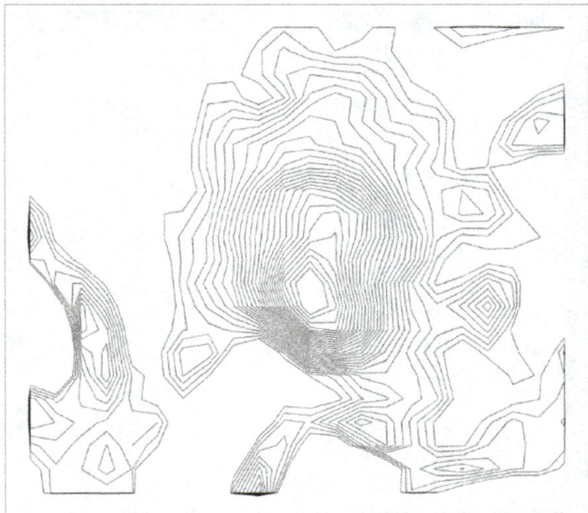

Figure 3 Iso-contour curves at 50 evenly spaced values. MACC searches for a pair of neighboring contours that are close together.

with the original ROI. The square root of the total area for all compliant contours at a given contour level, SqrtArea (L_n), is calculated where L_n represents the nth evenly spaced level value (starting from low to high). The level, L_n, that minimizes (SqrtArea(L_n)–SqrtArea(L_{n+1})) is chosen by the program, Figure 4, and the compliant contours at this level are used as the output "MACC" ROI, Figure 5. Using the square root of the contours' areas was motivated by the desire to find the minimum overall "radial" distance between neighboring ROIs, as would be the case if the set of conforming ROIs were concentric circles. A center could use another metric in place of the radial metric we present provided adequate testing was performed to ensure that it conforms well to how their raters contour lesions. The value should be unique and be efficiently calculated for contours of any shape.

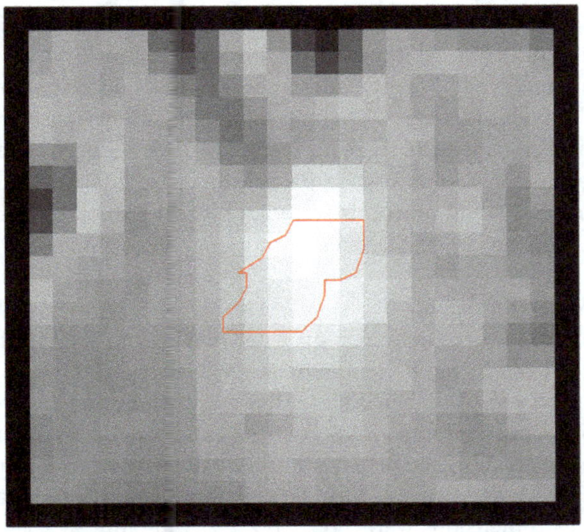

Figure 2 Close-up view of the hand-drawn ROI from Figure 1; the entire image displayed represents the rectangular region to bound the MACC ROI.

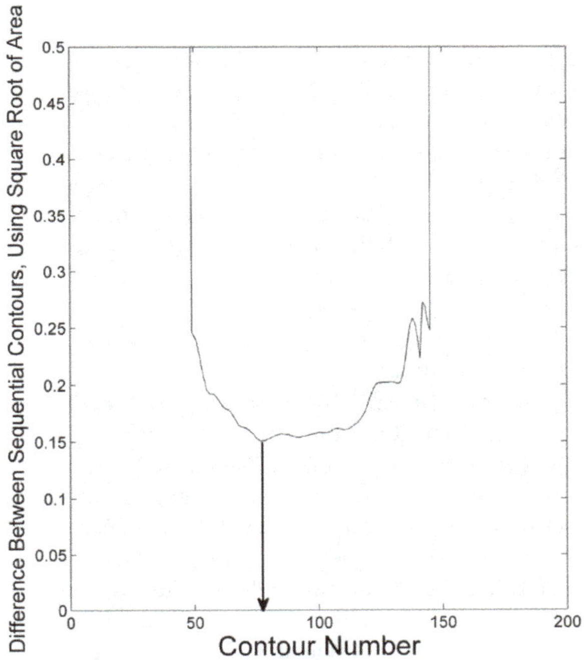

Figure 4 Graph of contour index number (from low to high) and SqrtArea(L_n)-SqrtArea(L_{n+1}). The arrow passes through the minimum of the graph, and points to the value of n that is selected by the algorithm.

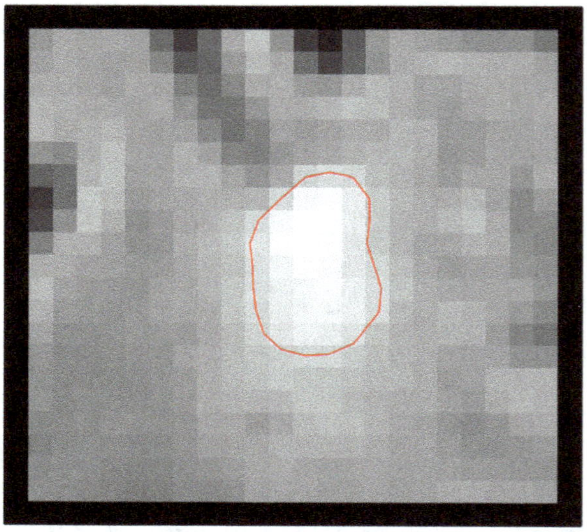

Figure 5 Close-up view of the MACC ROI for lesion displayed in Figures 1 and 2.

Around a hyper-intense lesion, higher valued contours will be nested within lower valued contours. For a given value, there may be more than one contour, which could be due to high intensity "peaks" found within a lesion. To have multiple ROIs formed from one input ROI is acceptable by the algorithm. Conversely, multiple input ROIs may lead to the same MACC ROI, which would typically fully contain those input ROIs.

Since MACC is dependent on the topography of the image around a lesion, it is possible for it to fail in finding any conforming ROIs. In this case, for purposes of evaluating calculations, the MACC program does not return an ROI. However, our implementation has two other "Failed" ROI modes: one, which returns the original ROI; the other returns a rectangular ROI roughly double the size of the original ROI, which enables quick identification by the operator.

Algorithm parameters

The area of a MACC ROI was restricted to being greater than 1/3 and less than three times the input ROI. This and selecting how to handle a "Failed" ROI are the only external "tuning" parameters. Remaining parameters are seldom changed and are internal. The MACC algorithm was run with an ROI bounding window that was twice the width and height of the smallest rectangle containing the ROI (with a minimum of 4 mm and maximum of 10 mm padding of the original ROI in any direction). The MACC program selected the best contour curve originating from 250 equally spaced contour values between the median and maximum pixel intensity values within the bounding rectangle.

Datasets

Human operators

To assess the amount by which MACC can improve agreement between operators (requirement 2), a pair of raters (both neurologists) was used who had spent approximately three months in our lab and had over 3 years' experience in lesion analyses at the time they performed their analyses. No effort was made to optimize inter-rater reliability between the pair of raters, and they should be considered independent experts. The ROIs from the pair of raters were also used in testing whether MACC ROIs were in close agreement with the original raters' ROIs (requirement 1). To assess whether MACC produces ROIs that are in close agreement with the original raters' ROIs on both the baseline and follow-up scans (requirements 1 and 3), a single rater was used who has several years of experience in our imaging laboratory. All raters were physicians with several years of experience working with MS scans. ROIs were drawn using JIM software and created 2D outlines of lesions on each scan slice.

Participants

Two separate datasets were used in testing the algorithm. In Dataset 1, a set of 17 FLAIR MRI images fulfilling the criteria for clinically definite MS were used as in Di Perri et al. [14] and Wack et al. [5], which allowed comparison between a pair of human operators' ROIs with and without the use of MACC (requirements 1 and 2). In Dataset 2, a set of 12 baseline and matching 12 month follow-up FLAIR MRI scans of relapsing-remitting MS patients were used to assess the agreement between MACC ROIs and the original raters' ROIs (requirements 1 and 3). To avoid any potential bias in data analysis, we placed images in a halfway space during co-registration. Briefly, we used FSL's FLIRT linear registration tool (http://www.fmrib.ox.ac.uk/) [15,16] to estimate a forward transform from baseline to follow-up, and a backward transform from follow-up to baseline. We then took the halfway transforms for each, and used these to re-sample their respective images into a common space. Participants gave informed consent and study protocols were approved by the University at Buffalo's Health Sciences Institutional Review Board.

Scanning protocol

All scans were acquired on a GE 3 T Signa Excite HD 12.0 Twin Speed 8-channel scanner (General Electric, GE, Milwaukee, WI). The scanner has a maximum slew rate of 150 T/m/s and maximum gradient amplitude of 50 mT/m in each orthogonal plane. A multi-channel Head and Neck (HDNV) coil was used for all sequence acquisitions. Scan voxel dimensions were $.86 \times .86 \times 2.92$ mm and $.94 \times .94 \times 3.0$ mm for the first and second sets of scans, respectively. Scans were collected in a clinical setting with a standardized protocol including double-echo proton density (PDw) and T2-weighted (T2w) spin echo (SE), a FLAIR, and T1-weighted (T1w) SE pre- and post-contrast injection, all prescribed axial with subcallosal alignment. Acquisition parameters were defined as follows: for the PD-T2 repetition time (TR) = 3000 ms, first/second Echo time (TE) = 12/95 ms, FA = 90°, echo train length (ETL) = 14, Bandwidth (BW) = 20.83 Hz/pix, field of view (FOV) = 240 mm, acquisition matrix = 256 × 256, phase field of view (pFOV) = 0.75 for an in plane resolution of 0.94 × 0.94 mm, slice thickness = 3 mm for 46 slices, NEX = 1 for an acquisition time of 4:31 min; for the FLAIR TR = 8500 ms, TE = 120 ms, FA = 90°, BW = 27.78 Hz/pix, FOV = 240 mm for the first dataset and FOV = 220 mm for the second one, acquisition matrix = 256 × 256, pFOV = 0.75 for an in plane resolution of respectively 0.94 × 0.94 mm and 0.83 × 0.83, slice thickness respectively of 3 mm and 2.92, for 46 slices, NEX = 1 for an acquisition time of 4:16 min; for the T1w SE pre- and post-contrast injection TR = 550 ms, TE = 12 ms, FA = 60°, FOV = 240 mm, acquisition matrix = 256 × 256, pFOV = 0.75 for an in plane resolution of 0.94 × 0.94 mm, slice thickness = 3 mm for 46 slices, NEX = 1 for an acquisition time of 3:47 min.

Assessment measures

In addition to the Similarity Index (SI) we use the measures of Detection Error (DE) and Outline Error Rate (OER) [5], to compare ROIs. We define a connected region as a single region (blob) contained in the union of raters' ROIs. We label each connected region, as CR1, CR2, or CR12 based on whether it is composed of ROIs solely from rater 1, rater 2, or from both raters 1 and 2, respectively. For a given connected region, *cr*, we denote the ROIs created by rater 1 contained within *cr* as R1(cr). Similarly, R2(*cr*) represents the ROIs created by rater 2 within *cr*, and hence $R1(cr) \cup R2(cr) = cr$. DE is the total area of ROIs of lesions that were marked by either, but only one, of the raters, and is sensitive to whether raters mark the same hyper-intense regions as a lesion:

$$DE = \sum_{cr \in CR1 \text{ or } CR2} |cr|,$$

where $|cr|$ represents the area of the connected region, *cr*; and $cr \in CR1$ *or* $CR2$ represents the set of connected regions that can be labeled as either CR1 or CR2.

OE is the difference in area between the union and intersection of ROIs of lesions that were marked by both raters, and is sensitive to how well two raters agree in determining and marking the edge of a lesion:

$$OE = \sum_{cr \in CR12} (|cr| - |R1(cr) \cap R2(cr)|)$$

where $|R1(cr) \cap R2(cr)|$ represent the area of the intersection of rater 1 and rater 2's ROIs within *cr*, respectively.

We calculate the mean total area (MTA) of the two raters ROIs as: MTA = (1/2)(|R1| + |R2|), where |R1| and |R2| represent the total area of rater 1 and rater 2's ROIs, respectively.

Similarity Index (SI) is commonly defined as 2 times the area of the intersection of the raters' ROIs, divided by sum of the area of the raters ROIs [17]. Defining $OER = \frac{OE}{MTA}$, SI is related to DE, OER, and MTA as (see appendix):

$$SI(R1, R2) = 1 - \left(\frac{1}{2}\right) OER - \left(\frac{1}{2}\right) \frac{DE}{MTA}$$

We expect OER to be very sensitive to the changes in ROIs in the presented experiments because MACC attempts to improve agreement between ROI sets through the re-contouring (outlining) of ROIs. We do not expect much change in DE, since MACC attempts to create an ROI at each location given by the input ROI. Hence, given SI's dependence on both DE and OER, we expect SI to be less sensitive than OER to measuring the changes in ROIs made by MACC.

We will also plot the histogram of $\frac{(|R2(cr)| - |R1(cr)|)}{|cr|}$ for all connected regions that can be labeled as CR12 regions, which we term the Outline Error Distribution (OED) graph. If MACC draws the majority of ROIs as either larger or smaller than the original set of ROIs, the OED graph will be biased to one side of 0. If operators draw most ROIs identically, there will be a large peak at 0.

Software assessment

We use r_1 and r_2 to denote the two raters used on Dataset 1, and r to denote the single rater used on Dataset 2. We use im to denote an image from Dataset 1 (single time point, with 17 participants), and im_b, and im_f to denote the baseline and follow-up images from Dataset 2. The ROIs created by rater r on the baseline image (im_b) from Dataset 2 (with 12 participants) are denoted as ROI(r, im_b). ROIs created by MACC on the follow-up image (im_f) are denoted as MACC(ROI(r, im_b), im_f). Other combinations will follow this same convention. We evaluate our software based on four assessments that correspond to our four requirements.

1) MACC ROIs are acceptable replacements for the original ROIs:
   Requirement: Differences between ROIs drawn by MACC and the operators' original ROIs should be similar to (or smaller than) the differences found between two operators.
   Assessment: Measure the agreement using DE, OER, and SI for all three raters between their original ROI and the MACC ROI created on the same image. That is, using Dataset 1 compare ROI(r_1, im) vs. MACC(ROI(r_1, im), im), and ROI(r_2, im) vs. MACC (ROI(r_2, im), im). With Dataset 2 compare the

agreement between: ROI(r, im_b) vs. MACC(ROI (r, im_b), im_b). All comparisons using MACC will then be compared with the agreement seen between two expert raters without MACC: ROI(r_1, im) vs. ROI(r_2, im).We will show the OED graph for the comparisons and inspect for signs of asymmetry or bias.

2) MACC improves inter-rater agreement:
Requirement: ROIs outlined by two operators and reanalyzed by MACC should be significantly closer to each other than the comparison between the operator's original hand-drawn ROIs.
Assessment: Using Dataset 1, measure the agreement using DE, OER, and SI between MACC(ROI(r_1, im), im) and MACC(ROI(r_2, im), im), and compare with the agreement seen between the two expert raters without MACC: ROI(r_1, im) vs ROI(r_2, im). Create, inspect, and compare the outline error distribution graph for both agreement comparisons.

3) MACC can propagate ROIs to follow-up images:
Requirement: If MACC is used to create ROIs for a follow-up image (from the ROIs of the previous scan), differences between ROIs re-contoured by MACC (on the follow-up image) and the operator's hand-drawn ROIs (on the follow-up image) should be similar to differences found between the two operators.
Assessment: Using Dataset 2, measure the agreement using DE, OER, and SI between ROI (r, im_f) and MACC(ROI(r, im_b), im_f). Additionally, measure the agreement between MACC(ROI (r, im_f), im_f) and MACC(ROI(r, im_b), im_f).

4) MACC executes quickly:
Requirement: MACC should process a set of ROIs fast enough to be routinely used by an operator.
Assessment: Measure the mean time for MACC to process the ROIs in assessment 3.

Post-hoc analysis

We examined the ROI files from 424 follow-up FLAIR scans of patients with MS, where the original follow-up ROI file was created by MACC, and subsequently edited by an expert. We then determined the percentage of ROIs that MACC produced that were found acceptable without adjustment, and the percentage of the final number of ROIs that were either edited or created by the expert.

Results

Assessment 1: MACC ROIs are acceptable replacements for the original ROIs

For Dataset 1, 1710 ROIs were drawn by either rater from 17 scans with mean LV of 15,084 mm^3. Values for DE, OER, and SI for the two raters' original ROIs and the corresponding MACC ROIs from Dataset 1 (Rows 2 and 3 of Table 1) were better than those found between two raters without MACC (Row 1, Table 1). Mean lesion volumes (LVs) measured from the rater and MACC processed ROIs were 8443 mm^3 and 7817 mm^3, respectively, for Dataset 2. ROIs from this dataset using the single rater were also processed with MACC and compared—using DE, OER, and SI—to the originals, see Row 1, Table 2. In total 1135 2D ROIs were evaluated from 12 scans. The program failed in creating a MACC contour for two ROIs that were both smaller than 10 mm^2 in size. The average DE, OER, and SI values between the original and MACC ROIs were in each case better than the corresponding values found in the comparison between the two raters (Row 1, Table 1). The distribution of sizes between ROIs drawn by the operator and the MACC program were evenly distributed as shown by the OED graph, Figure 6; coefficient of variation (COV) of MTA between the original and MACC ROIs was COV = .10. The Pearson correlation of the individual ROI areas of the original and MACC programs = .99 ($p << .0001$).

Assessment 2: MACC improves inter-rater agreement

Using Dataset 1, ROIs from two raters were processed through MACC together with the original image (same for both raters), on which the ROIs were created. 579 ROIs had a detection error with the other operator. The median ROI size having a detection error was 12 mm^2. DE, OER, and SI for both pre- and post-MACC processing are reported in Table 1. While DE remained roughly the same, both OER and SI, measured between the two raters ROIs (Row 4 vs. Row1, Table 1), improved for *all* 17 ROI sets after MACC processing. OER was approximately cut in half, with min/mean/max decreases of .05/.19/.35, ($p < .0001$, paired t-test). SI increased on average 12.5%, with min/mean/max increases of .01/.08/.16, ($p < .0001$, paired t-test).

The OED graph between the operators' original ROIs and the MACC ROIs is shown in Figure 7. MACC has over

Table 1 Cross-sectional Data, Dataset 1

ROI sets	Detection error (mm^2)	Outline error rate	Similarity index
ROI(r_1, im) v. ROI(r_2, im)	747	.41	.64
ROI(r_1, im) v. MACC(ROI(r_1, im), im)	1	.40	.80
ROI(r_2, im) v. MACC(ROI(r_2, im), im)	1	.39	.80
MACC(ROI(r_1, im), im) v. MACC(ROI(r_2, im), im)	714	.21	.72

Table 2 Longitudinal Data, Dataset 2

ROI sets	Detection error (mm^2)	Outline error rate	Similarity index
MACC(ROI(r, im_b), im_b) v. ROI(r, im_b)	~0 (.24)	.37	.82
MACC(ROI(r, im_b), im_f) v. ROI(r, im_f)	473	.41	.63
MACC(ROI(r, im_b), im_f) v. MACC(ROI(r, im_f), im_f)	450	.18	.74

six times the number of ROIs between raters with near zero differences, and has fewer ROIs with size mismatches except for extreme ROI size differences, where MACC and the original ROIs are roughly evenly distributed.

Assessment 3: MACC can propagate ROIs to follow-up images

An example of MACC used for lesion propagation is given in Figure 8. Mean LV as measured by the unprocessed raters' ROIs for the follow-up scans in Dataset 2 was 5822 mm^3. Mean values for DE, OER and SI between MACC(ROI(r, im_b), im_f) and ROI(r, im_f) are also given in Table 2. The average OER was .41 (Row 2, Table 2) and was the same as between two raters (Row 1, Table 1). Average DE was better (37% lower) than between two raters, however, SI was similar, .63 vs. .64.

When MACC ROIs originating from the baseline image but processed with the follow-up image were compared to MACC processed ROIs created from the rater's original ROIs from follow-up image, SI improved for *all* 12 comparisons (Row 3, Table 2), compared to using the original rater ROIs from the follow-up scan ($p < .0001$, paired t-test). That is SI was better between MACC(ROI(r, im_b), im_f) and MACC(ROI(r, im_f), im_f) than between MACC(ROI(r, im_b), im_f) and ROI(r, im_f). The min/mean/max improvement of SI were 05/.11/.26, respectively. Likewise, OER improved for *all* scans with min/mean/max decreases of .08/.23/.41 ($p < .0001$, paired t-test).

Assessment 4: MACC executes quickly

Average running time for the MACC software on the 34 trials performed in Assessment 3 was 23.5 seconds. For this calculation the program did not make use of parallelization, and was performed on a Dell (Round Rock, TX) R610 server.

Assessment post-hoc: MACC propagated ROIs are predominately acceptable

For an illustration of MACCs real-world utility, an analysis was performed of ROIs drawn on 424 follow-up FLAIR MRI scans of patients with MS where MACC was used to create initial sets of ROIs that were subsequently edited so every ROI was compliant with our center's standards. In total, the MACC program generated 56,656 ROIs, of which 91% needed no modification by the trained operator to meet our center's standards.

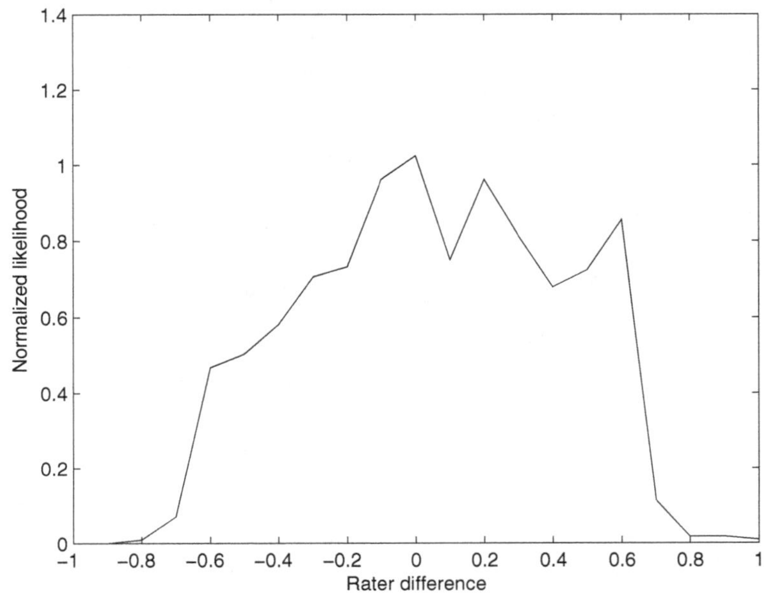

Figure 6 The Outline Error Distribution graph comparing ROI(r, im_b) and MACC (ROI(r, im_b), im_b). Negative abscissa values indicate the original ROIs are larger than the MACC ROIs, and positive values indicate the opposite.

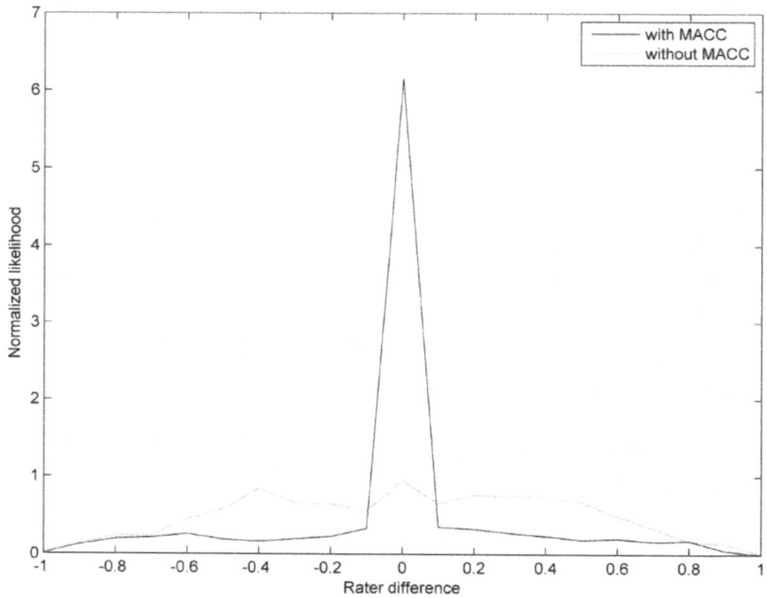

Figure 7 The graph with the sharp peak is the Outline Error Distribution (OED) graph of MACC (ROI(r_1, im), im) and MACC (ROI(r_2, im), im), and indicates that most compared ROIs have near zero area disagreement. The flatter graph is the Outline Error OED graph of ROI (r_1, im) and ROI(r_2, im), and indicates a broad range of area disagreement between corresponding ROIs. Negative abscissa values indicate that operator 1's ROIs are larger than operator 2's ROIs, and positive values indicate the opposite.

The final edited set consisted of 56,615 ROIs, of which only 9% were drawn by the operator. The plan for this analysis was made after the final ROI sets were created, and hence the operator was not biased to accept MACC ROIs, nor was the operator acting under time constraints.

Discussion

Incorporating MACC in the analysis of MS lesions not only achieves the more important goal of improving inter-operator agreement; but can also provide a significant time savings for the neuroimager. The above assessments of MACC established that: 1) MACC-created ROI's can be used in place of ROIs drawn by an expert operator; 2) inter-operator agreement between MACC-created ROIs is improved compared to the original ROIs; 3) significant time savings can be achieved for the lesion analysis of follow up scans; 4) MACC can be routinely used by any MS MRI reading center since the computational burden is low. Our post-hoc analysis on 424 follow-up scans showed that the vast majority of MACC propagated ROIs (91%) need no further expert adjustment.

MACC ROIs are acceptable replacements for the original ROIs

ROIs that have been created by MACC are in close agreement with ROIs that were used as input. The comparison measures between the rater-drawn ROIs and the output MACC ROIs, when the rater ROIs are used as input, were better for all three raters (Rows 2 and 3, Table 1; Row 1, Table 2), than between the two expert raters' original ROIs (Row 1, Table 1). DE in these comparisons is the total size of the rater-drawn ROIs for which MACC failed to produce an ROI, and is near zero. Given the dependence SI has on OER and DE, SI = 1-1/2*OER–½* DE/MTA, the high values for SI are largely attributable to the low DE.

A crucial point is that for MACC ROIs to be useful as a replacement for the original ROIs, the differences in ROIs (un-processed and MACC-processed ROIs) should be less than the expected difference between (un-processed) ROIs drawn by two experts. This is confirmed by OER being slightly higher (worse) for the two expert raters. Furthermore, the OED graph between the rater-drawn ROIs and the MACC ROIs is roughly symmetric and does not reveal an obvious bias (Figure 6). This demonstrates that MACC does not favor the creation of ROIs that are in general either larger or smaller than the expert rater's ROIs used as input. We conclude that MACC ROIs are an acceptable replacement for the operators' ROIs.

MACC improves inter-operator agreement

The use of MACC improves inter-operator agreement when applied to the ROIs from two different raters on the same scans (Assessment 2). MACC in this assessment reduced average OER from .41 to .21 ($p < .0001$, paired t-test), resulting in the average SI value increasing from .64 to .72, ($p < .0001$, paired t-test). MACC improved operator agreement for all 17 ROI sets in the assessment. If raters already

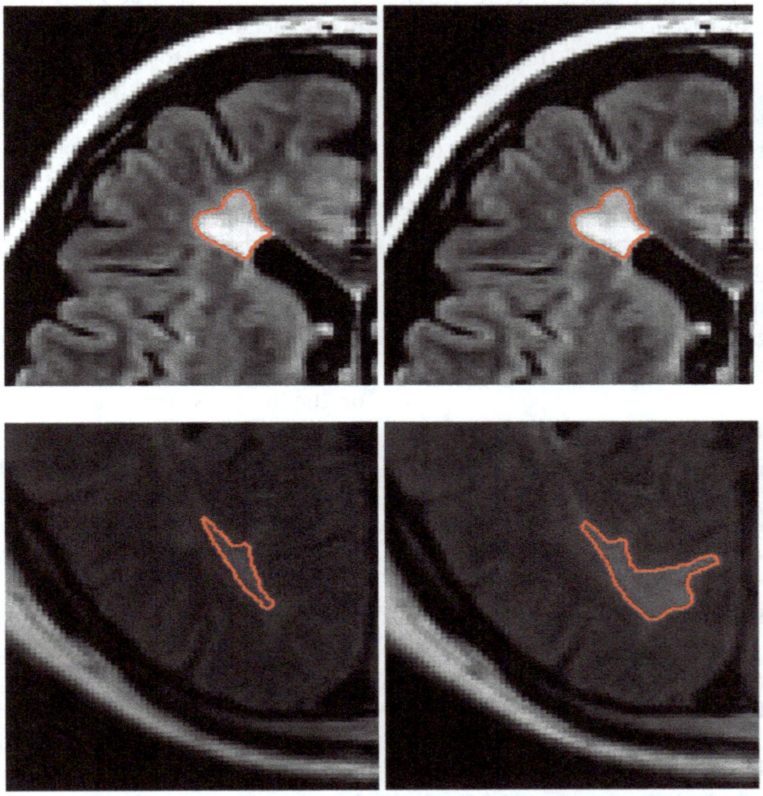

Figure 8 The left images are from a FLAIR MRI baseline scan of a patient with MS, and the right images are the matching planes at 3 month follow-up. MACC was used to propagate ROIs drawn of the lesions on the baseline scan to automatically create the ROIs on the follow-up scan. Since MACC creates the lesion ROIs based on the underlying image topography (in this case the follow-up scan), the automatically drawn follow-up ROIs accurately reflect both the changes in the size and shape of the lesion.

had perfect agreement, then MACC obviously would not be able to provide any improvement. However, we note that the closer the ROIs of two raters are to each other, the higher the likelihood that MACC will settle on the identical ROI (note the spike of 0 disagreements in Figure 7 after using MACC). Therefore, we consider it a strength of our study that we did not make an attempt to calibrate the raters prior to the study, and is an indication that MACC could likely be utilized effectively in multi-center studies to reduce rater variability.

MACC can propagate ROIs to follow-up images

Rater-drawn ROIs on the follow-up image are in close agreement with MACC ROIs created from the baseline ROIs together with the follow up image as input, MACC (ROI(r, im_b), im_f). That is, the baseline ROIs are re-contoured to account for the changes in the size and shape of the lesions seen on the follow-up image. DE was roughly half that observed between the two independent raters, while OER was the same (.41). The lower value for DE reflects the advantage a single rater has in agreeing on the identification of lesions on baseline and follow-up scans compared to two independent raters identifying the same region as a lesion on the same scan. We believe the most relevant value for this comparison is OER, which indicated an equal performance.

Significantly closer agreement is seen between MACC (ROI(r, im_b), im_f) and MACC(ROI(r, im_f), im_f) rather than ROI(r, im_f). The OER value for this new comparison (Row 3, Table 2) is lower (.18) and results in the higher SI value of .74 because DE remains essentially unchanged. To put the low value of OER = .18 into perspective, if DE equaled zero then SI would equal .91.

That DE is lower (better) for the follow-up image using one-rater than between the two-raters on a single image is not a relevant comparison. DE for the follow-up image mainly represents the area of new or disappearing lesions and is driven by pathology, whereas DE between the two raters represents their disagreement on which regions to mark as lesion. The important point about DE for the longitudinal study is that after editing the follow-up image, DE should be near zero. In fact, DE can be made to equal 0 by only adding or deleting ROIs (i.e., without having to change the shapes of any MACC propagated ROIs). To have DE equal zero after editing, is only to say that the same rater would choose all of the same regions to mark as lesion whether starting from propagated MACC ROIs, or starting from scratch. In practice, of course, operators should add, delete, and modify ROIs until they are 100% satisfied. Our argument above is to indicate that propagated MACC ROIs provide a good starting point for doing so. MACC was designed to be a simple and effective tool that improves rater agreement through the improvement of OE and the propagation of lesions. MACC does not delineate new lesions, nor does it automatically remove the ROIs of those that have disappeared. This aspect is left entirely to the expert human rater, or could be addressed with other software designed to improve DE.

MACC executes quickly

The improved inter-rater reproducibility should be worth MACC's short execution time, which averaged less than 24 seconds, and time needed to inspect the final ROIs. Our post-hoc analysis on a high number of scans indicates that the vast majorities of MACC ROIs are of use to an expert, and only a small percentage of ROIs needed to be created or edited for the final analysis, hence providing a time savings.

Choice of MACC parameters

An advantage of MACC is that it has few "tuning" parameters, and in fact only two settings are typically used, and *these will only affect a small percentage of ROIs*. The first parameter *only bounds* the size of an output ROI based on the size of the input ROI. In the presented assessments, MACC ROIs were constrained to be at least 1/3 and less than three times the input ROI. These values were chosen prior to testing as reasonable bounds that would handle the vast majority of lesions. The second parameter determines the output ROI if MACC does not find a solution otherwise. In these instances, MACC is designed to "fail" in one of three modes by returning: no ROI, the original ROI, or an easily identifiable rectangular ROI. This study chose to have MACC "fail" by producing no ROI, to enable some study calculations. The major precondition for MACC to be used to propagate ROIs between longitudinal scans is that the scans must be aligned with each other.

For an analysis center to improve inter-operator reproducibility, which is a concern in large studies requiring multiple operators, we recommend using MACC as a final pass after operators have created their ROIs. In this case, we suggest that MACC be run so the area of the output ROI is at least within the bounds of 1/2 and two times the original; if MACC fails to find a solution, the original ROI should be returned. The MACC ROIs should be inspected by the operator to ensure conformance with the center's standards, but used in this way very few ROIs should require any modifications. If MACC is used to propagate ROIs to a follow-up scan we recommend that MACC in this case be run in the failure mode that produces rectangular ROIs to mark locations where the software was unable to find a proper MACC ROI. Afterwards, an operator can quickly identify, examine, and fix the rectangular ROI. Locations where a lesion disappeared will often be locations where MACC is unable to produce a conforming ROI and will be marked with a rectangle.

An imaging center could use another metric in place of the radial metric we presented, provided adequate testing was performed to ensure that it conforms well to how their raters contour lesions. We choose this "radial" metric for its simplicity. The contour curves are evenly spaced based on intensity values, but are physically closer on the image as the image gradient increases. Varying the parameters for MACC will have only small effects, which we believe is desirable. The main purpose in *bounding* the extent to which a lesion can grow or shrink is to provide an easy way to avoid consideration of other strong image gradients such as the outline of the brain, or a small single spot of the lesion that has very high intensity. We did not try to optimize parameters such as the parameter limiting the extent to which the lesion can grow or shrink. That is, the results that we present represent what one could reasonably expect by implementing the MACC method themselves; the results are not from specialized modification of tuning parameters for our particular set of data. An investigator implementing the MACC method may want to test other bounds, perhaps including additional minimum or maximum sizes, etc.

Comparison automated lesion segmentation algorithms

We classify MACC as a lesion "propagation" tool, *not* an automated lesion segmentation algorithms (ALSAs) [18], and in this capacity it is only useful for determining ROIs for follow-up images in a longitudinal study. In contrast ALSAs are usually but not always tested on single time point images [19]. ALSAs, in essence, attempt to solve a harder problem: detect and outline lesions, without knowledge of where previous lesions were marked for that patient. But, if one considers a longitudinal study with four time points, then on ¾ of the scans traditional ALSAs are not using the very valuable information of how previous scans were marked. Region growing (RG) and fuzzy connectivity (FC) methods [20-22] have perhaps the closest similarity to MACC software, in that they can start with a selection of lesion and non-lesion voxels. The resulting segmentation of a lesion using FC or RG will be the collection of voxels that best optimizes the algorithms selection criteria. As with ALSAs methods, these have been evaluated in terms of SI values or calculation of total lesion volume, on datasets from the individual researcher's labs. This makes comparison between methods difficult. One difficulty is that agreement in terms of SI is better on high lesion load images than on low lesion load images

[5,23-25]. This is a benefit in breaking SI into OER and DE as SI = 1-.5 OER-.5 (DE/MTA), noting that MTA is an assessment of lesion load. Many ALSA methods have reported similar performance in terms of SI than we observed between our two raters [23-25]. Note that, since MACC provides contours that delineate lesions with sub-voxel accuracy, SI, OER, and DE for MACC are calculated at a sub-voxel level. In contrast, ALSAs typically work at a voxel level. For lesions with a high contrast between edge and background tissue, MACC, FC, and RG methods should have similar results. We view MACC as complementary to ALSAs, and speculate it could be applied as a post-processing step to give better agreement with a human rater whose ROIs were also processed by MACC.

Finally in our post-hoc assessment performed on 424 follow-up FLAIR images and over 55,000 ROIs, MACC was able to produce 91% of the required ROIs such that they did not need further editing to meet our centers stringent standards. Having to only draw/edit only ~9% of the ROIs represents a significant time savings for an analysis center.

Assessment indices

We included SI as a performance index for MACC because SI is commonly used for comparing image masks. We prefer DE and OER values because they are descriptive of how MACC improves agreement and are more resistant to the influence of the underlying ROI set's MTA. MACC was designed to improve OER and not DE. SI reflects the proportional size difference between ROI sets. That MACC performs well as measured by SI reflects the overall dominance of OER over DE in the calculation of SI, especially for ROI sets with high MTA. Despite the low impact DE may have on SI, DE is an important measure. For instance, DE will be much more sensitive than SI for determining whether raters agree in marking the same small lesions, which is important if an outcome for an analysis is the number of "new" lesions.

Uses of MACC

We have demonstrated using MACC to both improve inter-operator agreement in creating ROIs, and for efficiency when ROIs on follow-up scans are required. Furthermore, the concept of MACC can be readily used in other medical imaging scenarios. MACC was shown to improve measurement reliability and reproducibility of cerebral spinal fluid flow [26]. MACC could potentially be used for evaluation of "blackholes" [27], however because of the greatly reduced number of contours per image, the time savings would not be significant.

Conclusion

We have introduced a method that is both well-defined and easy to implement, which drastically reduces the error associated with multiple operators performing lesion analysis. The method also provides significant time savings for operators creating ROIs on follow up scans, assuming the spatial registration of MR images. The method is fast and enables better precision in subsequent steps of lesion activity analysis.

Appendix

Letting I be the intersection of both raters' ROIs, U be the union of the rater ROIs, SI can be expressed as SI = 2I / (U + I). By adding and subtracting U to the numerator, SI = ((U + I)-(U-I)) / U + I. Since DE + OE = U-I (i.e., total error equals the total difference between ROIs), MTA = ½(U + I), and OER = OE/MTA:

$$\mathrm{SI}(\mathrm{R1,R2}) = 1-\frac{\mathrm{U\text{-}I}}{\mathrm{U+I}} = 1-\frac{\mathrm{OE+DE}}{2\mathrm{MTA}} = 1-\left(\frac{1}{2}\right)\mathrm{OER}\text{-}\left(\frac{1}{2}\right)\frac{\mathrm{DE}}{\mathrm{MTA}}$$

We represent OE/MTA as a single variable (OER) since we expect OE to increase as MTA increases. That is, the total outline error area (OE) of two sets of ROIs increases with the number and sizes of ROIs in the sets. We do not necessarily believe that raters will misidentify a region as being a lesion is strongly dependent on the lesion load, hence the contribution to SI from DE is -.5 (DE/MTA). For this reason, we expect higher SI between raters of algorithms evaluated on higher lesion load images, as is consistently observed.

Competing interests

The authors declared that they have no competing interests.

Authors' contributions

Algorithm development: DSW; study design: DSW, MGD, NB, SH, RZ; image analysis: DR, CDP, LR, SH; image processing: DSW, MGB, NB, CM, KS; initial manuscript draft: DSW; manuscript review and revision: All authors read and approved the final manuscript.

Acknowledgements

The authors wish to thank Turi Dalaker, M.D. for many insightful comments in review of this manuscript; and Heather Yanofsky and Eve Salczynski for their review and technical assistance in the preparation of this manuscript. Additionally, Guy Poloni PhD is thanked for his expertise.

Author details

[1]Buffalo Neuroimaging Analysis Center, Department of Neurology, School of Medicine and Biomedical Sciences, University at Buffalo, State University of New York at Buffalo, Buffalo, NY, USA. [2]Department of Nuclear Medicine, University at Buffalo, State University of New York at Buffalo, Buffalo, NY, USA. [3]Department of Neuroradiology, IRCCS, C. Mondino, University of Pavia, Pavia, Italy. [4]MR Imaging Clinical Translational Research Center, School of Medicine and Biomedical Sciences, University at Buffalo, State University of New York, Buffalo, NY, USA. [5]School of Medicine and Biomedical Sciences, State University of New York at Buffalo, Buffalo, NY, USA.

References

1. Achiron A, *et al*: **Brain MRI lesion load quantification in multiple sclerosis: a comparison between automated multispectral and semi-automated thresholding computer-assisted techniques.** *Magnetic resonance imaging* 2002, **20**(10):713–720.
2. Filippi M, *et al*: **Effect of training and different measurement strategies on the reproducibility of brain MRI lesion load measurements in multiple sclerosis.** *Neurology* 1998, **50**(1):238–244.
3. Jackson EF, *et al*: **Accuracy and reproducibility in volumetric analysis of multiple sclerosis lesions.** *Journal of computer assisted tomography* 1993, **17**(2):200.
4. Rovaris M, *et al*: **Reproducibility of brain MRI lesion volume measurements in multiple sclerosis using a local thresholding technique: effects of formal operator training.** *European neurology* 1999, **41**(4):226–230.
5. Wack DS, *et al*: **Improved assessment of multiple sclerosis lesion segmentation agreement via detection and outline error estimates.** *BMC Med Imaging* 2012, **12**(1):17.
6. Hamarneh G, *et al*: *3D live-wire-based semi-automatic segmentation of medical images.* Proc. SPIE 5747, Medical Imaging 2005: Image Processing, 1597: Citeseer; 2005.
7. Schenk A, Prause G, Peitgen H: ***Efficient semiautomatic segmentation of 3d objects in medical images.*** **in** ***Medical Image Computing and Computer-Assisted Intervention - MICCAI.*** *Publisher: Springer-Verlag Berlin Heidelberg* 2000, **1935:**186–195.
8. Derraz F, *et al*: **Semi-automatic segmentation of multiple sclerosis lesion based active contours model and variational Dirichlet process.** *CMES* 2010, **67**(2):95–118.
9. Cuadra M, *et al*: **Atlas-based segmentation of pathological MR brain images using a model of lesion growth.** *IEEE Trans Med Imaging* 2004, **23**(10):1301–1314.
10. Rovaris M, *et al*: **A comparison of conventional and fast spin-echo sequences for the measurement of lesion load in multiple sclerosis using a semi-automated contour technique.** *Neuroradiology* 1997, **39**(3):161–165.
11. Freifeld O, Greenspan H, Goldberger J: **Multiple sclerosis lesion detection using constrained GMM and curve evolution.** *Journal of Biomedical Imaging* 2009, **2009:**1–13.
12. Chao M, *et al*: **Automated contour mapping with a regional deformable model.** *Int J Radiat Oncol Biol Phys* 2008, **70**(2):599–608.
13. Lu W, *et al*: **Automatic re-contouring in 4D radiotherapy.** *Phys Med Biol* 2006, **51:**1077.
14. Di Perri C, *et al*: **Signal abnormalities on 1.5 and 3 Tesla brain MRI in multiple sclerosis patients and healthy controls: a morphological and spatial quantitative comparison study.** *Neuroimage* 2009, **47**(4):1352–1362.
15. Jenkinson M, Smith S: **A global optimisation method for robust affine registration of brain images.** *Medical image analysis* 2001, **5**(2):143–156.
16. Jenkinson M, *et al*: **Improved optimization for the robust and accurate linear registration and motion correction of brain images.** *Neuroimage* 2002, **17**(2):825–841.
17. Zijdenbos A, *et al*: **Morphometric analysis of white matter lesions in mr images: methodand validation.** *IEEE Trans Med Imaging* 1994, **13**(4):716–724.
18. Lladó X, *et al*: **Segmentation of multiple sclerosis lesions in brain MRI: a review of automated approaches.** *Information Sciences* 2011, **186:**164–185.
19. Lladó X, *et al*: **Automated detection of multiple sclerosis lesions in serial brain MRI.** *Neuroradiology* 2011, **54:**787–807.
20. Udupa JK, *et al*: **Multiple sclerosis lesion quantification using fuzzy-connectedness principles.** *Medical Imaging, IEEE Transactions on* 1997, **16**(5):598–609.
21. Sajja B, *et al*: ***A unified approach for lesion segmentation on MRI of multiple sclerosis.*** **in** ***Engineering in Medicine and Biology Society, 2004. IEMBS'04. 26th Annual International Conference of the IEEE.*** *IEEE* 2004, **1:**1778–1781.
22. Alfano B, *et al*: **Automated segmentation and measurement of global white matter lesion volume in patients with multiple sclerosis.** *J Magn Reson Imaging* 2000, **12**(6):799–807.
23. Admiraal-Behloul F, *et al*: **Fully automatic segmentation of white matter hyperintensities in MR images of the elderly.** *Neuroimage* 2005, **28**(3):607–617.
24. Anbeek P, *et al*: **Probabilistic segmentation of white matter lesions in MR imaging.** *Neuroimage* 2004, **21**(3):1037–1044.
25. Khayati R, *et al*: **Fully automatic segmentation of multiple sclerosis lesions in brain MR FLAIR images using adaptive mixtures method and Markov random field model.** *Computers in biology and medicine* 2008, **38**(3):379–390.
26. Magnano C, *et al*: **Cine cerebrospinal fluid imaging in multiple sclerosis.** *J Magn Reson Imaging* 2012, **36**(4):825–834.
27. Datta S, *et al*: **Segmentation and quantification of black holes in multiple sclerosis.** *Neuroimage* 2006, **29**(2):467–474.

Quantification of cervical spine muscle fat: a comparison between T1-weighted and multi-echo gradient echo imaging using a variable projection algorithm (VARPRO)

James M Elliott[1*], David M Walton[2], Alfred Rademaker[3] and Todd B Parrish[4,5]

Abstract

Background: Previous data using T1-weighted MRI demonstrated neck muscle fat infiltration (MFI) in patients with poor functional recovery following whiplash. Such findings do not occur in those with milder symptoms of whiplash, chronic non-traumatic neck pain or healthy controls, suggesting traumatic factors play a role. Muscle degeneration could potentially represent a quantifiable marker of poor recovery, but the temporal constraints of running a T1-weighted sequence and performing the subsequent analysis for muscle fat may be a barrier for clinical translation. The purpose of this preliminary study was to evaluate, quantify and compare MFI for the cervical multifidus muscles with T1-weighted imaging and a more rapid quantitative 3D multi-echo gradient echo (GRE) Dixon based method in healthy subjects.

Methods: 5 asymptomatic participants with no history of neck pain underwent cervical spine MRI with a Siemens 3 Tesla system. The muscle and fat signal intensities on axial spin-echo T1-weighted images were quantitatively classified for the cervical multifidii from C3-C7, bilaterally. Additional axial GRE Dixon based data for fat and water quantification were used for comparison via paired t-tests. Inter-tester reliability for fat and water measures with GRE images were examined using 1) Pearson's Intra-class correlation coefficient 2) Bland-Altman Plots and 3) Lin's-Concordance Coefficient. $P < 0.05$ was used to indicate significance.

Results: Total mean (SD) MFI (C3-C7) for the multifidii obtained with T1-weighted imaging and GRE were 18.4% (3.3) (range 14-22%) and 18.8% (2.9) (range 15-22%), respectively. The Pearson correlation coefficients for inter-tester reliability on the GRE sequences for the C3-C7 multifidii ranged from .83 - .99, indicating high levels of agreement with segmental MFI measures. Bland-Altman Plots revealed all data points were within 2 SDs and concordance was established between 2-blinded raters, suggesting good agreement between two raters measuring fat and water with GRE imaging.

Conclusions: Results of this preliminary study demonstrate reliability between 2 raters of varying experience for MRI analysis of MFI with 3D GRE MRI. The quantification of MFI for healthy cervical musculature is comparable to T1-weighted images. Inclusion of larger samples of symptomatic data and histological comparison with the reference standard biopsy is warranted.

* Correspondence: j-elliott@northwestern.edu
[1]Department of Physical Therapy and Human Movement Sciences, Feinberg School of Medicine, Northwestern University, 645 North Michigan Avenue, Suite 1100 room 1139, Chicago, IL 60611, USA
Full list of author information is available at the end of the article

Background

Magnetic resonance imaging (MRI) has been used to quantify muscular fatty infiltrates (MFI) in patients with acute and chronic neck disorders [1-4], low back pain [5-8] and a number of neuromusculoskeletal conditions [9-11]. Cross-sectional investigations have determined significantly lower magnitudes of neck MFI in those with non-traumatic, insidious onset pain when compared to those with chronic whiplash related pain [3], suggesting traumatic factors play a role in their development. Using conventional T1-weighted MRI in prospective fashion, MFI were shown to develop between 4-weeks and 3-months post whiplash injury in patients with moderate to severe levels of pain and disability but not in those with lower levels of acute pain [2]. Findings of muscle degeneration in those with higher levels of pain and disability following whiplash injury from a motor vehicle crash could potentially represent a quantifiable marker of poor recovery. As such, the early radiological observation and quantification of MFI may prove informative for clinical practice. However, a potential challenge in translating such findings remains the temporal constraints of running the longer T1-weighted sequence and performing a quantitative analysis for MFI especially when considering patient throughput in a busy radiology practice.

There are however a number of other more rapid methods for quantifying the water and fat composition of a voxel when compared to T1-weighted imaging. These include a dual acquisition method, where the water frequency is selectively excited (water image) [12] and a standard image is collected (fat and water image). This however relies on the uniform frequency difference between water and fat across the whole volume of excitation, which is often difficult to obtain at higher magnetic fields. A fat suppressed acquisition using a short-tau inversion recovery (STIR) sequence is possible, but the T1 of fat has to be assumed, which may vary depending on the evolution of the infiltration of the muscle [13]. An alternative is the Dixon method [14], where one collects data at an echo time when water and fat are in-phase and at an echo time when the phases are opposed. The data can be combined to generate a fat and water image but is prone to errors in the presence of field inhomogeneities. Collecting multiple echo time data can improve the estimation of the fat and water images and this technique has been applied successfully in the musculoskeletal system [15], adrenal glands [16], kidneys [17] and liver [18,19]. The measure has recently expanded to include the quantification of intramuscular fat of the lower extremity in patients with myopathy [9] and in the lumbar paraspinals of a large population of patients with low back pain [20]. The proposition solicits that such rapid 3D imaging methods could be used to quantify fat content of the neck muscles. It is not possible however to offer physiological interpretation of such data without producing normative reliability data as a foundation.

The intent of this preliminary study was to 1) compare the measurement of cervical muscle fat using 3D Gradient Echo (GRE) multi-echo fat/water acquisitions to a previous measure using T1-weighted sequences and 2) establish inter-rater reliability for measuring cervical muscle fat and water using 3D fat/water separation MRI. We chose the GRE sequence because of the more time efficient data collection of the GRE sequence. We expect that the fat and water measure will provide valid quantification of muscle fat compared to that of the previously established and reliable T1-weighted measure [1], while offering the important clinical advantages of ease and efficiency.

Methods

Study population

3 healthy male and 2 female volunteers (mean age (SD) [range]- 35 (8.6) [26–48]), with no previous history of neck pain or trauma to the cervical spine, were sought for the study. Only males and females aged 18–55 years were considered in this first instance. There were several criteria that excluded potential participants, which related to their neuromusculoskeletal status and institutional guidelines for the safe application of MRI to asymptomatic volunteers. They included: a previous history of neck pain, vertiginous symptoms, a history of a motor vehicle accident, neurological conditions, inflammatory joint disease or systemic disease e.g. diabetes. In relation to the MRI scan, volunteers were not considered if they suffered claustrophobia, had a pacemaker, aneurysm clip or any small implanted metal hardware or wires that could move or be affected when introduced to a magnetic field. Furthermore, subjects were not considered if they were pregnant or if, in the absence of an effective form of contraception, they could possibly have conceived since the first day of their last normal menstrual period.

Healthy subjects were recruited from the university community in urban Chicago, Illinois, USA. Eight volunteers responded to the appeals for participants. In total, 3 out of 8 potential participants were excluded secondary to a previous motor vehicle accident (1), claustrophobia (1) and pregnancy (1). Thus, 5 healthy subjects were included (2 males and 3 females).

Ethical clearance was obtained from the Northwestern University Institutional Review Board, Chicago, Illinois, USA. All subjects provided written informed consent to participate. All data were stored in a secured database and de-identified.

Measurements

Demographic and anthropometric data

Subjects completed a baseline questionnaire that included details on their age, height, weight, and an institutional checklist of absolute and relative contraindications for MRI.

MRI examinations

All examinations were performed with a 3.0 T MRI scanner (Trio, Siemens, Erlangen, Germany). Each participant underwent MR examination of the cervical spine (from the cephalad portion of C2 to the caudal portion of C7). In addition to the standard 12-channel head coil, a dedicated neck coil of the manufacturer was used as a receiver coil. Once positioned in the magnet, a localizer scan and a T2-weighted sagittal turbo spin echo sequence were performed.

T1-Weighted MRI

The T1-weighted axial scan of the cervical spine was planned from the T2-weighted sagittal sequence and the slab was manually angled perpendicular to the normal lordotic curve of each subject using the middle of the C2/3 intervertebral disc as a reference point. The slab was then manually positioned from the cephalad portion of C2 through the caudal portion of the C7 vertebral end plate to ensure proper capture of the cervical extensor musculature. Parameters consisted of: slices = 24, slice thickness of 4 mm and a gap of 0.8 mm, FOV = 200 × 200 mm, TR = 448 ms, TE = 14 ms, matrix size = 256*256, in plane resolution of 0.9 mm × 0.9 mm, acquisition time TA = 8:42 seconds.

This established measure of relative fat within the muscle [1,3,4,21] was used to quantify a pixel intensity profile for both muscle and fat with AnalyzeDirect software (V. 11.0). The measure, based on the contrasting signal intensities of fat and water on T1-weighted imaging, allows for the simple process of quantifying relative amounts of intramuscular fat compared to a recognized area of intermuscular fat at the C2 level [21]. Analysis consisted of manually tracing user-defined regions of interest (ROI) over the bilateral multifidii muscles on the axial T1-weighted images at the most cephalad portion of the vertebral bodies of C3 – C7.

Histograms were created from the summated user-defined ROI, displaying each particular image pixel intensity profile. A numerical representation of each image muscle and intermuscular fat pixel intensity profiles were created and the text file was exported to an Excel ® spreadsheet for calculation of the MFI for T1-weighted imaging. Dividing the mean pixel intensity of the muscle ROI by the mean pixel intensity of the intermuscular fat ROI created the MFI value.

3D Multi-echo Dixon fat/water imaging

A number of imaging techniques, based on the different precessional frequencies of fat and water protons can be used to quantify fat and water concentration. We used a three-dimensional multi-echo gradient echo acquisition to collect the data required for the analysis of phase related to the precessional differences in fat and water. The Fast Low Angle Shot (FLASH) based axial gradient echo sequence parameters were TR = 23.81 ms, 8 echo times with a spacing of 1.78 ms starting at 1.36 ms. A single slab was placed over the cervical spine with 36 partitions and a partition thickness of 3 mm and slab oversampling of 22% to prevent aliasing in the 3D direction. The in-plane resolution was 1.4 mm using a rectangular field of view of 75% resulting in an acquisition time of 2:06 minutes. This scan also covered the cephalad portion of C2 through the caudal portion of the C7 vertebral end plate.

Fat/water quantification

The water separation algorithm uses the variable projection (VARPRO) method to find an iterative solution for the entire image [22]. The VARPRO algorithm can use four or more echoes with non-uniformly spaced echo times (phase shifts between water and fat) to solve the nonlinear problem with a globally optimized solution. The reconstruction process was automated in the Siemens sequence environment so that fat-only, water-only, and calculated in-phase and opposed-phase images were created. The MFI from 3D fat/water separation imaging was created from the mean pixel intensity of fat-only (Fat) and the mean pixel intensity of water-only (Water) images with the following equation:

$$\mathrm{Fat}/(\mathrm{Fat}+\mathrm{Water})*100$$

Procedure

Subjects were requested to lie supine inside the magnet with a foam pad under their knees and foam padding placed on top of the head as well as on the right and left of the head to position the cervical spine in the neutral position and reduce any head movement during the exam. They were asked to lie completely still during the examination with communication between subject and operator occurring between each sequence to ensure participant comfort.

Two raters, one with 10 years of experience measuring muscle structure and one with 3-months, were tasked with establishing repeatability of MFI measures in the bilateral cervical multifidus muscle at C3 through C7 with the fat/water images. Regions of interest were drawn using AnalyzeDirect Software (V. 11.0) of the bilateral multifidii muscles at the most cephalad portion of each respective vertebral level (C3-C7). The right and left sides were combined for the analysis. The rater with less experience (rater 2) was trained by the investigator with more experience (rater 1). Each rater measured

Table 1 The age and BMI (Means ±SD [range]) of the asymptomatic cohort (n = 5)

	Age (years)	BMI (lbs/in^2)
Total population (n = 5)	35.0 ± 8.6	27.4 ± 2.4
	[26 – 48]	[24.4 – 30.5]

the MFI independently and this data was used for analysis. Repeatability of the T1-weighted measure has been established previously [1,21].

Statistical analysis

Data analysis was performed with the procedures implemented by using SPSS statistical software (Version 20.0 for Mac; Chicago, IL). Participant demographic data are presented as proportions or means ± SD (range). The inter-rater reliability for the 3D fat/water measurements of MFI was tested using the Intraclass Correlational Coefficient ($ICC_{3,1}$ - *which is used when all subjects are rated by the same raters who are assumed to be the entire population of raters*), Bland & Altman plots and Lin's Concordance Coefficients to assess and confirm levels of consistency and agreement of MFI. Because the calculated MFI's on both sequences were found to be normally distributed using the Kolmogorov-Smirnov method, the differences in MFI between the measures were evaluated by a parametric paired *t*-test with a level of significance set at $\alpha = 0.05$. The inter-rater reliability for the T1-weighted measure of MFI was tested using the $ICC_{3,1}$.

Table 2 The average measures intra-class correlation coefficients [95% CI] of the inter-observer reliability of cervical multifidii MFI on 3D Multi-Echo GRE Imaging

	Rater 1 vs. Rater 2 ICC [95% CI]	p - value
C3	.97 [.78 - .99]	0.001
C4	.95 [.55 - .99]	0.006
C5	.94 [.43 - .99]	0.009
C6	.83 [.60 - .98]	0.05
C7	.99 [.97 - .99]	0.001

Sample size

Walter and colleagues have presented a robust mathematical algorithm for predicting adequate sample size for reliability studies [23]. Assuming a minimum agreement (ICC) of 0.80, with a null hypothesis (level below which we would deem the tool not reliable) of 0.4, a minimum of 9 independent observations provides an acceptable 5% alpha error rate ($p < 0.05$) and 20% beta error rate. In order to produce a more robust estimate, right and left multifidus was measured from C3-C7 by each rater. As such, each image represented 10 data points (5 pairs of data). The images were presented in a randomized fashion and thus, error was also random.

Results

The subjects' characteristics in relation to age and BMI are presented in Table 1. The ICCs for the inter-rater reliability using the fat/water sequence of the multifidus ranged from .83 - .99 indicating good to excellent inter-rater reliability and consistent with previously established

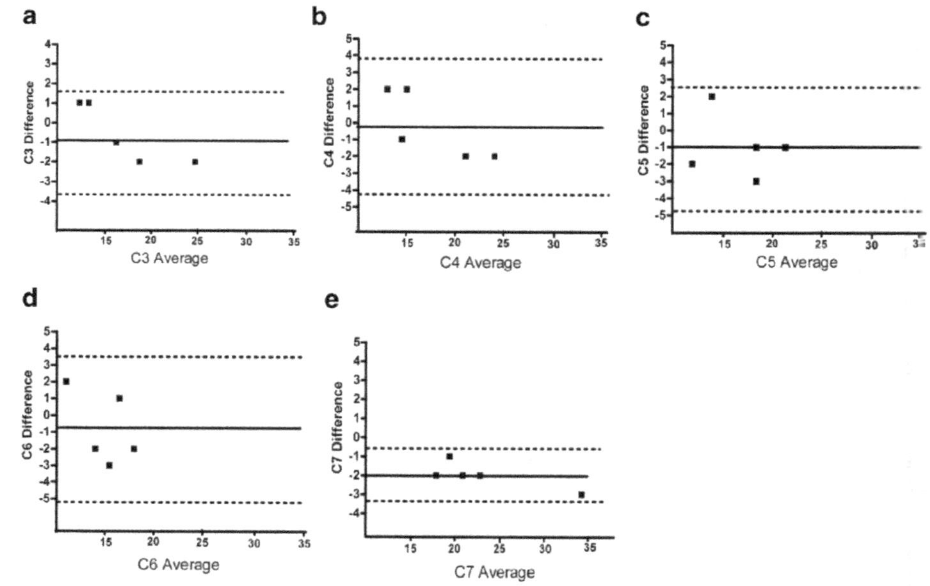

Figure 1 Bland-Altman Plots of C3-C7 multifidus MFI difference vs. average between 2-raters: a) C3, b) C4, c) C5, d) C6 and e) C7. Data was acquired from the 3D multi-echo GRE fat/water separation sequence.

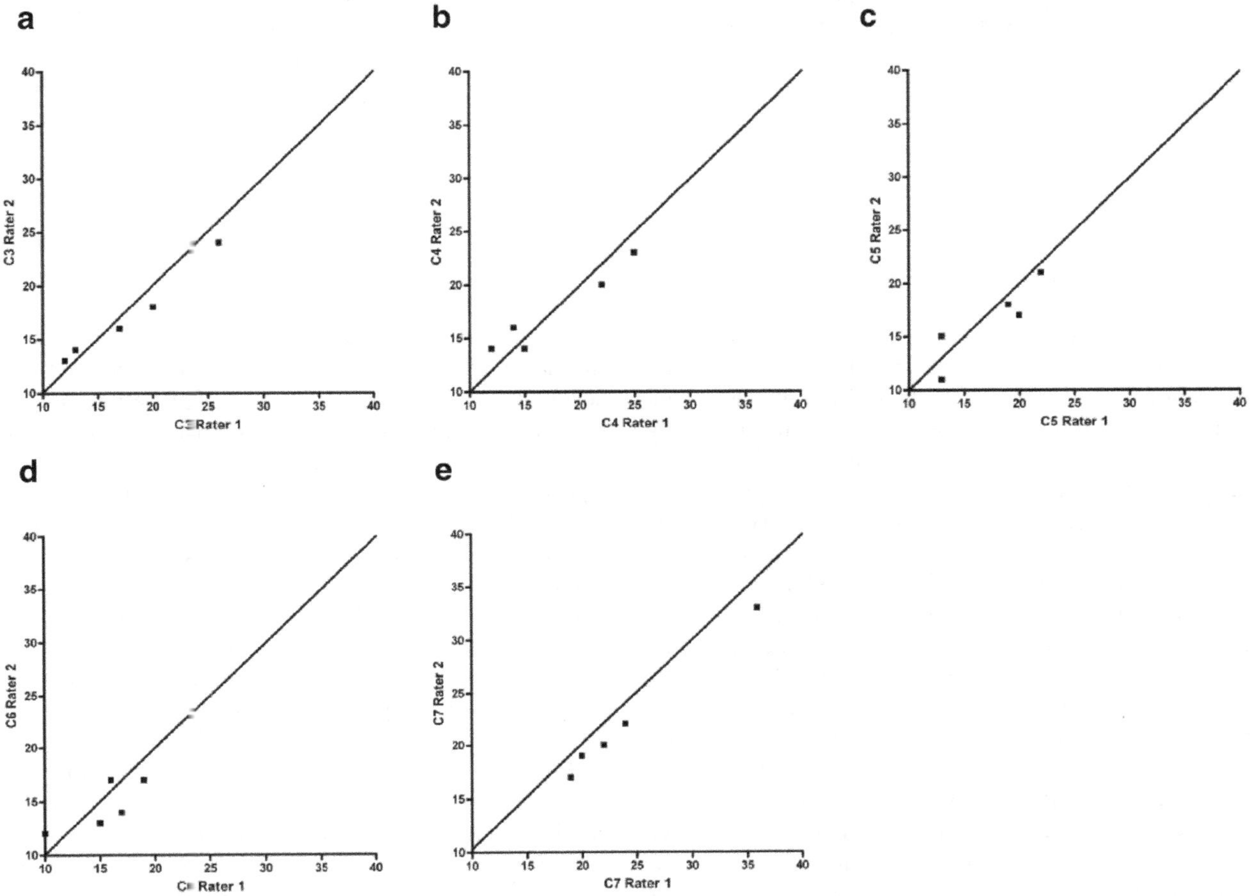

Figure 2 Lin Concordance Coefficients for segmental multifidus MFI between 2-raters: a) C3, b) C4, c) C5 d) C6 and e) C7. Data was acquired from the 3D multi-echo GRE fat/water separation sequence.

data (Table 2) [1,21]. Figure 1a-e details the results from Bland & Altman Plots for the fat/water imaging measure, which reveals that both rater differences for MFI were within +/− 2 standard deviations and Figure 2a-e details Lin Concordance Coefficients, confirming concordance between 2 raters for segmental MFI of the cervical multifidus as measured by fat/water imaging. The values from Lin Concordance Coefficients are presented in Table 3.

The MFI values (mean (SD) [Range]) within the cervical multifidus with T1-weighted and fat/water separation MRI are presented in Table 4. There were no significant differences between the MRI findings of segmental (C3, C4, C5 and C6) or total MFI (C3-C7 combined) within the multifidus muscle with both sequences, demonstrating little discrepancy between the two measures ($p = 0.47$). There was however a significant difference in MFI at the C7 level where the fat/water measure was significantly higher when compared to the T1-weighted measure ($p = 0.04$).

Discussion

The results of this preliminary study involving a small sample ($n = 5$) asymptomatic participants indicates that the rapid acquisition 3D fat/water separation technique is comparable to T1-weighted imaging in detecting the relative fat content in the healthy cervical multifidii musculature (Figure 3). In addition, the inter-rater reliability was good to excellent for the fat/water technique,

Table 3 Means for rater 1 and rater 2 (+/− SD) from Lin Concordance Coefficients for MFI of the cervical multifidus with 3D Multi-Echo GRE Imaging

	Mean (SD) 3D GRE - MFI		concordance	p – value	95% CI
	Rater 1	Rater 2			
C3	17.6 (5.6)	17 (4.4)	.95	< 0.001	.82 - .98
C4	17.6 (5.6)	17.4 (3.9)	.90	< 0.001	.69 - .98
C5	17.4 (4.2)	16.4 (3.7)	.86	0.018	.22 - .98
C6	15.4 (3.4)	14.6 (2.3)	.69	0.08	−0.10 - .94
C7	17.6 (5.6)	17 (4.4)	.94	< 0.001	.82 - .98

Table 4 Mean MFI (C3-C7) from T1-weighted and 3D Multi-Echo GRE Imaging ((SD) [Range])

	Mean T1-weighted MFP (SD) [Range %]	Mean 3D GRE MFP (SD) [Range %]	p - value
C3	19.6% (2.4) [17 - 23]	17.6% (5.7) [12 - 26]	0.25
C4	19.2% (3.9) [13 - 24]	17.6% (5.6) [12 - 25]	0.44
C5	19.8% (2.4) [18 - 24]	17.4% (4.2) [13 - 22]	0.15
C6	17.4% (1.8) [15 - 19]	15.4% (3.4) [10 - 19]	0.09
C7	17.8% (7.4) [12 - 30]	24.2% (6.8) [19 - 36]	0.04*
TOTAL	18.8% (2.9) [15 - 22]	18.4% (3.3) [14 - 22]	0.47

* Indicates significance at $p < 0.05$ (two-tailed).

suggesting this method is reliable between a finite set of 2-raters of varying experience ($ICC_{3,1}$) but it needs to be determined if it would be readily and rapidly replicated by different examiners (or raters) outside our laboratory ($ICC_{2,1}$). As can be seen in Tables 2 and 3 and Figures 1 and 2, the measure of MFI with fat/water separation is repeatable between two blinded raters with varying levels of experience. Altogether, the more experienced rater 1 consistently measured higher levels of MFI when compared to rater 2. The clinical significance of this difference between raters is however unknown at this time. While experience could factor into a more liberal inclusion of musculofascial borders for the cervical multifidus on axial images, larger numbers of raters with varying levels of experience would be required before deriving definitive conclusions on the influence of experience. Furthermore, precise reasons into the significantly higher MFI at the C7 level with the 3D fat/water measure when compared to the T1-weighted measure is unknown at this time but could result from field inhomogeneities or RF profile induced signal changes at the outer edge of the excitation volume.

There is support for establishing equivalence between different methods on the basis of their ability to quantify measured samples, all of which however carry some limitations. Lin first proposed the Concordance Coefficient in 1989 for assessment of concordance in continuous data as an alternative way of assessing agreement between alternative methods, such as the Pearson correlation coefficient *r*, paired *t*-tests, coefficient of variation, and the ICC [24]. In addition, the Lin concordance coefficient has shown to be robust for small samples of data [24], such as reported in this preliminary study. Accordingly, we chose to include the Lin Concordance Coefficient in tandem with $ICCs_{3,1}$ and Bland Altman Plots to ensure a robust statistical analysis of our repeatability when producing multiple measures for MFI in the cervical multifidus in a small healthy sample of five subjects.

Considerable evidence exists to support a relationship between muscle fatty infiltrates and painful symptoms in patients with neck [1,2,4,25-27] and low back pain as well as a host of other neuromususculoskeletal disorders [7-11,20,28,29]. A recent longitudinal study of whiplash provides preliminary evidence that the manifestation of fatty degeneration, between 4-weeks and 3-months post injury, is associated with higher levels of initial pain and signs of post-traumatic stress [2]; a robust predictor of poor-functional recovery [30,31]. Such muscle changes were not expressed in those with lower levels of initial pain suggesting their presence is unique to those who transition to chronic pain following whiplash [2] and that the observation of their development could be important in clinical MR imaging studies. However, the routine quantification of such muscle changes following

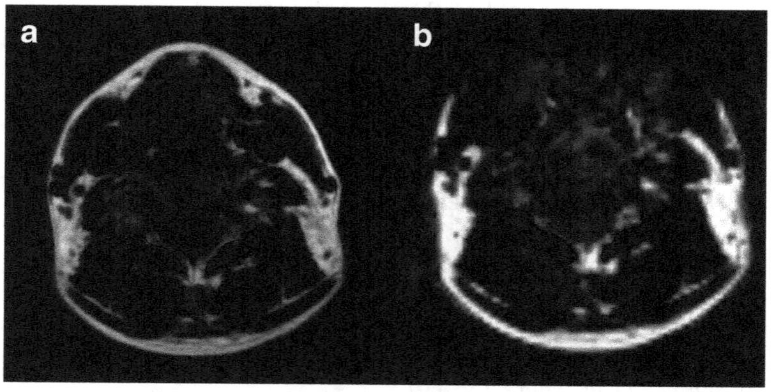

Figure 3 Regions of interest measures of right and left multifidus muscle at the C5 segmental level; a) T1-weighted magnetic resonance image **b)** fat-only image derived from the 3D VARPRO acquisition. Images were co-registered.

whiplash is unlikely when one considers the time-constraints of currently available clinical measures. The use of rapid acquisition 3D multi-echo fat/water imaging provides a potential clinical alternative and results of this small study provide foundation for its use in quantifying the temporal degeneration of soft-aqueous neck muscles following whiplash injury in prospective fashion. Positive findings would help to translate the use of such imaging sequences to the clinical setting whereby the exploration and development of more informed (and early) management strategies could be explored and realized.

The results of this preliminary study were obtained in a small sample of asymptomatic subjects. Larger sampled studies involving symptomatic subjects are required before the findings can be generalized to patient populations and this is well underway in our laboratory. Furthermore, repeated measures experiments are required to determine repeatability error with the MRI measures over time.

Conclusions

3D multi-echo fat/water MR imaging provides for an accurate and rapid measure of MFI for the cervical multifidus in a small sample of healthy subjects. We found excellent agreement in a small sample of healthy subjects between two-raters across multiple analysis strategies supporting the use of this method in longitudinal evaluation of temporal changes in muscle tissue structure, particularly following traumatic whiplash injury. An advantage of the 3D acquisition method is that a further time reduction could be obtained if the coverage of interest was reduced to a single level, which is not true for spin echo based imaging methods. For the future, inclusion of other muscles beyond the multifidii is required to compare MFI within and between different muscular regions. Finally, comparison of MFI with 3D multi-echo fat/water separation MR to the reference standard, muscle biopsy, is also required and this validation is underway.

Abbreviations

MFI: Muscle fatty infiltrate; STIR: Short tau inversion recovery; GRE: Gradient echo; FLASH: Fast low angle shot magnetic resonance imaging; VARPRO: Variable projection algorithm; ICC- Intra: Class correlation coefficient; MFI: Muscle fat percentage.

Competing interests

The authors declare that they have no competing interests.

Authors' contributions

Guarantor of integrity of the entire study- JE, TP, DW. Study concepts and design- JE, TP, DW. Literature research- JE, TP, DW. Clinical studies- JE, TP. Experimental studies/data analysis – JE, FR, TP. Statistical analysis- JE, FR, DW. Manuscript preparation- JE, FR, TP, DW. Manuscript editing- JE, FR, TP, DW. All authors read and approved the final manuscript.

Acknowledgements

We wish to thank Saurabh Shah, PhD for implementing the VARPRO algorithm and acquisition sequence in the Cardiovascular Research & Development team located at Northwestern University. Currently this feature is a WIP at VB17 software. We also wish to thank Tobey Demott Yeates, PT, for her time, assistance and attention to detail in completing this study. James Elliott is supported by NIH KL2 RR025740.

Author details

[1]Department of Physical Therapy and Human Movement Sciences, Feinberg School of Medicine, Northwestern University, 645 North Michigan Avenue, Suite 1100 room 1139, Chicago, IL 60611, USA. [2]School of Physical Therapy, Western University, London, Ontario, Canada. [3]Department of Preventive Medicine, Feinberg School of Medicine, Northwestern University, Chicago, IL, USA. [4]Department of Biomedical Engineering, McCormick School of Engineering, Northwestern University, Evanston, IL, USA. [5]Department of Radiology, Feinberg School of Medicine, Northwestern University, Chicago, IL, USA.

References

1. Elliott J, Jull G, Noteboom JT, Darnell R, Galloway G, Gibbon WW: **Fatty infiltration in the cervical extensor muscles in persistent whiplash-associated disorders: a magnetic resonance imaging analysis.** *Spine (Phila Pa 1976)* 2006, **31**(22):E847–E855.
2. Elliott J, Pedler A, Kenardy J, Galloway G, Jull G, Sterling M: **The temporal development of Fatty infiltrates in the neck muscles following whiplash injury: an association with pain and posttraumatic stress.** *PLoS One* 2011, **6**(6):e21194.
3. Elliott J, Sterling M, Noteboom JT, Darnell R, Galloway G, Jull G: **Fatty infiltrate in the cervical extensor muscles is not a feature of chronic, insidious-onset neck pain.** *Clin Radiol* 2008, **63**(6):681–687.
4. Elliott JM, O'Leary S, Sterling M, Hendrikz J, Pedler A, Jull G: **Magnetic resonance imaging findings of fatty infiltrate in the cervical flexors in chronic whiplash.** *Spine (Phila Pa 1976)* 2010, **35**(9):948–954.
5. Ali I, Ulbricht C, McGregor AH: **Degeneration of the extensor muscle group in a surgical low back and leg pain population.** *J Back Musculoskelet Rehabil* 2011, **24**(1):23–30.
6. Kader DF, Wardlaw D, Smith FW: **Correlation between the MRI changes in the lumbar multifidus muscles and leg pain.** *Clin Radiol* 2000, **55**(2):145–149.
7. Mengiardi B, Schmid MR, Boos N, Pfirrmann CW, Brunner F, Elfering A, Hodler J: **Fat content of lumbar paraspinal muscles in patients with chronic low back pain and in asymptomatic volunteers: quantification with MR spectroscopy.** *Radiology* 2006, **240**(3):786–792.
8. Campbell WW, Vasconcelos O, Laine FJ: **Focal atrophy of the multifidus muscle in lumbosacral radiculopathy.** *Muscle Nerve* 1998, **21**(10):1350F–1353F.
9. Gaeta M, Scribano E, Mileto A, Mazziotti S, Rodolico C, Toscano A, Settineri N, Ascenti G, Blandino A: **Muscle fat fraction in neuromuscular disorders: dual-echo dual-flip-angle spoiled gradient-recalled MR imaging technique for quantification–a feasibility study.** *Radiology* 2011, **259**(2):487–494.
10. Gerber C, Schneeberger AG, Hoppeler H, Meyer DC: **Correlation of atrophy and fatty infiltration on strength and integrity of rotator cuff repairs: a study in thirteen patients.** *J Shoulder Elbow Surg* 2007, **16**(6):691–696.
11. Fleckenstein JL, Watumull D, Conner KE, Ezaki M, Greenlee RG Jr, Bryan WW, Chason DP, Parkey RW, Peshock RM, Purdy PD: **Denervated human skeletal muscle: MR imaging evaluation.** *Radiology* 1993, **187**(1):213–218.
12. Haase A, Frahm J, Hänicke W, Matthaei D: **1H NMR chemical shift selective (CHESS) imaging.** *Phys Med Biol* 1985, **30**:341–344.
13. Bydder GM, Steiner RE, Blumgart LH: **MR imaging of the liver using short TI inversion recovery.** *J Comput Assist Tomogr 1985* 1985, **9**:1084–1108.
14. Dixon W: **Simple proton spectroscopic imaging.** *Radiology* 1984, **153**:189–194.
15. Gerdes CM, Kijowski R, Reeder SB: **IDEAL imaging of the musculoskeletal system: robust water fat separation for uniform fat suppression, marrow evaluation, and cartilage imaging.** *AJR Am J Roentgenol* 2007, **189**(5):W284–W291.
16. Savci G, Yazici Z, Sahin N, *et al*: **Value of chemical shift subtraction MRI in characterization of adrenal masses.** *AJR Am J Roentgenol* 2006, **186**:130–135.
17. Israel GM, Hindman N, Hecht E, *et al*: **The use of opposed phase chemical shift MRI in the diagnosis of renal angiomyolipomas.** *AJR Am J Roentgenol* 2005, **184**:1868–1872.

18. Reeder SB, Wen Z, Yu H, Pineda AR, Gold GE, Markl M, Pelc NJ: **Multicoil Dixon chemical species separation with an iterative least squares estimation method.** *Magn Reson Med 2004* 2004, **51**:35–45.
19. Reeder SB, Pineda AR, Wen Z, Shimakawa A, Yu H, Brittain JH, Gold GE, Beaulieu CH, Pelc NJ: **Iterative decomposition of water and fat with echo asymmetry and least-squares estimation (IDEAL): application with fast spin-echo imaging.** *Magn Reson Med* 2005, **54**:636–644.
20. Paalanne N, Niinimäki J, Karppinen J, Taimela S, Mutanen P, Takatalo J, Korpelainen R, Tervonen O: **Assessment of association between low back pain and paraspinal muscle atrophy using opposed phase magnetic resonance imaging a population-based study among young adults.** *Spine* 2011, **36**(23):1961–1968.
21. Elliott JM, Galloway GJ, Jull GA, Noteboom JT, Centeno CJ, Gibbon WW: **Magnetic resonance imaging analysis of the upper cervical spine extensor musculature in an asymptomatic cohort: an index of fat within muscle.** *Clin Radiol* 2005, **60**(3):355–363.
22. Hernando D, Haldar JP, Sutton BP, Ma J, Kellman P, Liang Z-P: **Joint estimation of water/Fat images and field inhomogeneity Map.** *Magn Reson Med* 2008, **59**:571–580.
23. Walter SD, Eliasziw M, Donner A: **Sample size and optimal designs for reliability studies.** *Stat Med* 1998, **17**(1):101–110.
24. Lin IK: **A concordance correlation coefficient to evaluate reproducibility.** *Biometrics* 1989, **45**(1):255–268.
25. Andary MT, Hallgren RC, Greenman PF, Rechtien JJ: **Neurogenic atrophy of suboccipital muscles after a cervical injury: a case study.** *Am J Phys Med Rehabil* 1998, **77**(6):545–549.
26. Hallgren RC, Greenman PF, Rechtien JJ: **Atrophy of suboccipital muscles in patients with chronic pain: a pilot study.** *J Am Osteopath Assoc* 1994, **94**(12):1032–1038.
27. McPartland JM, Brodeur RR, Hallgren RC: **Chronic neck pain, standing balance, and suboccipital muscle atrophy–a pilot study.** *J Manipulative Physiol Ther* 1997, **20**(1):24–29.
28. Fritz RC, Domroese ME, Carter GT: **Physiological and anatomical basis of muscle magnetic resonance imaging.** *Phys Med Rehabil Clin N Am* 2005, **16**(4):1033–1051.
29. McDonald CM, Carter GT, Fritz RC, Anderson MW, Abresch RT, Kilmer DD: **Magnetic resonance imaging of denervated muscle: comparison to electromyography.** *Muscle Nerve* 2000, **23**(9):1431–1434.
30. Sterling M, Jull G, Kenardy J: **Physical and psychological factors maintain long-term predictive capacity post-whiplash injury.** *Pain* 2006, **122**(1-2):102–108.
31. Sterling M, Jull G, Vicenzino B, Kenardy J, Darnell R: **Physical and psychological factors predict outcome following whiplash injury.** *Pain* 2005, **114**(1–2):141–148.

16

Dynamic contrast enhanced magnetic resonance imaging in chronic Achilles tendinosis

Anna Gärdin[1,2*], Torkel B Brismar[1,2], Tomas Movin[1,3] and Adel Shalabi[1,4]

Abstract

Background: Chronic Achilles tendinosis is a common problem. When evaluating and comparing different therapies there is a need for reliable imaging methods. Our aim was to evaluate if chronic Achilles tendinosis affects the dynamic contrast-enhancement in the tendon and its surroundings and if short-term eccentric calf-muscle training normalizes the dynamic contrast-enhancement.

Methods: 20 patients with chronic Achilles tendinopathy were included. Median duration of symptoms was 31 months (range 6 to 120 months). Both Achilles tendons were examined with dynamic contrast enhanced MRI before and after a 12- week exercise programme of eccentric calf-muscle training. The dynamic MRI was evaluated in tendon, vessel and in fat ventrally of tendon. Area under the curve (AUC), time to peak of signal, signal increase per second (SI/s) and increase in signal between start and peak as a percentage (SI%) was calculated. Pain and performance were evaluated using a questionnaire.

Results: In the fat ventrally of the tendon, dynamic contrast enhancement was significantly higher in the symptomatic leg compared to the contralateral non-symptomatic leg before but not after treatment. Despite decreased pain and improved performance there was no significant change of dynamic contrast enhancement in symptomatic tendons after treatment.

Conclusion: In Achilles tendinosis there is an increased contrast enhancement in the fat ventrally of the tendon. The lack of correlation with symptoms and the lack of significant changes in tendon contrast enhancement parameters do however indicate that dynamic enhanced MRI is currently not a useful method to evaluate chronic Achilles tendinosis.

Background

Chronic Achilles tendinosis is common especially in athletes but also in non- athletes [1,2]. Deranged vasculature is thought to be involved in the pathogenesis [3]. A pathologic vascularity not only inside the tendon but also outside, ventrally of the tendon, has been shown [4]. Several treatment approaches have been applied [5-9]. When evaluating and comparing different therapies there is a need of reliable imaging methods since evaluation with clinical examination and questionnaires cannot be fully blinded. By using ultrasound tendon thickening, hypoechoic areas and neovascularisation can be visualized and quantified [4,10,11]. Unfortunately ultrasound is user dependent and reproducibility is limited [12]. MRI techniques focus on measuring tendon thickening and on quantifying areas of intratendinous high signal [10,11,13]. By also administering intravenous gadolinium contrast media the intratendinous signal changes have been shown to be more pronounced [11]. After histopathological correlates it was hypothesized that the increased enhancement of the affected tendons from intravenous gadolinium might be explained by a local pathologically increased amount of glycosaminoglycans, a macromolecule with high water containing capacity.

In a previous publication we have shown that the absolute signal intensity was increased in symptomatic tendons before training and that it decreases towards normal values after three months of eccentric training [14]. Comparison of intratendinous signal between different occasions is however not fully reliable due

* Correspondence: anna.gardin@karolinska.se

[1]Department of Clinical Science, Division of Medical Imaging and Technology, Intervention and Technology at Karolinska Institutet, Stockholm SE-141-86, Sweden

[2]Department of Radiology, Karolinska University Hospital in Huddinge, Stockholm SE-141-86, Sweden

Full list of author information is available at the end of the article

to its arbitrary scaling with different extrinsic factors, such as placement of coils, temperature and normal T1/T2 fluctuations affecting the signal intensity. To avoid that methodological error a semi-quantitative scale was used when performing a follow-up of these patients 4 years after training [15]. The intratendionous signal of the previously affected tendons was then comparable to that of the non-symptomatic tendons. Use of semi-quantitative scales does however have a lower sensitivity than quantitative measurements due to influence from inter- and intra-observer variation. Further improvements of techniques to quantify Achilles tendinosis are therefore needed.

At dynamic contrast-enhanced MR imaging (DEMRI) of the Achilles tendon several images are obtained at fixed time-points after the injection of an MRI contrast agent. By analyzing the changes in signal intensity it is possible to calculate the physiologic kinetics. This gives information about tissue vascularity, perfusion and capillary permeability [16,17]. This technique should in theory be ideal to quantify the histopathological changes that have been observed in chronic Achilles tendinosis including increased vascularity, abnormal fiber structure, focal variation in cellularity and increased areas of non-collagen extracellular matrix [18,19]. The micro vascularisation in Achilles tendinosis has been evaluated during one year in a pilot study using MRI time-intensity curves together with power Doppler ultrasound [20].

The aim of this study was to evaluate the dynamic contrast-enhancement in Achilles tendinosis and if an altered dynamic contrast-enhancement is normalized after a short-term eccentric calf-muscle training. We also evaluated if the dynamic contrast-enhancement is correlated to the subjective symptoms.

Patients

This study consists of a subgroup of a previously published patient material [14]. In that study intratendinous MRI signal, tendon volume and pain and performance before and after three months of eccentric training was evaluated. That study and the present study were approved by the local ethics committee at Karolinska Institutet and informed consent was obtained from each patient.

Because of technical problems when performing the DEMRI (three cases of incorrect contrast injection timing, one with extravasation and in one case intolerance of the contrast agent) only 20 patients of the original 25 patients participated in this dynamic contrast study.

The 20 patients (14 male and 6 females) were aged 28 to 70 years (median 51). Achilles tendinosis was defined as pain and local tenderness of the midportion of the Achilles tendon 2 to 7 cm proximal to the tendon insertion. Median duration of symptoms was 31 months (range 6 to 120 months). In 9 of the 20 patients the Achilles tendon symptoms were sports related; at the time when symptoms appeared 7 patients practiced recreational running and one of them also practiced skiing and another also basketball. One patient practiced golf and one patient related the symptoms to snowboard skiing. The remaining 11 were regarded as idiopathic. Previous corticosteroid injections and systemic diseases such as rheumatic disease constituted exclusion criteria. 14 of the 20 patients had unilateral symptoms whereas 6 of the patients also had a history of symptoms in the contralateral Achilles tendon. In patients with bilateral symptoms, the Achilles tendon with most symptoms was considered as the symptomatic tendon. One of the 20 patients had had an operation in the contralateral tendon 5 years previous to this study. None of the other patients had had any previous treatment other than pain medication.

Treatment

The eccentric exercise programme followed a model developed by Alfredson et al. [5]. Eccentric loading of the calf was done in two ways; with the knee straight and with the knee bent. The eccentric loading was performed with all body weight on the symptomatic side. Each of the two exercises was done with 15 repetitions in 3 sets (3 × 15 repetitions) twice a day for 12 weeks. The patients were instructed to train their symptomatic side, but it is possible that some patients might have also trained the non-symptomatic side. To ensure compliance the patients saw a physiotherapist on two occasions and were contacted once on telephone. Symptoms were evaluated using a questionnaire, modified from a classification by Curwin and Stanish, grading pain on a six-level scale and performance on a four-level scale [21] (Table 1).

MRI acquisition

Both Achilles tendons were examined with Dynamic MRI at two occasions, before (DEMRI 1) and after three months of heavy loaded eccentric calf-muscle training (DEMRI 2) using a 1.5 Tesla Magnetom Vision (Siemens, Erlangen, Germany). Both Achilles tendons were examined simultaneously using a commercially available CP-flexible 21 × 52 cm coil centered over the Achilles tendons. The patients were examined in a supine position with the feet in a resting position in the coil. The sequence used for the dynamic MRI series was a sagittal Flash 2D with 3 mm slice thickness, TR/TE 50/9 ms, flip angle 40°, FOV 180 × 180 mm, matrix 128 × 256 mm, time of acquisition 31 seconds. The contrast agent (gadopentetate dimeglumine, Magnevist®, Schering or gadodiamid, Omniscan®, Nycomed Amersham), 0.2 mmol/kg body weight, was injected by an auto-injector, 2 ml/second, via a catheter

Table 1 Classification of the level of pain and functional impairment

Intensity	Level	Pain	Level	Performance
Mild	1	None	1	Normal
	2	With extreme exertion only, not intense	1	Normal
Moderate	3	Starts with activity, lasts for 1–2 hours after activity	2	Performance may be affected
	4	With any athletic activity, increase during activity	3	Performance level significantly decreased
Severe	5	Immediately upon any activity involving tendon. Sudden increase in pain if activity is continued, lasts for 12–24 hours	3	Performance markedly curtailed or prevented
	6	During daily activities	4	Unable to participate

Modified from Curwin & Stanish [18].

in the cubital vein followed by 20 ml of saline. The acquisition of the Dynamic MR series was started at the same time as the contrast injection. The Dynamic MR series lasted 5 minutes and 20 seconds, consisting of 5 sets with an interval of 40-seconds followed by two sets with an interval of 80 seconds. Every set had four sagittal slices, two from the symptomatic tendon and two from the contralateral tendon.

Evaluation of dynamic MRI

The Dynamic MRI series of the symptomatic and the contralateral tendons, before and after three months of eccentric training, were evaluated on a Hermes workstation (Nuclear Diagnostics, Stockholm, Sweden). From the two sagittal slices obtained from each Achilles tendon in every set, the most centered one was chosen by visual estimation. A circular ROI with a radius of 2 mm was placed in the thickest part of the tendon, and in the horizontal direction the area with the highest signal was chosen (Figure 1). In the case of no visible signal increase the ROI was placed in the centre of the thickest part of the tendon. The ROI's distance from the upper posterior margin of the calcaneal bone was noted to ensure correct placement of the ROI at the follow up examination. One ROI with a radius of 2 mm was placed in a vessel ventrally of the tendon. One ROI with a radius of 5 mm was placed in the fat ventrally of the tendon. The three ROI:s placed in the first image of the dynamic series were then copied and pasted into the following images of the dynamic series. The signal intensity of each ROI was then plotted as a function of time, reflecting the contrast enhancement. Since signal intensity is a relative value and changes proportionally, the signal intensity at each point of the dynamic series was normalized by dividing the signal intensity of all subsequent intensity values with that obtained at the start of contrast injection (SI_0) (i.e. so that $SI_0 = 1$). The area under the curve (AUC) was then calculated for each ROI from the start of contrast injection until 320 seconds later, using the trapezoid method [22].

$$\begin{aligned}\mathrm{AUC} = {} & (\mathrm{SI}_0 + \mathrm{SI}_1) \times 40\ \mathrm{seconds}/2 \\ & + (\mathrm{SI}_1 + \mathrm{SI}_2) \times 40\ \mathrm{seconds}/2 \\ & + (\mathrm{SI}_2 + \mathrm{SI}_3) \times 40\ \mathrm{seconds}/2 \\ & + (\mathrm{SI}_3 + \mathrm{SI}_4) \times 40\ \mathrm{seconds}/2 \\ & + (\mathrm{SI}_4 + \mathrm{SI}_5) \times 80\ \mathrm{seconds}/2 \\ & + (\mathrm{SI}_5 + \mathrm{SI}_6) \times 80\ \mathrm{seconds}/2 \\ & - \mathrm{SI}_0 \times 320\ \mathrm{seconds}\end{aligned}$$

In addition to AUC, time to peak (i.e. the time from start of contrast injection until maximum signal), SI/s (i.e. the increase of signal intensity per second until maximum signal) and SI% (i.e. the increase in signal between start and peak, expressed in percent) was calculated for each ROI.

Statistical methods and data management

Statistical comparisons in order to test differences between the symptomatic side and the contralateral side and between DEMRI 1 and DEMRI 2 was made by use of paired Student's *t*-test for correlated variables. The Spearman rank order correlation was used in order to test independence between variables. The study employs multiple hypothesis testing, where each hypothesis was analyzed separately and the existence of patterns in and the consistency of the results were considered in the analysis. Probability values (p-value) <0.05 were considered significant.

Results and discussion

Comparison between symptomatic and contralateral ankle in the 14 patients with unilateral symptoms

In the fat ventrally of the symptomatic tendon, AUC, SI/s and SI% was significantly higher than that of the asymptomatic side before, but not after, eccentric training (Table 2). In the tendons there was no statistically significant difference of mean AUC, SI/s, SI% or time to peak between the symptomatic and the contralateral asymptomatic tendons before or after eccentric training. After, but not before training, there was a significantly

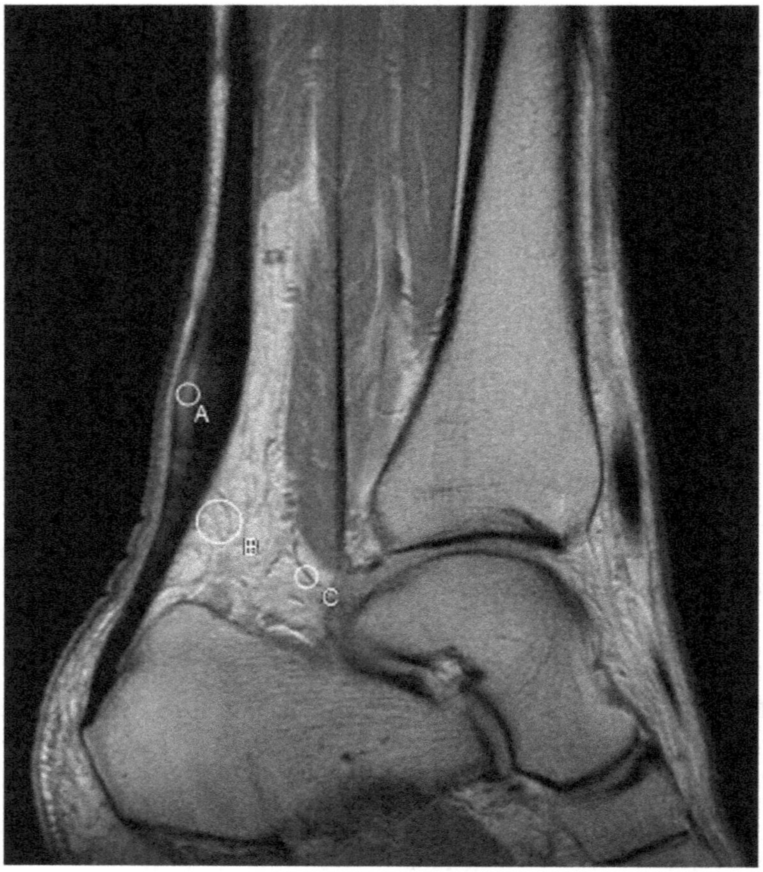

Figure 1 Proton density weighted turbo spin-echo image of the right Achilles tendon prior to eccentric training in a 45-year-old man with chronic Achilles tendinosis. There is a fusiform thickening of the mid-portion of the Achilles tendon with increased intratendinous signal. The measurement regions of interest were placed in: **A** = the tendon, **B** = the fat ventrally of the tendon and **C** = a vessel.

shorter mean time to peak in the vessel on the symptomatic tendon side compared to the asymptomatic side (238 seconds (SD 97) and 289 seconds (SD 59) respectively, $p < 0.05$).

Comparison between before and after eccentric training in 20 patients

Mean AUC, SI/s, and SI% in tendon, fat and vessel did not change during eccentric training. Neither was there any significant change in time to peak in the symptomatic tendons. In the tendon of the contralateral side (the asymptomatic or the least symptomatic tendon) there was a significantly shorter time to peak after training (Table 3).

Pain and performance

The median level of pain decreased from 5 to 3 after training ($p < 0.01$ in all 20 patients and $p < 0.05$ in 14 patients with unilateral symptoms). The median level of performance improved from 4 to 3 after training ($p < 0.01$ in all 20 patients and $p < 0.001$ in 14 patients with unilateral symptoms).

Correlation to pain and performance

Tendon

AUC, time to peak, SI/s, or SI% in the symptomatic tendons ($n = 20$) did not correlate to the level of performance or pain neither before nor after the exercise programme. In the 14 contralateral non-symptomatic tendons, AUC and time to peak correlated to pain before training ($r = 0.53$ and $r = 0.59$ respectively, $p < 0.05$ both) but not after. SI/s or SI% in the 14 contralateral non-symptomatic tendons had no correlation to pain or performance.

Fat

In the 20 symptomatic sides, time to peak in the fat ventrally of the tendon correlated both to pain ($r = 0.61$, $p < 0.01$) and performance ($r = 0.50$, $p < 0.05$) after, but not before, training. Time to peak in the fat had an inverted correlation to performance after training

Table 2 Dynamic contrast enhancement in tendon and in fat ventrally of tendon

	Symptomatic Before training	Contralateral Before training	Symptomatic After training	Contralateral After training
AUC tendon	80 (65) NS	66 (59)	76 (53) NS	52 (65)
SI/s 10^3 tendon	1.8 (1.5) NS	1.6 (0.8)	1.9 (1.2) NS	3.0 (4.7)
SI% tendon	41 (21) NS	38 (18)	38 (19) NS	33 (26)
AUC fat	31 (15)***	20 (11)	26 (15) NS	22 (13)
SI/s x 10^3 fat	0.44 (0.24)*	0.32 (0.13)	0.43 (0.20) NS	0.34 (0.16)
SI% fat	14.5 (7.4)**	9.5 (4.9)	12.1 (6.3) NS	10.6 (5.4)

Mean AUC, SI/s and SI% in the symptomatic and contralateral side measured in the tendon and in the fat ventrally of the tendon before and after eccentric training, in 14 patients with unilateral symptoms. One standard deviation is provided within parenthesis. The significance of mean difference between the symptomatic and contralateral side has been noted. *** = $p < 0.001$, ** = $p < 0.01$, * = $p < 0.05$, NS = Not Significant.

($r = -0.68$, $p < 0.01$) in the 14 contralateral non-symptomatic sides.

Vessel

In the 20 symptomatic sides SI/s in vessel correlated to performance before ($r = 0.4$, $p < 0.05$) but not after training. Time to peak had an inverted correlation to performance in the 20 symptomatic sides ($r = -0.52$, $p < 0.05$). In the 14 contralateral non-symptomatic sides AUC and SI/s in vessel had an inverted correlation to pain after training ($r = -0.53$ and $r = -0.57$ respectively, $p < 0.05$ both).

Discussion

In this study dynamic contrast-enhanced MR imaging was performed in 20 patients with Achilles tendinosis before and after three months of eccentric calf-muscle training. In the fat ventrally of the tendon there was a significantly increased contrast enhancement in the symptomatic side compared to the contralateral non-symptomatic side before treatment but not after three months of treatment. However, in contradiction to this result there was no difference when comparing before to after treatment. Inside the tendon there was no difference of contrast enhancement in the symptomatic tendon compared to the contralateral tendon before or after the training programme. This finding is in disagreement with a previous study by Shalabi et al [23], and a study by Richards et al [20], where both these studies could show an increased AUC on the symptomatic tendon before treatment. This difference might be due to differences in duration of symptoms. The patients in Shalabi's study had a median symptom duration of 12 months compared to the 31 month median duration in our study. In Richards' study the duration was not reported. It might therefore be that the AUC had already returned to baseline due to the relatively long duration of the symptoms in our chronic tendinosis patients at the time of inclusion in our study.

In the present study a stronger contrast enhancement in the fat ventrally of the tendon in the symptomatic compared to the contralateral non-symptomatic tendon side was observed before, but not after three months of treatment. The observed contrast enhancement in the fat ventrally of the symptomatic tendon in the present study may be due to an increased vascularity but also to increased permeability because mean time to peak signal in the fat ventrally of the tendon in the symptomatic side was 40 seconds longer compared to the corresponding vessel (Table 3). Thus, it might be that the vascularity of the areas ventrally to the tendon [4], is an early marker of treatment effect, while the changes in the tendon need longer time to disappear. However, when evaluating the treatment effect by comparing the enhancement before with that of after training no significant effect could be observed, probably due to lack of statistical power. The clinical value of evaluating the vascularity of pretendinous fat is therefore low. The histopathological changes in Achilles tendinosis such as vascular proliferation, focal

Table 3 Mean time to peak contrast enhancement

	Symptomatic Before training	Contralateral Before training	Symptomatic After training	Contralateral After training
Tendon	240 (89)	250 (78)	240 (100) NS	190 (110)*
Vessel	260 (76)	270 (61)	240 (89) NS	270 (78) NS
Fat	300 (64)	300 (57)	290 (53) NS	300 (42) NS

Mean time in seconds from start of contrast injection to peak contrast enhancement in tendon, vessel and in the fat ventrally of the tendon in the symptomatic and contralateral ankle of 20 patients with chronic achilles tendinosis before and after three months of eccentric calf-muscle training. One standard deviation is provided within parenthesis. The p-value comparing time from start to peak contrast enhancement before and after three months of eccentric training has been noted. * = $p < 0.05$, NS = Not Significant.

variation in cellularity, rounded nuclei, abnormal fibre structure, and increased areas of non-collagen extra cellular matrix have previously been shown to correlate with increased intratendinous signal at MRI of the tendon [2,11,17,18,10]. An increased contrast enhancement at MRI in pathologic tissue is thought to reflect an increased vascularity and/or an increased capillary permeability [16,17]. By using ultrasound and colour Doppler an increased vascularity mainly inside but also outside ventrally of the symptomatic tendon has previously been shown [4]. The observed contrast enhancement in the fat ventrally of the symptomatic tendon observed in the present study may thus be due to an increased vascularity. However, in the study by Shalabi et al [23] no correlation between histological increase in vascularity and increased AUC of contrast enhancement could be shown.

In a recent review of loading treatment programmes the majority of studies did not find any association between improved imaging parameters and clinical outcome in Achilles tendinosis [24]. A pilot study evaluating longitudinal microvascularisation of Achilles tendinosis showed that pain is not invariably associated with microvascularity [20]. This may explain the lack of correlation with symptoms in our study. Despite of a significant clinical improvement with both improved performance and decreased pain during the training programme there were almost no significant correlations between dynamic contrast enhancement in the symptomatic tendons to pain or performance. AUC and time to peak measured in the fat ventrally of the tendon at three months after treatment were related to pain and there was a relationship between AUC and SI/s measured in vessel before treatment to performance. There was no significant change of contrast enhancement in tendon, fat or vessel before compared to after 3 months of eccentric training.

In this study 20 patients with chronic achilles tendinosis were studied. In nine of those the tendinosis was sports related, while 11 were idiopathic. Although most of the sports related were due to running (n = 7) the heterogenous material in our study is a limitation. When our study was planned and conducted the questionnaire by Curwin and Stanish was used at our institution. That questionnaire is easier to use for the patients, but to enable comparisons with other studies it might have been better if the VISA-A questionnaire had been used.

The lack of correlation with symptoms indicates that dynamic enhanced MRI is currently not a useful method to evaluate chronic Achilles tendinosis compared to MRI without contrast media. Further development of imaging methods to visualize the pathology at chronic Achilles tendinosis is necessary. For example, the use of ultra short echo time (UTE) at MRI makes it possible to demonstrate features that are not apparent with conventional MRI sequences [25] which may make it possible to quantify the subtle signal changes at Achilles tendinosis and its treatment.

Conclusion

In conclusion there was an increased contrast-media enhancement in the fat ventrally of the tendon in Achilles tendinosis that disappeared after three months of training, but otherwise dynamic contrast enhanced MRI did not show any additional value.

Competing interests

The authors declare that they have no competing interests.

Authors' contributions

Study design was made by AG, AS and TM. Data acquisition was made by AG. Data analysis was made by AG and TB. The manuscript was drafted by AG and all authors have revised it critically. All authors read and approved the final manuscript.

Acknowledgements

Financial support was provided through the regional agreement on medical training and clinical research (ALF) between Stockholm County Council and Karolinska Institutet.

Author details

[1]Department of Clinical Science, Division of Medical Imaging and Technology, Intervention and Technology at Karolinska Institutet, Stockholm SE-141-86, Sweden. [2]Department of Radiology, Karolinska University Hospital in Huddinge, Stockholm SE-141-86, Sweden. [3]Department of Clinical Science, Division of Orthopedics and Biotechnology, Intervention and Technology at Karolinska Institutet, Stockholm SE-141-86, Sweden. [4]Centre for Medical Imaging, Department of Radiology, Oncology and Radiation Sciences Akademiska University Hospital, Uppsala SE-751-85, Sweden.

References

1. Kvist M: **Achilles tendon injuries in athletes.** *Ann Chir Gynaecol* 1991, **80**:188–220.
2. Rolf C, Movin T: **Etiology, histopathology and outcome of surgery in achillodynia.** *Foot Ankle Int* 1997, **18**:565–569.
3. Pufe T, Petersen WJ, Mentlein R, Tillmann BN: **The role of vasculature and angiogenesis for the pathogenesis of degenerative tendons disease.** *Scand J Med Sci Sports* 2005, **15**:211–222.
4. Öhberg L, Lorentzon R, Alfredson H: **Neovascularisation in Achilles tendons with painful tendinosis but not in normal tendons: an ultrasonographic investigation.** *Knee Surg, Sports Traumatol, Arthrosc* 2001, **9**:233–238.
5. Alfredson H, Pietilä T, Jonsson R, Lorentzon R: **Heavy-load eccentric calf muscle training for the treatment of chronic Achilles tendinosis.** *Am J Sports Med* 1998, **26**:360–366.
6. Paavola M, Kannus P, Paakkala T, Pasanen M, Järvinen M: **Long-term prognosis of patients with Achilles tendinopathy. An observational 8-year follow-up study.** *Am J Sports Med* 2000, **28**:634–642.
7. McLauchlan GJ, Handoll HHG: **Interventions for treating acute and chronic Achilles tendinitis.** *Cochrane Database Syst Rev* 2001, **2**:CD000232. 10.1002/14651858.CD000232.
8. Öhberg L, Lorentzon R, Alfredson H: **Ultrasound guided sclerosis of painful neovessels in painful chronic Achilles tendinosis: pilot study of a new treatment.** *Br J Sports Med* 2002, **36**:173–177.
9. Rompe JD, Nafe B, Furia JP, Maffulli N: **Eccentric loading, shock-wave treatment, or a wait-and-see policy for tendinopathy of the main body of tendo Achillis: a randomized controlled trial.** *Am J Sports Med* 2007, **35**:374–383.

10. Åström M, Gentz CF, Nilsson P, Rausing A, Sjöberg S, Westlin N: **Imaging in chronic Achilles tendinopathy: a comparison of ultrasonography, magnetic resonance imaging and surgical findings in 27 histologically verified cases.** *Skeletal Radiol* 1996, **25:**615–620.
11. Movin T, Kristoffersen-Wiberg M, Shalabi A, Gad A, Aspelin P, Rolf C: **Intratendinous alterations as imaged by ultrasound and contrast medium-enhanced magnetic resonance in chronic achyllodynia.** *Foot Ankle Int* 1998, **19:**311–317.
12. O'Connor PJ, Grainger AJ, Morgan SR, Smith KL, Waterton JC, Nash AFP: **Ultrasound assessment of tendons in asymptomatic volunteers: a study of reproducibility.** *Eur Radiol* 2004, **14:**1968–1973.
13. Neuhold A, Stiskal M, Kainberger F, Schwaighofer B: **Degenerative Achilles tendon disease: assessment by magnetic resonance and ultrasonography.** *Eur J Radiol* 1992, **14:**213–220.
14. Shalabi A, Kristoffersen-Wiberg M, Svensson L, Aspelin P, Movin T: **Eccentric training of the gastrocnemius-soleus complex in chronic Achilles tendinopathy results in decreased tendon volume and intratendinous signal as evaluated by MRI.** *Am J Sports Med* 2004, **32:**1286–1296.
15. Gärdin A, Movin T, Svensson L, Shalabi A: **The long-term clinical and MRI results following eccentric calf muscle training in chronic Achilles tendinosis.** *Skeletal Radiol* 2010, **39:**435–442.
16. Brasch R: **New directions in the development of MR imaging contrast media.** *Radiology* 1992, **183:**1–11.
17. Verstraete K, De Deene Y, Roels H, Dierick A, Uyttendaele D, Kunnen M: **Benign and malignant musculoskeletal lesions: dynamic contrast-enhanced MR imaging parametric "first-pass" images depict tissue vascularization and perfusion.** *Radiology* 1994, **192:**835–843.
18. Åström M, Rausing A: **Chronic Achilles tendinopathy: a survey of surgical and histopatological findings.** *Clin Orthop* 1995, **316:**151–164.
19. Movin T, Gad A, Reinholt FP, Rolf C: **Tendon pathology in long standing achillodynia. Biopsy findings in 40 patients.** *Acta Orthop Scand* 1995, **68:**170–175.
20. Richards P, McCall I, Day C, Belcher J, Maffulli N: **Longitudinal microvascularity in Achilles tendinopathy (power Doppler ultrasound, magnetic resonance imaging time-intensity curves and the Victorian Institute of Sport Assessment-Achilles questinnaire): a pilot study.** *Skeletal radiology* 2010, **39:**509–521.
21. Curwin SL, Stanish WD: *Tendinitis: its etiology and treatment.* DC Heath Lexington, MA: Collamore Press; 1984.
22. Ashton M, Björkman I, Emanuelsson B-M: *Grunderna i biofarmaci farmakokinetik.* Uppsala, Sweden: Institutionen för Biofarmaci: Uppsala Universitets Biomedicinska Centrum; 1984.
23. Shalabi A, Kristoffersen-Wiberg W, Papadogiannakis N, Aspelin P, Movin T: **Dynamic contrast-enhanced MR imaging and histopathology in chronic Achilles tendinosis. A longitudinal MR study of 15 patients.** *Acta Radiol* 2002, **43:**198–206.
24. Malliaras P, Barton C, Reeves N, Langberg H: **Achilles and patellar tendinopathy loading programmes. A systematic review comparing clinical outcomes and identifying potential mechanisms for effectiveness.** *Sports Med* 2013, **43:**267–286.
25. Syha R, Martirosian P, Ketelsen D, Grosse U, Claussen CD, Schick F, Springer F: **Magnetization transfer in human Achilles tendon assessed by a 3D ultrashort echo time sequence: Quantitative examinations in healthy volunteers at 3 T.** *ROFO* 2011, **183:**1043–1050.

17

Application of mean-shift clustering to Blood oxygen level dependent functional MRI activation detection

Leo Ai[1*], Xin Gao[2] and Jinhu Xiong[3]

Abstract

Background: Functional magnetic resonance imaging (fMRI) analysis is commonly done with cross-correlation analysis (CCA) and the General Linear Model (GLM). Both CCA and GLM techniques, however, typically perform calculations on a per-voxel basis and do not consider relationships neighboring voxels may have. Clustered voxel analyses have then been developed to improve fMRI signal detections by taking advantages of relationships of neighboring voxels. Mean-shift clustering (MSC) is another technique which takes into account properties of neighboring voxels and can be considered for enhancing fMRI activation detection.

Methods: This study examines the adoption of MSC to fMRI analysis. MSC was applied to a Statistical Parameter Image generated with the CCA technique on both simulated and real fMRI data. The MSC technique was then compared with CCA and CCA plus cluster analysis. A range of kernel sizes were used to examine how the technique behaves.

Results: Receiver Operating Characteristic curves shows an improvement over CCA and Cluster analysis. False positive rates are lower with the proposed technique. MSC allows the use of a low intensity threshold and also does not require the use of a cluster size threshold, which improves detection of weak activations and highly focused activations.

Conclusion: The proposed technique shows improved activation detection for both simulated and real Blood Oxygen Level Dependent fMRI data. More detailed studies are required to further develop the proposed technique.

Keywords: Mean-shift, fMRI, BOLD, Clustering

Background

Functional Magnetic Resonance Imaging (fMRI) is a technique that is used to identify regions of activations in the brain. Techniques based on cross-correlation analysis (CCA) and the General Linear Model (GLM) is commonly used for fMRI data analysis [1-7], however these techniques are not without drawbacks. Both techniques typically perform its calculations on a per voxel basis. This means that each calculation does not take into consideration any relationship that neighboring voxels may have with each other. This has the effect of lowering the sensitivity of the technique when looking for activations. This is especially true in low contrast to noise ratio (CNR) situations.

There has been interest in enhancing fMRI data analysis with cluster size tests. Various techniques have been examined with that intention in mind. Cluster analysis (based on random field theory) is commonly used to help isolate activations [8-10]. K-means clustering [11] is a method where observations are partitioned into "k" number of clusters where each observation belongs to the cluster with the closest mean. Fuzzy clustering [12] is similar to k-means clustering, except that fuzzy clustering takes into consideration that a single observation can belong to more than one cluster. Both K-means and Fuzzy clustering have been examined for improving fMRI data analysis [13-16]. Mean-shift clustering (MSC) is another technique to consider for the same purpose.

* Correspondence: leo-ai@uiowa.edu
[1]Department of Biomedical Engineering, University of Iowa, 200 Hawkins Drive C721 GH, Iowa City, IA 52242, USA
Full list of author information is available at the end of the article

The MSC technique was first introduced by Fukunaga et al. [17] for examining pattern recognition, but the technique was mostly unexplored until more recently [18,19]. The technique has found uses in image processing and vision tasks. Image segmentation has also been explored with this technique on brain images [20]. MSC revolves around a density estimation that is done on a predetermined feature space. Intuitively, the technique works by calculating the mean shift vector, then shifting the kernel as dictated by the mean shift vector. This process is repeated as appropriate until convergence at which time a cluster in the feature space can be identified. By selectively choosing the features used for the feature space, it would be possible to incorporate characteristics of the data that normally would not be part of the analysis with CCA and GLM based techniques. MSC also offers some other advantages with regards to implementation. The technique does not require assumptions to be made about noise distribution. Compared to typical cluster analysis, no hard cut-off in cluster size is required with MSC. Since MSC is based on density estimation of a feature space, it does not make any assumption on the shape of the clusters either as well as allowing different feature spaces to be used to incorporate different characteristics of the data into analysis. These advantages with MSC may allow higher sensitivity when detecting activations for improved results.

To the best knowledge of the authors, MSC has not been closely explored in the application of fMRI activation analysis. As a first step, this study investigates a straight forward application of MSC to fMRI data analysis.

Methods

The proposed MSC technique was evaluated using both simulated and real fMRI data. The data analysis was performed using Cross Correlation Analysis (CCA) to generate a statistical parametric image (SPI). The mean-shift clustering was then applied to a feature space constructed using selected characteristics of the SPI. Comparisons were made among CCA, CCA plus cluster analysis (CCA + CA), and CCA + MSC to examine the application of MSC.

Simulated data

The simulated data was designed to emulate fMRI data using one hundred images, 128 × 128 matrix size, and with a block design of two and a half off/on cycles (20 images per off or on cycle). Activations of various sizes (20 × 20, 10 × 10, 2 × 2 voxels) were inserted onto the data for analysis. Gaussian noise at different CNRs (0.20, 0.40, 0.06, and 0.80) was generated and inserted into the simulated data.

fMRI data

Ten subjects (5 females, 5 males, age 22–32) gave informed written consent with the approval of the University of Iowa's (USA) Institutional Review Board. All subjects reported that they were right-handed, not using medications at the time of scanning, healthy, and had no history of any mental or psychiatric conditions. All ten subjects were scanned at the University of Iowa's Medical Education and Research Facility.

Blood Oxygen Level Dependent (BOLD) fMRI data were acquired on a Siemens 3 T Trio scanner (Siemens Medical Solutions, Erlangen, Germany). A gradient echo EPI pulse sequence was used with the following parameters: TR = 2000 ms, flip angle = 90 degrees, TE = 30 ms, matrix = 64 × 64, FOV = 220 mm, slice thickness = 5 mm with 20% gap, 180 images per run. Each scanning session was composed of seven six-minute runs, though only the first run was used for the purpose of this study. A T1 anatomical scan was also performed with the following parameters: TR = 1590 ms, flip angle = 10 degrees, TE = 3.39 ms, matrix = 128 × 128, FOV = 220 mm, slice thickness = 2 mm.

Unilateral electrical stimulation was delivered to the subject's right median nerve using a Grass S48 stimulator (Grass Technologies, West Warwick, Rhode Island, USA). The stimulation voltage used was 15 volts above the motor threshold, which was individually defined as the minimum voltage required to obtain a thumb twitch. The delivered stimulations were square wave pulses with 0.2 ms duration. A block design of four and a half off/on cycles (40 seconds off, 40 seconds on) with a randomized inter-stimulation interval (ISI) between 1.0-2.0 seconds was used. A randomized ISI was used to reduce any effect that expecting a stimulation occurring with a fixed inter stimulation interval might have on the resulting BOLD signal. The volunteers were asked to passively feel the stimulation, stay still, stay awake, and not actively perform anything else for the duration of the scan.

Mean shift clustering

MSC is based on density estimation of a predetermined multi-modal feature space of image characteristics. Previously used feature spaces, such as perceived color [21,22], are generally not applicable to fMRI analysis since color is not a feature that would be of interest. For this study, a feature space of the estimated Z values of the SPI and the mean voxel values surrounding a voxel (eight neighboring voxels in 2D and twenty six neighboring voxels in 3D) was used as they can be features of interest and incorporating them in the analysis may help with activation detection. The estimated Z values were used because it relates directly to statistical significance, and the mean voxel value of the surrounding voxels were used to take into consideration neighboring effects.

The image features are mapped into a point in a multi-dimension space. The density is calculated within a defined kernel on the feature space. The kernel is moved based on the density gradient in the feature space until the local maximum is found. Points in the feature space associated with the same local maximum are considered to belong to the same cluster, and the calculation is repeated until all points are assigned to a cluster.

Using the Parzen window technique [23], the kernel density estimation at point x can be described by:

$$\hat{f}(x) = \frac{c_k}{nh^d}\sum_{i=1}^{n} k\left(\left\|\frac{x-x_i}{h}\right\|^2\right) \tag{1}$$

where n is the number of data points, c_k is a constant, k is the kernel, h is the kernel size, and d is the number of dimensions in the feature space. The local maximum density is identified at $\nabla\hat{f}(x) = 0$ by moving the kernel based on the gradient ascent in the feature space. Equation 1 can be rewritten as:

$$\nabla\hat{f} = \frac{2c_k}{nh^{d+2}}\sum_{i=1}^{n}(x-x_i)k'\left(\left\|\frac{x-x_i}{h}\right\|^2\right) \tag{2}$$

Assuming g(x) = –k'(x), the gradient density estimator can then be described as:

$$\nabla\hat{f} = \frac{2c_k}{nh^{d+2}}\sum_{i=1}^{n}(x_i-x)g\left(\left\|\frac{x-x_i}{h}\right\|^2\right) \tag{3}$$

$$\nabla\hat{f} = \frac{2c_k}{nh^{d+2}}\left[\sum_{i=1}^{n} g\left(\left\|\frac{x-x_i}{h}\right\|^2\right)\right] \times \left[\frac{\sum_{i=1}^{n} x_i g\left(\left\|\frac{x-x_i}{h}\right\|^2\right)}{\sum_{i=1}^{n} g\left(\left\|\frac{x-x_i}{h}\right\|^2\right)} - x\right] \tag{4}$$

The first term of Equation 4 is proportional to the density estimate computed with the kernel. The second term:

$$m(x) = \frac{\sum_{i=1}^{n} x_i g\left(\frac{x-x_i}{h}\right)}{\sum_{i=1}^{n} g\left(\frac{x-x_i}{h}\right)} - x \tag{5}$$

is the mean shift vector where g is the kernel, h is the kernel size, x is the mean estimate inside the kernel, and x_i is the element inside the kernel. The mean shift vector, m(x), defines how the kernel will move along the density gradient towards the local maximum which corresponds with dense regions in the feature space. This calculation is performed at each data point, shifted by m(x) along the density gradient, and repeated until convergence is reached when local maximum is found. This procedure allows the mean shift clustering technique to identify such locations without having to estimate the probability density function of the associated data. Points associated with the same local maximum belong to the same cluster.

Within the mean-shift vector equation, the parameter that likely has the largest effect on the analysis is the kernel size, h, as differences in kernel sizes can change the density estimates calculated which the MSC technique is based on. While adaptive techniques do exist, a range of kernel sizes will be used to examine how the technique will behave.

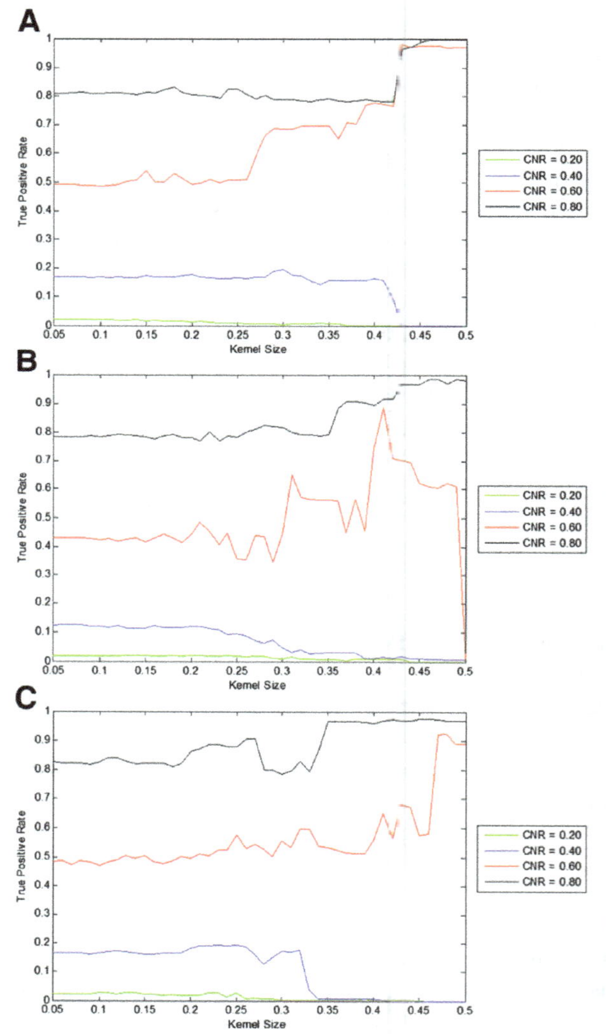

Figure 1 Effect of kernel size on true positive rates for various activation sizes with simulated data. The statistical threshold was held constant at z = 3. A range of kernel sizes was used from 0.05 to 0.50. CNRs used are 0.20, 0.40, 0.60, and 0.80. **A**: 20 × 20 activation size. **B**: 10 × 10 activation size. **C**: 2 × 2 activation size.

Data analysis

The general approach to the proposed MSC analysis method is applying MSC to a feature space constructed using selected characteristics of the SPI generated using CCA. CCA was chosen over GLM because (1) which technique used to generate the SPI is less important for the purposes of this study; (2) the CCA technique allows easy control over the significance level while it is more difficult to do so with GLM.

The real fMRI images were processed using Analysis of Functional NeuroImages (AFNI) [24] and custom Matlab software. As part of the CCA analysis, three-dimensional motion correction was performed to minimize motion effects. All images were normalized to Talairach space (www.bic.mni.mcgill.ca). Constant, linear, and quadratic trends were removed. To investigate the effect of a Gaussian filter on activation detection with MSC, no Gaussian filter and a Gaussian filter with full width half maximum (FWHM) of 4 mm was applied. SPIs were generated for individual subjects.

Comparisons

The proposed method (CCA + MSC) was compared with typical CCA and CCA plus cluster analysis (CCA + CA) procedure using the same simulated data. Activations of sizes 20 × 20, 10 × 10, and 2 × 2 were inserted onto the data to identify how the techniques behave with different sized activations. The total area of all test patterns were maintained to be the same by varying the number of inserted activations. The 2 × 2 activation size can be considered to be a simulation for highly focused activations. Gaussian white noise was generated and inserted into the simulated data at several CNRs (0.20, 0.40, 0.60, 0.80) for examination on how the technique reacts to noise. No additional smoothing filter was applied to the simulated data.

The proposed technique was assessed based on sensitivity and specificity and compared with the performances of the aforementioned techniques (CCA, CCA + CA, CCA + MSC) on simulated data. True positive rate comparisons were used to examine how the different kernel sizes affect the outcomes at various CNRs, and false positive rate comparisons were used to examine the amount of noise that appear in the results of each technique. Since simulated data was used, the ground truth is known, so identifying true and false positive rates is a simple task by comparing detected activations with true activations. Receiver operating characteristic (ROC) curves were drawn to allow a direct comparison of performance between the techniques.

The real fMRI data from ten subjects was analyzed for evaluating CCA, CCA + CA, and CCA + MSC. The three

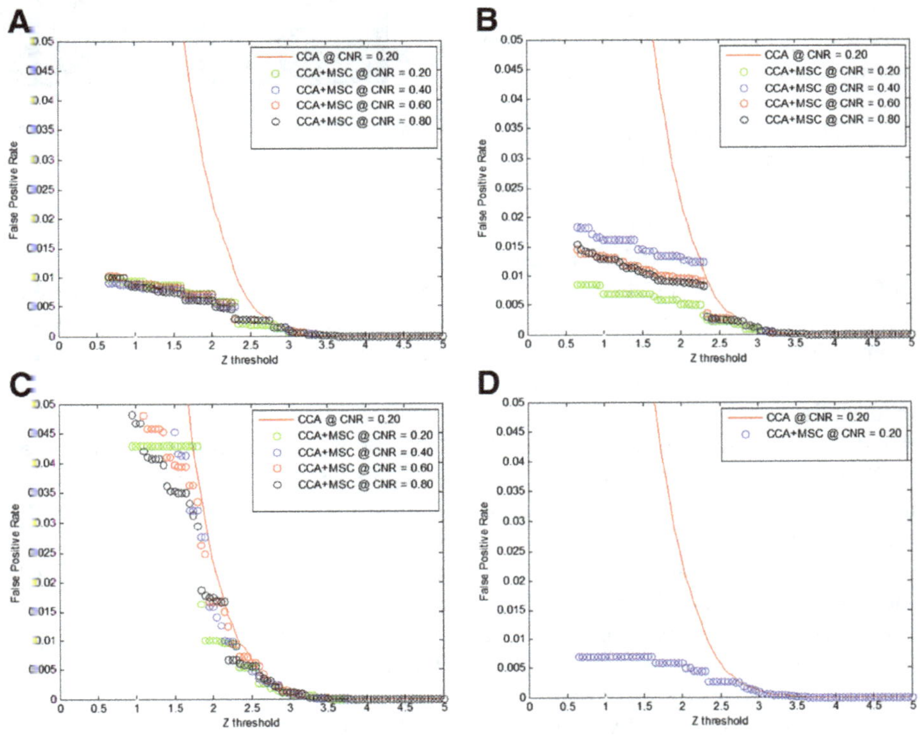

Figure 2 Change of false positive rates at different z thresholds using various activation sizes with simulated data. Kernel size was held constant at 0.20. The z thresholds were varied from 0 to 5. CNRs used are 0.20, 0.40, 0.60, and 0.80. **A**: 20 × 20 activation size. **B**: 10 × 10 activation size. **C**: 2 × 2 activation size. **D**: Activation map consisting of noise only.

techniques are evaluated using both individual fMRI data and averaged fMRI data while controlling significance level at p = 0.01. Different statistical thresholds were determined and applied in order to set the significance level to p = 0.01 for comparison purposes. The threshold for CCA was calculated to be z = 4.8 for the filtered and z = 4.9 for the unfiltered (Bonferroni corrected). The CCA + CA used a threshold of z = 2.6 which was calculated based on a study performed by Xiong et al. [10] with a cluster of threshold of 6 voxels for FWHM = 4 mm and 4 voxels for the unfiltered dataset. The CCA + MSC used a threshold of z = 2 for both filtered and unfiltered data. The z threshold for CCA + MSC was selected based on the results of simulations to achieve an approximate significance level of p = 0.01 (see Results section).

Results

True positive rate comparison

Using the proposed CCA + MSC technique, true positive rates were plotted to examine the behavior of the technique at various kernel sizes. The statistical threshold was applied at Z = 3. The kernel sizes used were in the range of 0.05 to 0.50. The CNRs of the simulated data are 0.20, 0.40, 0.60, and 0.80. The results show the true positive rate is dependent on the kernel size (Figure 1). For low CNRs (0.20, 0.40), the true positive rates start to decline at a kernel size of 0.25. For very high CNR (0.80), the true positive rate remains high across the range of kernel sizes used. The true positive rates also fluctuates as the kernel size is changed, but this is expected as the noise is being randomly generated and changing the kernel size likely has an effect on the cluster assignment of the voxels. Figure 1 indicates that the kernel size can be optimized for enhanced activation detection. A kernel size of 0.20 was used for the rest of the simulated data comparisons as it seems to be an appropriate choice for all CNR and activation sizes.

False positive rate comparison

False positive rates of the proposed CCA + MSC technique were examined while varying the z threshold (0.1 to 5.0) using simulated data. The same CNRs were used. A kernel size of 0.20 was selected based on the true positive rate comparisons (Figure 1). The false positive rate shows significant improvements over CCA at all simulated activation sizes, especially at lower z thresholds (Figure 2). The false positive rate for all activation sizes except 2 × 2 are relatively flat at low z thresholds. It slightly increases as z threshold decreases until z = 0.05 where it increases beyond the figure cap of 0.05 and thus not shown. The 2 × 2 case follows the CCA curve, but an improvement was still seen. The comparison was also made without an activation map (only Gaussian noise), and the result is similar with the 20 × 20 case. Figure 3 shows representative activation maps generated by CCA and CCA + MSC with a z = 1 threshold at CNR = 0.80 with a 0.20 kernel size. It can be visually observed that there are less false activations in the case with CCA + MSC, which agrees with the results from Figure 2.

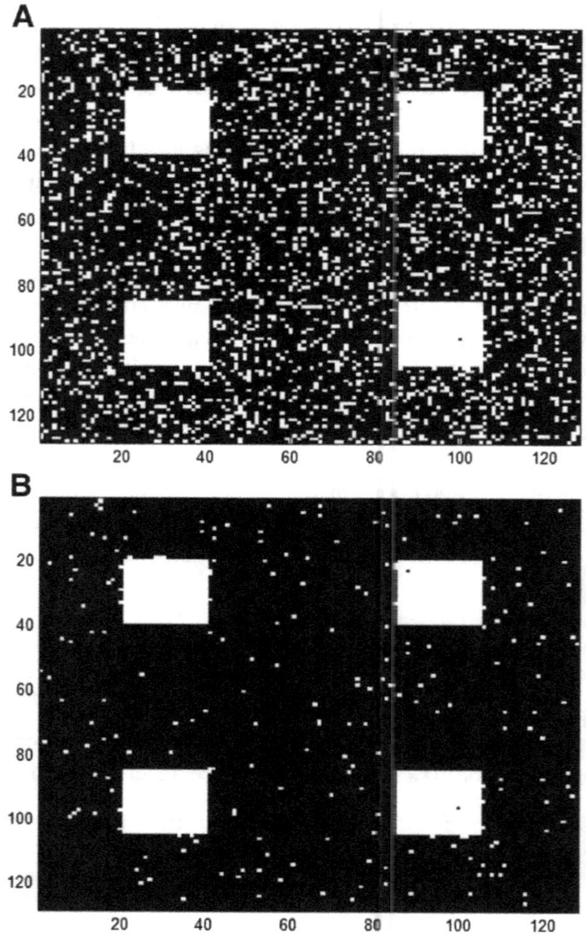

Figure 3 Activation map of CCA and CCA + MSC. A threshold of Z = 1 was applied. CNR of 0.80 was used with kernel size of 0.20. **A**: CCA activation map. **B**: CCA + MSC activation map

ROC comparison of different kernel sizes

A comparison was made with ROC curves between CCA, CCA + CA, and the proposed CCA + MSC at the same CNRs as before, and on the same simulated data set (Figure 4). Simulated data was used for this comparison with the statistical threshold varied from Z = 0.1 to 5.0 and the kernel size being set at 0.10, 0.20, and 0.50. The ROC curves indicate that a properly chosen kernel size, in this case 0.20, show an improvement over both CCA and CCA + CA. If the kernel size (e.g., 0.50) used is too large, essentially no activations are detected using CCA + MSC. If the kernel size (e.g., 0.10) is too small, the CCA + MSC technique is inferior to CCA + CA and

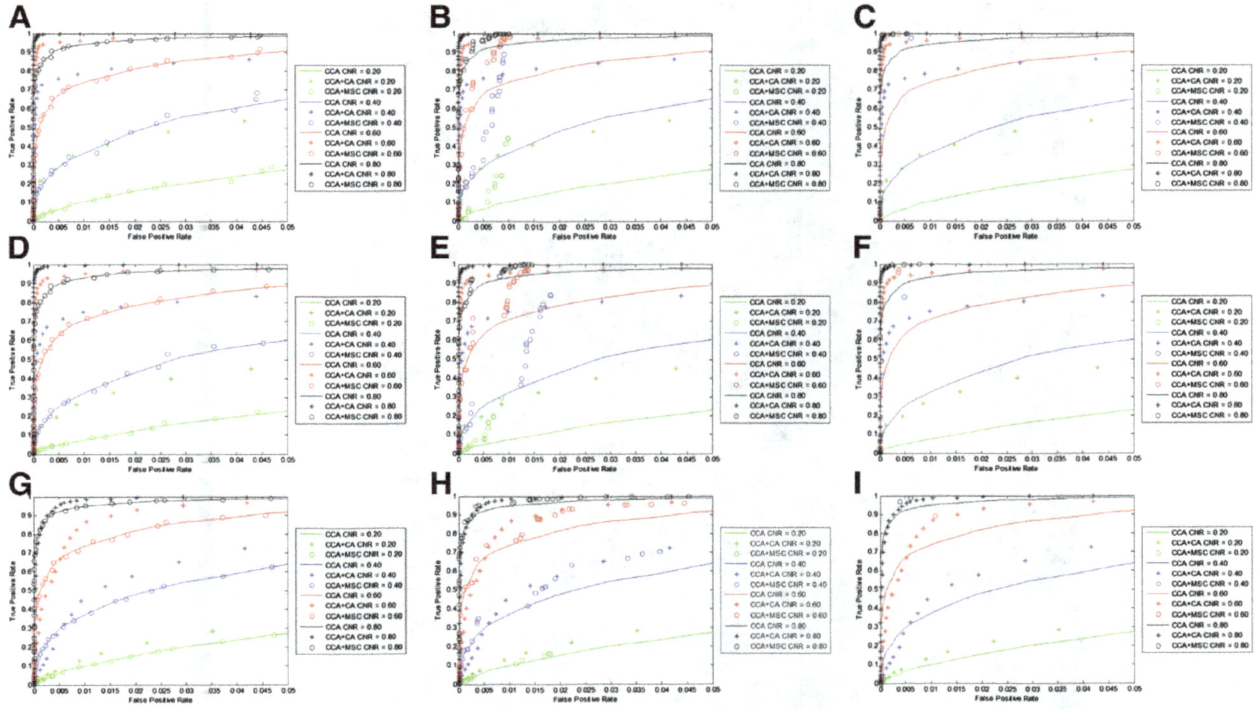

Figure 4 ROC curves for CCA, CCA + CA, CCA + MSC with different kernel sizes and different activation sizes using simulated data. Kernel sizes are 0.10, 0.20, and 0.50. Activation sizes used are 20 × 20, 10 × 10, and 2 × 2. CNRs used are 0.20, 0.40, 0.60, and 0.80. **A**: 20 × 20 activation size, kernel size = 0.10 **B**: 20 × 20 activation size, kernel size = 0.20 **C**: 20 × 20 activation size, kernel size = 0.50 **D**: 10 × 10 activation size, kernel size = 0.10 **E**: 10 × 10 activation size, kernel size = 0.20 **F**: 10 × 10 activation size, kernel size = 0.50 **G**: 2 × 2 activation size, kernel size = 0.10 **H**: 2 × 2 activation size, kernel size = 0.20 **I**: 2 × 2 activation size, kernel size = 0.50.

performs similarly with CCA. This would be consistent with the true positive rate comparison (Figure 1).

The relative performance of CCA + MSC and CCA + CA shows a rather complex relationship. In the 20 × 20 and 10 × 10 cases at kernel size = 0.20, CCA + MSC is better than CCA + CA when the false positive rates range from 0.01 and 0.05. It is inferior to CCA + CA when the false positive rate is below 0.01. Considering that significance levels of p = 0.05 and p = 0.01 are commonly used for activation detection, CCA + MSC should show improvement over CCA + CA in a practical situation. In the 2 × 2 case, CCA + MSC appears to be better than CCA + CA up to a false positive rate of about 0.01, then becomes worse until about 0.02, and the two techniques perform similarly after that.

CCA vs CCA + MSC vs CCA + CA on real data

The real fMRI data was analyzed using CCA, CCA + CA, and CCA + MSC (Figure 5). Activations are expected to be seen on the left M1/S1 region due to the right median nerve stimulation. The CCA + MSC was applied with different kernel sizes of 0.05, 0.10, 0.15, and 0.20. Based on Figure 2, a threshold of z = 2 was applied to achieve a significance of p = 0.01. As shown in Figure 4, the expected activations can be detected using CCA + CA and CCA + MSC with or without a filter in the expected areas while no activation can be seen with standard CCA. Table 1 summarizes the activation volume and average z-scores of the averaged data of both filtered and unfiltered fMRI data. The optimal kernel size for real fMRI is 0.05 and 0.10, which is smaller than the kernel size of 0.20 for the simulated data. Both kernel sizes of 0.05 and 0.10 cases show activations with the 0.10 case showing slightly smaller activations than CCA + CA and the 0.05 case showing larger activations when compared to CCA + CA. In the cases with no filter applied, the detected activations are smaller than their filtered counterparts (Table 1) likely due to the filter enhancing CNR of the SPI, but the non-filtered results generally show the same trends as the filtered results. Individual results are summarized in Table 2 and essentially follow the same trends seen in Table 1. The results show that CCA, CCA + CA, and CCA + MSC (kernel size = 0.10) are statistically different when unfiltered (ANOVA, F = 15.4, $p < 0.05$) or filtered (ANOVA, F = 10.9, $p < 0.05$). The Tukey test further reveals that CCA + MSC is significantly better than CCA in both filtered and unfiltered cases (p = 0.05). The performance of CCA + MSC is statistically similar with CCA + CA (p = 0.05).

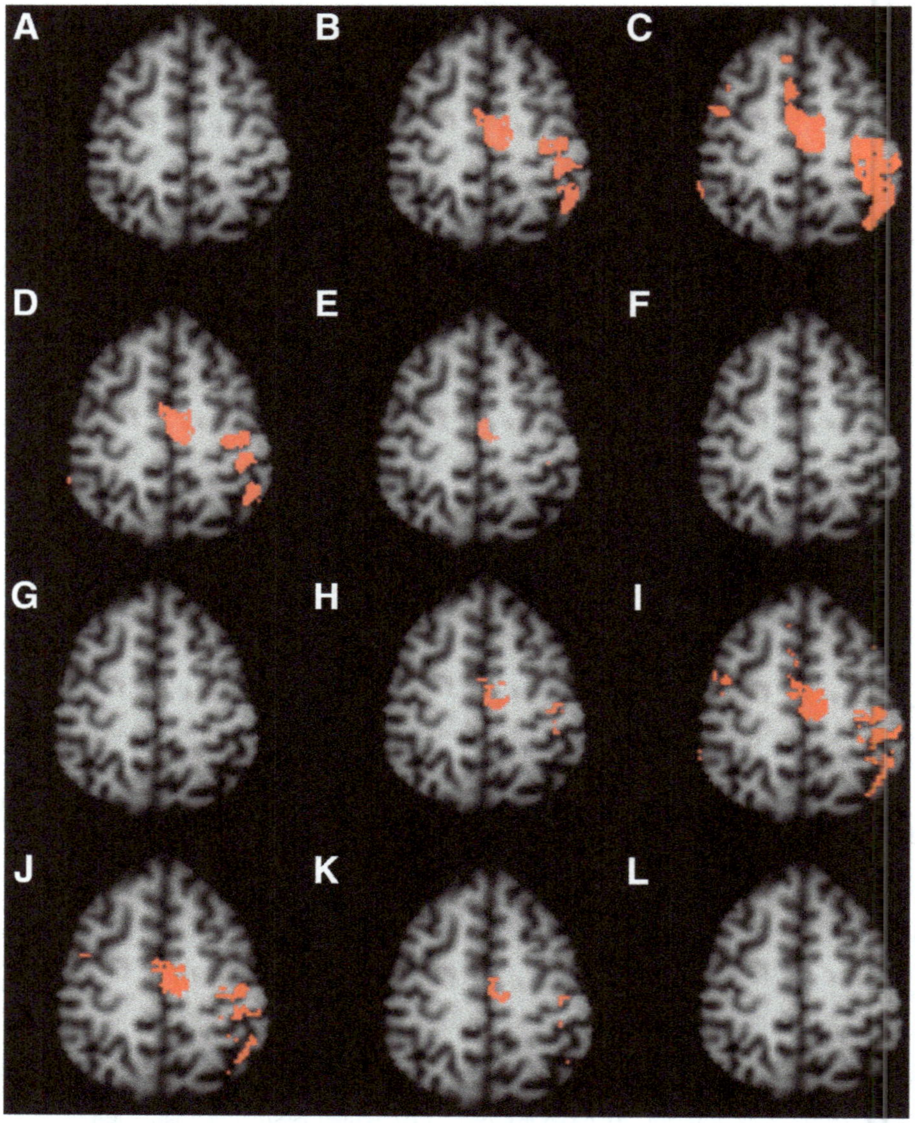

Figure 5 Activation of median nerve stimulation detected with CCA, CCA + CA, CCA + MSC. Significance levels were controlled at p = 0.01 for all images. Z thresholds were changed for each technique based on the significance level. **A**: CCA, Z = 4.8, FWHM = 4 mm **B**: CCA + CA, Z = 2.6, cluster size threshold = 6 voxels, FWHM = 4 mm **C**: CCA + MSC, Z = 2, kernel size = 0.05, FWHM = 4 mm **D**: CCA + MSC, Z = 2, kernel size = 0.10, FWHM = 4 mm **E**: CCA + MSC, Z = 2, kernel size = 0.15, FWHM = 4 mm **F**: CCA + MSC, Z = 2, kernel size = 0.20, FWHM = 4 mm **G**: CCA, Z = 4.8, no filter applied **H**: CCA + CA, Z = 2.6, cluster size threshold = 4 voxels, no filter applied **I**: CCA + MSC, Z = 2, kernel size = 0.05, no filter applied **J**: CCA + MSC, Z = 2, kernel size = 0.10, no filter applied **K**: CCA + MSC, Z = 2, kernel size = 0.15, no filter applied **L**: CCA + MSC, Z = 2, kernel size = 0.20, no filter applied.

Discussion

In this study, the adoption of MSC into fMRI analysis was examined by comparing it to CCA and CCA + CA. The ROC curves (Figure 4) indicate that the proposed MSC technique show an improvement over CCA and an improvement over CCA + CA when the false positive rate is above 0.01 in most cases. The false positive rate comparisons (Figure 2) showed significant improvement over CCA which indicates that CCA + MSC controls noise very well. This allows a lower statistical threshold to be used when identifying activations (Figure 3). Another potential benefit of MSC is for highly focused activation detection since no cluster threshold is applied.

The performance of CCA + MSC depends on the kernel size being used (Figure 1), but determining an optimal range of kernel sizes is not a trivial issue. If the kernel size used is too large, no activations would be detected. Conversely, if the kernel size used is too small, the proposed technique does not show an improvement when compared to CCA and CCA + CA. A proper kernel size needs

Table 1 Activation volume and average Z-scores for averaged real fMRI data

	FWHM = 0 mm		FWHM = 4 mm	
	Volume	Z mean	Volume	Z mean
CCA	0	0.0	0	0.0
CCA + CA	18	3.1	134	3.1
CCA + MSC 0.05	27	2.4	311	2.6
CCA + MSC 0.10	54	2.5	109	3.1
CCA + MSC 0.15	6	3.0	1	4.0
CCA + MSC 0.20	0	0.0	0	0.0

Note: Volumes are measured in voxels.

to be used in order to see an improvement over CCA and CCA + CA. When tested with simulated data, the ROC curves and true positive comparison indicate that a kernel size of roughly 0.20 should show an improvement over CCA (Figure 4), but no activations were detected with real fMRI data if that kernel size is used. Real fMRI data showed activations at kernel size of 0.05 and 0.10 (Figure 5). The difference in optimal kernel sizes between the real and simulated data may be explained by the different noise characteristics of the data. The simulated data is the ideal situation with only Gaussian white noise. Real fMRI data will have multiple noise types such as movement artifacts, physiological noise, noise from the MRI machine itself, etc. It is likely that the optimal kernel size depends on the structure of noise in the data and needs optimized for each individual data set. Future studies are required to examine this issue in more detail.

Significant improvement is seen with CCA + MSC over CCA on the simulated data in the ROC curves in the 20 × 20 and 10 × 10 cases at a kernel size of 0.20 (Figure 4B and E), but this improvement is sudden and is concentrated in the region of false positive rates up to 0.02. While this type of improvement is typically unexpected, it is consistent with Figure 2 where false positive rates are shown to be well controlled (lower than 0.02) at a large range of z thresholds for all cases except the 2 × 2 case. This explains why the data is concentrated in the region of false positive rate up to 0.02.

The false positive rate comparison for the 2 × 2 test pattern showed a curve that is similar to the CCA curve, which does not follow the 10 × 10 and 20 × 20 cases (Figure 2). This may be due to the 2 × 2 case having many more neighboring voxels adjacent the test pattern than the other cases. Four 20 × 20 test patterns were inserted into simulated fMRI images which results in 320 neighboring voxels. To maintain the same total area of the test pattern, four hundred 2 × 2 activations were used, resulting in 3200 neighboring voxels. The 2 × 2 test image has ten times the number of voxels that are directly adjacent the inserted activations when compared to the 20 × 20 test image. It is more likely for falsely activated voxels to be detected by cluster analysis techniques if it is attached to the test pattern than when isolated. More falsely activated voxels are expected to be detected for the 2 × 2 test pattern, thus increasing the false positive rate. Regardless, the proposed technique still shows improvement when compared to CCA in the 2 × 2 case.

CCA + MSC can show an improvement over CCA + CA at a false positive rate of greater than about 0.01 with a kernel size of 0.20 (Figure 4), but this improvement is not seen in the 2 × 2 case where CCA + CA was either superior or about the same as CCA + MSC. A cluster threshold of 4 voxels was used to set the significance value at p = 0.01, which also happens to be the exact size of the simulated activations in the 2 × 2 case.

Table 2 Activation volume and average Z-score for individual subjects on real fMRI data

	FWHM = 0 mm						FWHM = 4 mm					
	CCA		CCA + CA		CCA + MSC		CCA		CCA + CA		CCA + MSC	
Subject	Volume	Z mean	Volume	Z mean	Volume	Z mean	Volume	Z mean	Volume	Z mean	Volume	Z mean
1	45	7.5	163	5.3	212	6.4	128	7.4	200	6.1	200	6.4
2	[illegible]0	6.1	114	4.0	169	3.6	18	6.8	106	3.7	181	3.8
3	5	5.8	106	3.9	136	3.5	18	5.8	181	3.6	258	3.2
4	0	0.0	58	3.3	98	2.9	0	0.0	23	3.4	135	2.9
5	102	6.4	251	4.9	265	4.9	182	6.4	390	5.1	395	5.1
6	78	6.6	159	5.2	165	5.1	137	6.7	285	5.2	301	5.1
7	[illegible]0	6.4	135	4.8	146	4.7	51	6.4	192	4.8	243	5.0
8	0	0.0	41	3.6	60	3.2	6	5.3	64	3.6	88	3.1
9	[illegible]1	6.3	66	5.0	70	4.9	60	6.3	181	4.6	180	4.5
10	239	8.4	292	7.7	299	7.6	402	9.0	424	8.7	423	8.7
Mean	55.9	5.4	138.5	4.8	162.0	4.7	100.2	6.0	204.6	4.9	240.4	4.8
Standard deviation	72.0	2.9	81.8	1.2	78	1.5	123.1	2.3	130.3	1.6	107.7	1.8

Note: Volumes are measured in voxels.

If the activation size was three voxels or a different significance level was used and the voxel cluster threshold was increased, the activations would have been removed by the cluster analysis. The CCA + MSC does not have a cluster threshold and has the potential of better detecting highly focused activations.

The selection of image characteristics used in the feature space should be examined in future studies as the feature space will likely have a large effect on the results as well as the range of acceptable kernel sizes. The image characteristics selected for the featured space used in this study was the estimated Z values found in the SPI and the mean voxel values surrounding a voxel. While there are many methods of constructing a feature space, the feature space used did show an improvement over CCA in the simulated and real fMRI data at the same significance level, it is unknown what image features or what combination of image feature will produce the best feature space for fMRI analysis. The feature space used in this study does not incorporate temporal features in the data or positional features for example. There may be other types and combinations of image features that can be used, and it would certainly be an area of further examination.

The proposed technique has the limitation that the significance levels cannot be easily theoretically calculated (or at least we have not been able to come up with a method of doing so). This presents a particular drawback when doing comparisons. Significance levels can be approximated using simulations as was done in this study, but still may present some challenges when very accurate comparisons are required.

Conclusion

The experiment performed in this study examines the application of MSC to CCA in fMRI activation detection. The results show that an improvement with CCA + MSC can be seen over the typical CCA and CCA + CA analysis technique. The proposed technique maintains a low false positive rate which allows the use of lower statistical thresholds while controlling for noise and helps activation detection in low CNR situations. This also helps in detecting small highly focused activations especially considering that CCA + MSC does not require the application of a cluster size threshold, which is required by most cluster analysis techniques. By nature, CCA + MSC also has the ability to incorporate different image characteristics into a feature space for analysis. These benefits can help to improve activation detection in fMRI data. However, studies in the optimization in kernel size and feature space are needed to further develop the proposed technique. Despite the aforementioned limitations, the proposed technique shows promise in improving fMRI activation detection.

Abbreviations

BOLD: Blood oxygen level dependent; CCA: Cross correlation analysis; CNR: Contrast to noise ratio; fMRI: Functional magnetic resonance imaging; GLM: General linear model; MSC: Mean shift clustering; ROC: Receiver operating characteristic; SPI: Statistical parametric image.

Competing interests

None of the authors have any conflict of interest or competing interests with regard to the findings presented in this manuscript, financial, or otherwise.

Authors' contributions

Study design; LA, GX, JX; Data collection: LA, JX; Analysis; LA, JX; Interpretation; LA, GX, JX. All authors read and approved the final manuscript.

Acknowledgements

Funding for this study was provided by National Institutes of Health (R21 MH 082187-01, R01 DC004290-11), the National Natural Science Foundation of China (81371640), and the International Science and Technology Cooperation Plan of Suzhou, China (SH201210). None of these organizations had a further role in study design, data collection, data analysis, data interpretation, the writing of this manuscript, or the decision to submit the manuscript for publication.

Author details

[1]Department of Biomedical Engineering, University of Iowa, 200 Hawkins Drive C721 GH, Iowa City, IA 52242, USA. [2]Department of Medical Imaging, Suzhou Institute of Biomedical Engineering and Technology, Suzhou, China. [3]Department of Radiology, University of Iowa, Iowa, USA.

References

1. Bandettini P, Jesmanowicz A, Wong E, Hyde J: **Processing strategies for time-course data sets in functional MRI of the human brain.** *Magn Reson Med* 1993, **30**(2):161–173.
2. Boynton G, Engel S, Glover G, Heeger D: **Linear systems analysis of functional magnetic resonance imaging in human.** *J Neurosci* 1996, **16**(13):4207–4221.
3. Bullmore E, Brammer M, Williams SCR, Rabe-Hesketh S, Janot N, David A, Mellers J, Howard R, Sham P: **Statistical methods of estimation and inference for functional MR image analysis.** *Magn Reson Med* 1996, **35**(2):261–277.
4. Calhoun V, Adali T, McGinty V, Pekar J, Watson T, Pearlson G, fMRI Activation in a Visual-Perception Task: **Network of Areas Detected Using the General Linear Model and Independent Components Analysis.** *NeuroImage* 2001, **14**(5):1080–1088.
5. Cohen M: **Parametric Analysis of fMRI Data Using Linear Systems Methods.** *NeuroImage* 1997, **6**(2):93–103.
6. Friston K, Holmes A, Worsley K, Poline J, Frith C, Frackowaik R: **Statistical parametric maps in functional imaging: a general linear approach.** *Hum Brain Mapp* 2004, **2**(4):189–210.
7. Penny W, Friston K: **Mixtures of general linear models for functional neuroimaging.** *IEEE Trans Med Imag* 2003, **22**(4):504–514.
8. Foreman S, Cohen J, Fitzgerald M, Eddy W, Mintun M, Noll D: **Improved assessment of significant activation in functional magnetic resonance imaging (fMRI): use of a cluster-size threshold.** *Magn Res Med* 1995, **33**(5):636–647.
9. Worsley K, Evans A, Marrett S, Neelin P: **Three-dimensional statistical analysis for CBF activation studies in human brain.** *J Cereb Blood Flow Metab* 1992, **12**(6):900–918.
10. Xiong J, Gao J, Lancaster J, Fox P: **Clustered Pixel Analysis for Functional MRI Activation Studies of the Human Brain.** *Hum Brain Mapp* 1995, **4**(4):287–301.
11. MacQueen J: **Some Methods for Classification and Analysis of Multivariate Observatoins.** In *Proceedings of 5th Berkeley Symposium on Mathematical Statistics and Probability.* Berkeley, USA: University of California Press; 1967:281–297.
12. Bezdek J, Ehrlich R, Full W: **FCM: The fuzzy C-Means Clustering Algorithm.** *Comput Geosci* 1984, **10**(2):191–203.

13. Baumgartner R, Scarth G, Teichtmeister C, Somorjai R, Moser E: **Fuzzy Clustering of Gradient-Echo Functional MRI in the Human Visual Cortex Part I: reproducibility.** *J. Magn Reson Imag* 1997, **7**(6):1094–1101.
14. Baumgartner R, Windischberger C, Moser E: **Quantification in functional magnetic resonance imaging: fuzzy clustering vs correlation analysis.** *Magn Reson Imag* 1998, **16**(2):115–125.
15. Moser E, Diemling M, Baumgartner R: **Fuzzy clustering of gradient-echo functional MRI in the human visual cortex. Part II: quantification.** *J Magn Reson Imag* 1997, **7**(6):1102–1108.
16. Singh M, Patel P, Khosla D, Kim T: **Segmentation of functional MRI by K-Means Clustering.** *IEEE Trans Nucl Sci* 1996, **43**(3):2030–2036.
17. Fukunaga K, Hostetler L: **The Estimation of the Gradient of a Density Function, with Applications in Pattern Recognition.** *IEEE Trans Inf Theory* 1975, **21**(1):32–40.
18. Cheng Y: **Mean shift, Mode seeking, and Clustering.** *IEEE Trans Pattern Anal Mach Intell* 1995, **17**(8):790–799.
19. Dorin C, Peter M: **Mean shift: a robust approach towards feature space analysis.** *IEEE Trans Pattern Anal Mach Intell* 2002, **24**(5):603–619.
20. Mayer A, Greenspan H: **An Adaptive Mean-Shift Framework for MRI Brain Segmentation.** *IEEE Trans Med Imag* 2009, **28**(8):1238–1250.
21. Connolly C: **The relationship between colour metrics and the appearance of three-dimensional coloured objects.** *Color Res Appl* 1996, **21**:331–337.
22. Wyszecki G, Stilles W: *Color Science: Concepts and Methods, Quantitative Data, and Formulae.* New York: J Wiley; 1982.
23. Parzen E: **On Estimation of a Probability Density Function and Mode.** *Ann Math Statist* 1962, **33**(3):1065–1076.
24. Cox R: **AFNI: Software for Analysis and Visualition of Functional Magnetic Resonance Neuroimages.** *Comput Biomed Res* 1996, **29**(3):169–173.

Automatic segmentation of myocardium at risk from contrast enhanced SSFP CMR: validation against expert readers and SPECT

Jane Tufvesson[1,2], Marcus Carlsson[1], Anthony H. Aletras[1,3], Henrik Engblom[1], Jean-François Deux[4], Sasha Koul[5], Peder Sörensson[6], John Pernow[6], Dan Atar[7], David Erlinge[5], Håkan Arheden[1] and Einar Heiberg[1,2*]

Abstract

Background: Efficacy of reperfusion therapy can be assessed as myocardial salvage index (MSI) by determining the size of myocardium at risk (MaR) and myocardial infarction (MI), (MSI = 1-MI/MaR). Cardiovascular magnetic resonance (CMR) can be used to assess MI by late gadolinium enhancement (LGE) and MaR by either T2-weighted imaging or contrast enhanced SSFP (CE-SSFP). Automatic segmentation algorithms have been developed and validated for MI by LGE as well as for MaR by T2-weighted imaging. There are, however, no algorithms available for CE-SSFP. Therefore, the aim of this study was to develop and validate automatic segmentation of MaR in CE-SSFP.

Methods: The automatic algorithm applies surface coil intensity correction and classifies myocardial intensities by Expectation Maximization to define a MaR region based on *a priori* regional criteria, and infarct region from LGE. Automatic segmentation was validated against manual delineation by expert readers in 183 patients with reperfused acute MI from two multi-center randomized clinical trials (RCT) (CHILL-MI and MITOCARE) and against myocardial perfusion SPECT in an additional set ($n = 16$). Endocardial and epicardial borders were manually delineated at end-diastole and end-systole. Manual delineation of MaR was used as reference and inter-observer variability was assessed for both manual delineation and automatic segmentation of MaR in a subset of patients ($n = 15$). MaR was expressed as percent of left ventricular mass (%LVM) and analyzed by bias (mean ± standard deviation). Regional agreement was analyzed by Dice Similarity Coefficient (DSC) (mean ± standard deviation).

Results: MaR assessed by manual and automatic segmentation were 36 ± 10 % and 37 ± 11 %LVM respectively with bias 1 ± 6 %LVM and regional agreement DSC 0.85 ± 0.08 ($n = 183$). MaR assessed by SPECT and CE-SSFP automatic segmentation were 27 ± 10 %LVM and 29 ± 7 %LVM respectively with bias 2 ± 7 %LVM. Inter-observer variability was 0 ± 3 %LVM for manual delineation and -1 ± 2 %LVM for automatic segmentation.

Conclusions: Automatic segmentation of MaR in CE-SSFP was validated against manual delineation in multi-center, multi-vendor studies with low bias and high regional agreement. Bias and variability was similar to inter-observer variability of manual delineation and inter-observer variability was decreased by automatic segmentation. Thus, the proposed automatic segmentation can be used to reduce subjectivity in quantification of MaR in RCT.

(Continued on next page)

* Correspondence: einar.heiberg@med.lu.se
[1]Department of Clinical Physiology, Skåne University Hospital in Lund, Lund University, Lund, Sweden
[2]Department of Biomedical Engineering, Faculty of Engineering, Lund University, Lund, Sweden
Full list of author information is available at the end of the article

(Continued from previous page)

Keywords: Quantification, Myocardial salvage, Randomized clinical trials, Expectation maximization, A priori information, Surface coil correction

Background

Myocardium at risk (MaR) is defined as the ischemic myocardium during coronary artery occlusion, at risk of infarction if the blood flow in the occluded artery is not restored in time. The myocardial infarction evolves during time to treatment and if blood flow is not restored in time the whole region of MaR becomes myocardial infarction (MI). If both the size of MaR and final MI size is determined, the efficacy of reperfusion therapy can be assessed as myocardial salvage index (MSI = 1-MI/MaR). By using MSI instead of MI size alone the number of patients needed in clinical trials can be reduced [1] since MI size is related to MaR which is specific for each patient and coronary occlusion.

Cardiovascular magnetic resonance (CMR) is considered gold standard for assessment of infarct size by late gadolinium enhancement (LGE) [2]. Myocardial perfusion SPECT is considered gold standard for assessment of MaR but requires an radioactive isotope to be injected before the blood a flow is restored in occluded artery and imaging is performed only hours after the treatment. By CMR MaR can be assessed by either T2-weighted imaging [3] or contrast enhanced steady state free precession (CE-SSFP) [4] and both have been validated against SPECT for assessment of MaR up to one week after MI [4, 5]. Recently, both T2-weighted imaging and CE-SSFP have been used to determine myocardial salvage in two multi-center cardioprotective studies, CHILL-MI [6] and MITOCARE [7]. In these multi-center trials CE-SSFP was shown to provide significantly better diagnostic image quality than T2-weighted images and to be more robust across vendors [8]. CE-SSFP may therefore be more suitable than T2-weighted imaging for quantification of MaR in multi-center settings.

An automatic segmentation algorithm is preferable for objective quantification in order to reduce subjectivity as well as time required for image analysis. Several algorithms have been developed and validated for automatic segmentation of MI size in LGE images [3, 9, 10]. Two automatic algorithms have been developed and validated in T2-weighted images, one specifically for MaR [11] and one for edema [12]. However, no algorithm has been developed yet for quantification of MaR in CE-SSFP images. Automatic quantification of MaR in T2-weighted images has been shown to yield more accurate results when utilizing Expectation Maximization (EM) to classify myocardial intensities and adding an *a priori* model of the perfusion territories compared to thresholding methods such as two standard deviations (2SD) from remote, full width half maximum (FWHM) and Otsu's method for quantification of MaR in T2-weighted images [11]. Therefore, the aim of this study was to develop and validate this automatic segmentation algorithm for MaR in CE-SSFP.

Methods

Study population and design

For validation of the automatic algorithm, patients with first time ST-elevation myocardial infarction (STEMI) treated with percutaneous coronary intervention (PCI) who had undergone CMR examination with CE-SSFP and LGE images of diagnostic quality as a part of the recently published clinical cardioprotection trials CHILL-MI [6] ($n = 92$) and MITOCARE [7] ($n = 91$) were included ($n = 183$). Patients underwent CMR imaging within 2-6 days following acute MI treated with PCI. Inclusion and exclusion criteria for each of the clinical trials have been previously published [6, 13]. In short, all patients had clinical signs of acute myocardial infarction defined as clinical symptoms and ECG signs consistent with ST-elevation infarction or new onset of left bundle branch block (LBBB), were ≥ 18 years old and had symptom duration of less than 6 h. Patients with a history of previous myocardial infarction or history of coronary revascularization were excluded.

For validation against an independent reference method of imaging MaR, an additional set of patients who had undergone both CE-SSFP CMR and single photon emission computed tomography (SPECT) ($n = 16$) [4] were included in this study. Inclusion and exclusion criteria for this cohort have also been previously published [4]. In short, all patients had clinical signs of acute myocardial infarction defined as clinical symptoms and ECG signs consistent with ST-elevation infarction and chest pain ≥ 30 min and ≤ 9 h. Patients with a history of previous myocardial infarction or history of coronary revascularization were excluded.

Imaging

All CMR examinations were performed on 1.5 T scanners from Philips (Philips Healthcare, Best, The Netherlands), Siemens (Siemens AG, Erlangen, Germany) or GE (GE Healthcare, Waukesha, WI, USA). For visualization of

MaR and evaluation of left ventricular function, CE-SSFP cine images were obtained approximately 5 min after intravenous injection of 0.2 mmol per kilogram of body weight of an extracellular gadolinium-based contrast agent [4, 6, 13]. The slice thickness was 8 mm with no slice gap. In-plane resolution was typically 1.5 x 1.5 mm. Typically, 20-30 CE-SSFP images were acquired per cardiac cycle. For infarct visualization LGE images covering the entire left ventricle were acquired approximately 15 min after injection of the gadolinium-based contrast agent. The LGE-images were acquired using an inversion-recovery gradient-recalled echo sequence with a slice thickness of 8 mm with no slice gap [14]. In-plane resolution was typically 1.5 x 1.5 mm. Inversion time was manually adjusted to null the signal of viable myocardium. Surface coil intensity correction was not mandatory across vendors and sites.

SPECT was performed in the additional set of 16 patients. Prior to opening the occluded vessel an intravenous injection of ^{99m}Tc-tetrofosmin body weight adjusted (350-700 MBq) was administered to the patient. Myocardial perfusion SPECT imaging was performed within four hours to visualize and quantify MaR using either of two dual head cameras: GE (Ventri, GE Healthcare, Waukesha, WI, USA) or Sopha (DST-XL, Sopha Medical Vision, Bue, Cedex, France). Typical pixel size was 6.4 x 6.4 x6.4 mm (GE) and 3 x 3 x 3 mm (Sopha). Short axis images were reconstructed semi-automatically on the workstation for each camera.

Image analysis

Both CMR and SPECT images were analyzed using the software Segment (http://segment.heiberg.se) [15].

In CE-SSFP images, MaR was manually assessed from short-axis images according to previously described methods [4, 6, 7]. In short, the left ventricular myocardium was defined by manually delineating the epicardial and endocardial borders both at end-diastole and at end-systole as previously described. Hyper-intense regions within the myocardium in CE-SSFP images were manually delineated for assessment of MaR. Hypointense myocardium within the area of increased signal intensity was regarded as microvascular obstruction [16] and was included in the MaR. The delineation of each data set was performed by one of three primary observers with a quality control of the delineations by a second opinion for each case. Different opinions for the delineation were resolved in consensus between all three observers when necessary. All three observers had long experience in the field of CMR (HE, MC and HA with 14, 15 and 20 years of experience, respectively). MaR was expressed as percent of left ventricular mass (%LVM) [17]. In a subset of 15 patients from the multi-center studies, second observer analysis was performed to evaluate inter-observer variability (MC vs. HE).

In LGE images, infarct was delineated from the short-axis images according to a previously validated method [9]. In short, the endocardial and epicardial borders were traced manually with exclusion of the papillary muscles. The LGE myocardium was defined using a previously validated automatic segmentation algorithm [9] which is based on a 1.8SD from remote threshold, region analysis and a weighted summation according to pixel intensities to take partial volume effects into consideration. Manual adjustments were made when obvious image artefacts caused misinterpretation by the automatic algorithm and to include micro vascular obstruction when not detected by the algorithm. Hypointense regions within the region of LGE as a sign of microvascular obstruction [16], were included in the analysis as 100 % infarction.

In SPECT images, MaR was delineated by use of an 55 % threshold [18] and manual corrections after automatic delineation of epicardial and endocardial borders [19]. MaR was expressed as percent of left ventricular mass (%LVM).

Image quality was manually assessed as (1) non-diagnostic, (2) acceptable or (3) good. Acceptable and good images were considered to be of diagnostic quality and only CE-SSFP images with diagnostic quality and full coverage of the left ventricle were included in this study as test set ($n = 183$, Additional file 1: Figure S1) and additional set ($n = 16$). Patient characteristics of the test set and additional set are reported in Table 1.

Automatic segmentation algorithm

The automatic segmentation algorithm was originally developed for segmentation of MaR in T2-weighted images [11] and has in this study been developed for CE-SSFP images. Maximal extent models of perfusion territories for each coronary artery [11] were defined by expert observers and used to define remote and culprit region. The maximal extent models correspond to the MaR region of proximal occlusions and takes anatomy variations between patients into consideration. As input to the automatic algorithm, the manual delineation of

Table 1 Patient characteristics from test set $n = 183$

	Mean ± SD	(Min,max)
Heart rate [beats/min]	63 ± 12	(31, 111)
End diastolic volume [ml]	173 ± 43	(32, 336)
End systolic volume [ml]	94 ± 32	(20, 240)
Ejection fraction [%]	43 ± 9	(19, 70)
Left ventricular mass [g]	124 ± 28	(25, 252)
Infarct size [%LVM]	17 ± 10	(2, 47)
Microvascular obstruction [%LVM]	3 ± 5	(0, 27)

endocardial and epicardial borders is used and the user defines the culprit artery as either left anterior descending artery (LAD), left circumflex artery (LCx), right coronary artery (RCA), or left main artery (LM) based on the overall appearance of the hyper enhanced region and defines right ventricular insertion points in CE-SSFP and LGE images, to find how to rotate the maximal extent model.

The automatic algorithm consist of four processing blocks after user input as shown in Fig. 1, 1) surface coil intensity correction, 2) classification of myocardial intensities by Expectation Maximization (EM) [20], 3) definition of MaR region based on *a priori* regional criteria, and 4) incorporation of infarct region from LGE images. Surface coil intensity correction is applied as a second order linear correction based on the intensities in the blood pool and remote myocardium to be able to account for intensity gradient proportional to the squared coil distance. Classification of myocardial intensities is performed using the EM-algorithm to overcome varying contrast and noise level between patients, centers and vendors. The EM-algorithm estimates the mean and standard deviation of intensity for normal myocardium and myocardium at risk based on the intensity histogram and was initialized based on the maximal extent model. Myocardium at risk was defined as a continuous region within the maximal perfusion territory of the culprit artery and assumed to be transmural. These *a priori* regional criteria were implemented by applying the classification by EM sector wise for sectors within the maximal extent model. The myocardium is divided into 24 sectors circumferentially. Further *a priori* information was implemented by using the infarct region from LGE images to define possible regions of microvascular obstruction as MaR despite the hypoenhancement. The original algorithm for T2-weighted images [11] was based on intensity classification by Expectation Maximization (EM) and utilization of a priori information on MaR. Surface coil intensity correction and incorporation of the infarct region from LGE images was added in the new algorithm based on qualitative assessment of the CE-SSFP images. The new segmentation algorithm was named "Segment MaR CE-SSFP" and was implemented in the cardiac image analysis software Segment [9]. The algorithm will be made freely available at time of publication (http://segment.heiberg.se) and each processing block of the algorithm is further described in the Appendix.

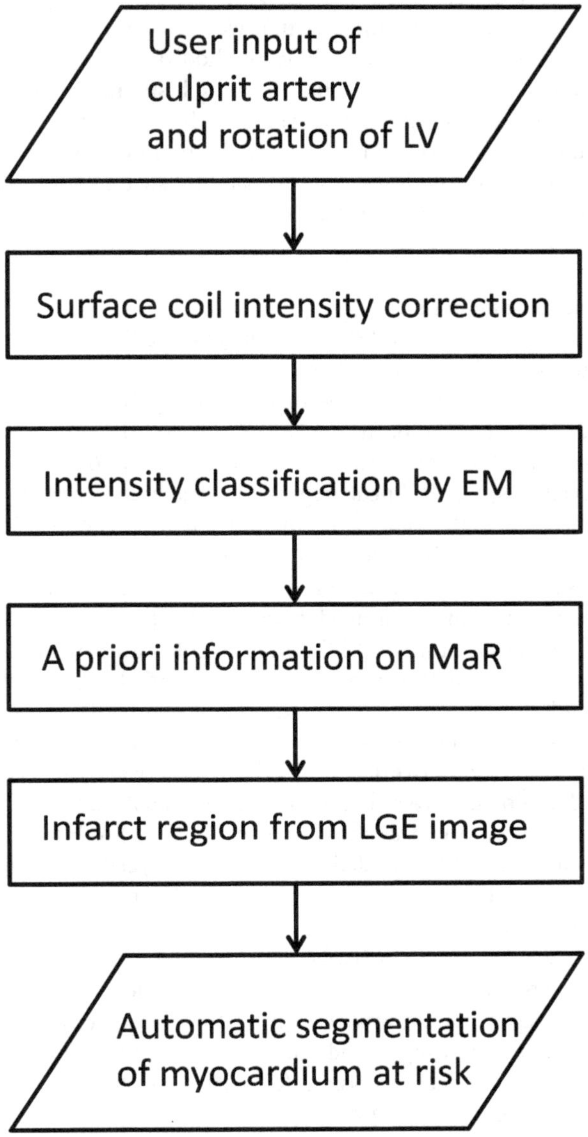

Fig. 1 Automatic segmentation algorithm. The new automatic algorithm for segmentation of myocardium at risk (MaR) in CE-SSFP lets the user define the culprit artery and the rotation of the left ventricle as input. The algorithm consists of four processing blocks, surface coil intensity correction, intensity classification by Expectation Maximization (EM), segmentation based on a priori information on MaR and incorporation of infarct region from LGE images

Comparison to other automatic threshold methods

The new automatic segmentation method was compared to three direct threshold methods which have been used for quantification of MaR in T2-weighted imaging [21, 22], two standard deviations from remote (2SD) [23, 24], full width half maximum intensity (FWHM) [25] and Otsu [26]. All methods used the same manual delineation of endocardium and epicardium. The 2SD threshold method estimates an intensity threshold from a remote region as the mean plus two standard deviations of the intensity within the remote region. The remote region was defined as the region outside the maximal extent model of the culprit artery [11]. The FWHM threshold method [27] estimates an intensity threshold from a remote region as midway between the mean intensity within the remote region and the maximal intensity within the myocardium. The remote region was defined in the same way as for 2SD. The threshold method of Otsu [28] estimates the intensity threshold from the histogram of all intensities to get minimal variance both above and below the threshold. For all three methods the intensity threshold was calculated and applied slice by slice as generally applied in T2-weighted images to account for the intensity gradient across slices.

Statistical analysis

In the test set ($n = 183$) quantification of MaR by the automatic Segment MaR CE-SSFP algorithm was compared to the manual delineation using Bland-Altman bias (mean ± standard deviation), limits of agreement ([mean - 1.96 standard deviations; mean + 1.96 standard deviations]), and linear regression analysis (correlation coefficient). Regional agreement to manual delineation was evaluated by calculating Dice similarity coefficient (DSC) [29] (mean ± standard deviation). Dice similarity coefficient can be derived from the kappa statistics for classification of pixels [30] and is calculated as two times the volume of the intersection of the MaR regions divided by the sum of the volumes of the MaR regions. The DSC is therefore 0 if the regions do not overlap and 1 if the regions overlap perfectly. Bias, linear regression and regional agreement was similarly analyzed for the three automatic threshold methods, 2SD, FWHM and Otsu. Bias to manual delineation was analyzed separately for each of the three camera vendors for the automatic algorithm.

In a subset of 15 patients from the multicenter studies, inter-observer analysis of manual delineation and automatic segmentation was performed. Inter-observer analysis was assessed using Bland-Altman bias (mean ± standard deviation), linear regression (correlation coefficient) and regional agreement DSC (mean ± standard deviation) for manual delineation and automatic segmentation. Bias, linear regression and regional agreement was also assessed for automatic segmentation against manual delineation in the subset for comparison to inter-observer variability.

In the additional set ($n = 16$), quantification of MaR in CE-SSFP images by the automatic Segment MaR CE-SSFP algorithm and manual delineation was compared to quantification of MaR in SPECT using bias (mean ± standard deviation) and linear regression analysis (correlation coefficient).

The added value of each of the four processing blocks in the automatic algorithm described above was analyzed using bias (mean ± standard deviation), linear regression analysis (correlation coefficient), regional agreement DSC (mean ± standard deviation) and visualized by box-whisker plot of median, upper quartile, lower quartile, minimum, maximum and outliers. Two sided paired t-test of bias and DSC were performed for each processing block in comparison to the first block and the previous block with Bonferroni correction.

Results

In the test set ($n = 183$) MaR assessed by manual delineation in CE-SSFP was 36 ± 10 % LVM and MaR assessed by Segment MaR CE-SSFP automatic segmentation was 37 ± 11 %LVM. Bias was 1 ± 6 %LVM [-11; 14] %LVM, R = 0.83 and regional agreement DSC 0.85 ± 0.08 when Segment MaR CE-SSFP was compared to manual delineation (Fig. 2, Table 2). Figure 3 shows MaR in CE-SSFP at end-distole and end-systole with manual delineation and automatic segmentation by Segment MaR CE-SSFP. The bias was lower, regression stronger and regional agreement higher for Segment MaR CE-SSFP than for the threshold methods of 2SD, FWHM and Otsu (Fig. 2, Table 2). Bias to manual delineation analyzed per scanner vendors was 0 ± 7 %LVM, 2 ± 6 %LVM, and 2 ± 7 %LVM, for automatic segmentation in images from GE ($n = 23$), Philips ($n = 76$), and Siemens ($n = 84$), respectively. Inter-observer variability for manual delineation in CE-SSFP ($n = 15$) was 0 ± 3 %LVM compared to a bias between manual delineation and Segment MaR CE-SSFP of 2 ± 6 %LVM and inter-observer variability of Segment MaR CE-SSFP of -1 ± 2 %LVM (Table 3).

In the additional set of patients ($n = 16$), MaR assessed by SPECT was 27 ± 10 %LVM. In CE-SSFP MaR was by manual delineation 28 ± 7 %LVM and by Segment MaR CE-SSFP 29 ± 7 %LVM. Bias against SPECT was 1 ± 5 %LVM (R = 0.90) for CE-SSFP by manual reference delineation and 2 ± 7 %LVM (R = 0.73) by Segment MaR CE-SSFP (Fig. 4).

A significant difference in regional agreement DSC was shown for each of the processing blocks of the Segment MaR CE-SSFP algorithm even though the difference in bias %LVM was not significant (Fig. 5, Table 4).

Discussion

This study has presented an automatic algorithm for quantification of MaR in CE-SSFP images, validated against manual delineation in 183 patients from two multi-center, multi-vendor studies and against SPECT, as reference method, in 16 patients. The proposed automatic segmentation, Segment MaR CE-SSFP, shows low bias and variability, strong correlation and high regional agreement compared to manual delineation and SPECT. The Segment MaR CE-SSFP algorithm was shown superior to thresholding methods (2SD, FWHM and Otsu).

Technical aspects

The added value of each processing block was shown significant by regional agreement DSC even though a significant difference in bias was only seen when bias

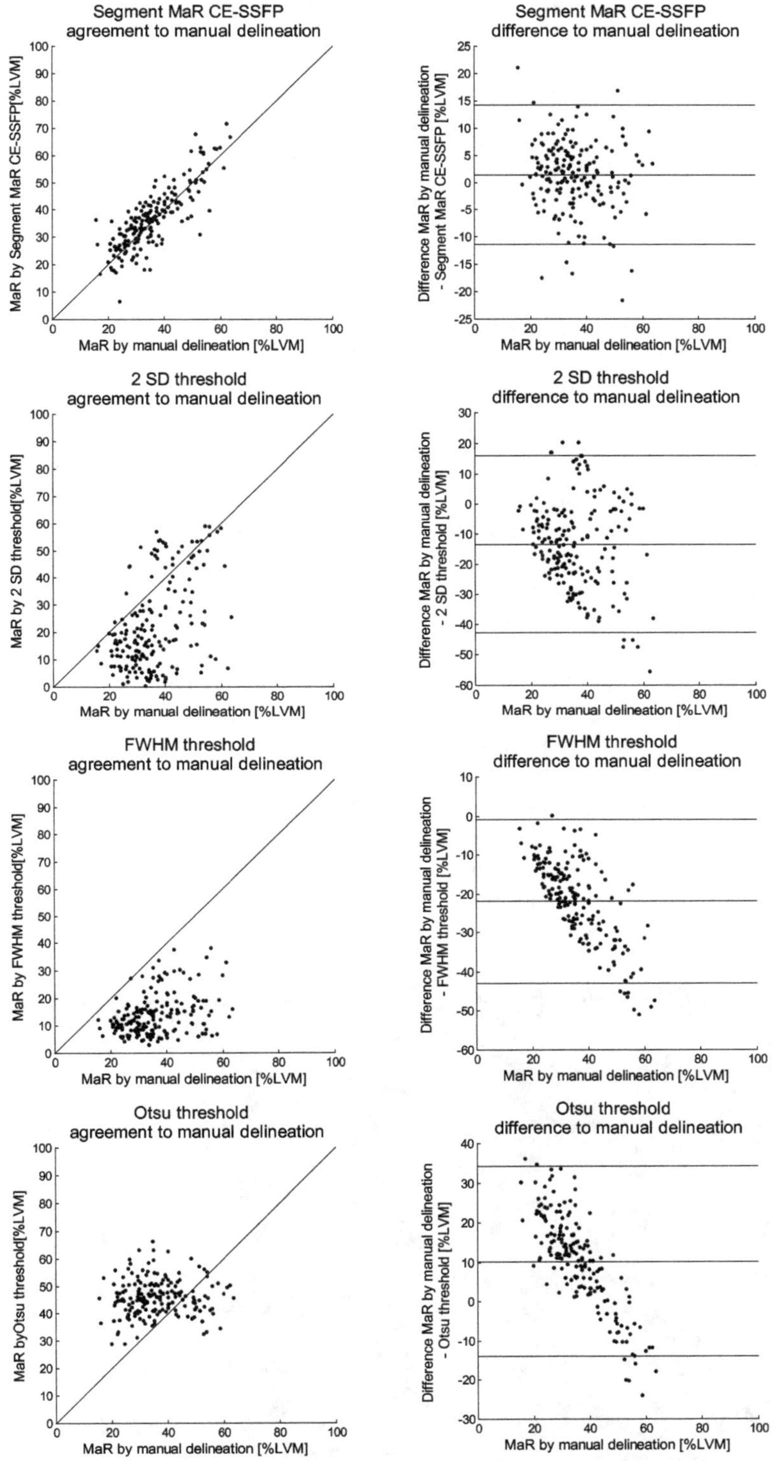

Fig. 2 Correlation and bias for automatic segmentation and threshold methods against manual delienation. Correlation of MaR as % of LVM (left column) and Bland-Altman plot of MaR bias as % of LVM (right column) for the automatic segmentation algorithm (first row), threshold of 2SD from remote (second row), FWHM (third row) and Otsu (fourth row), all against manual delineation. The line of identity is shown as a solid line for all correlations plots and mean bias (solid line) and mean ± two standard deviations (dashed line) is shown for all Bland-Altman plots

Table 2 Results from test set $n = 183$ for automatic Segment MaR CE-SSFP segmentation and threshold methods against manual delineation

	MaR bias [% of LVM]	Regression *R*-value	DSC
Segment MaR CE-SSFP	1 ± 6	0.83	0.85 ± 0.08
2SD threshold	-13 ± 15	0.47	0.54 ± 0.27
FWHM threshold	-22 ± 11	0.42	0.42 ± 0.21
Otsu threshold	10 ± 12	0.05	0.65 ± 0.12

MaR Myocardium at risk, *LVM* Left ventricular mass, *DSC* Dice similarity coefficient, *Segment MaR CE-SSFP* automatic segmentation proposed in this study, *2SD* two standard deviations from remote, *FWHM* full width half maximum intensity

changed from overestimation to underestimation adding use of *a priori* information on MaR. The significant change seen for DSC highlights the importance of analyzing regional agreement as a part of the validation in addition to bias.

Expectation Maximization was shown superior to 2SD, FWHM and Otsu, when considering regional agreement DSC, quantitative bias and correlation R-value. The EM-algorithm was used by Johnstone et al. [12] to find the mean and standard deviation of remote myocardium in T2-weighted black blood images, but the mean and standard deviation of edema was not used to define the threshold which may explain the lower regional agreement with DSC 0.50 ± 0.27. Gao et al. [31] also used the EM-algorithm to classify myocardial intensities in T2-weighted bright blood images, with the assumption of Rayleigh-Gaussian mixture model. Rayleigh distributed intensities were assumed due to nulling of remote myocardium [31] which is not done in CE-SSFP and therefore, in this study, Gaussian intensity distributions were assumed for both normal myocardium and MaR. Surface coil intensity correction was shown to increase regional agreement. The surface coil correction was based on intensities in remote myocardium and blood pool and thereby the bright blood property of CE-SSFP was advantageous to the black blood T2-STIR images in the original Segment MaR algorithm [11] where no intensity correction was applied. Surface coil correction was applied by the Segment MaR CE-SSFP algorithm if it resulted in reduced intensity variability in the remote myocardium and mean intensity in the culprit region higher than in the remote region. Surface coil correction was not mandatorily applied at the scanner and surface coil correction was applied by the Segment MaR CE-SSFP algorithm in a majority of the patients indicating that surface coil correction was either not applied at the scanner or not sufficient. Gao et al. [31] used intensity correction developed for the bright blood ACUT2E [32] images with use of proton density maps and achieved a DSC 0.7 ± 0.06 before applying feature analysis. By incorporating *a priori* regional criteria in the definition of the MaR region the regional agreement was further increased from 0.74 to 0.81. This is in line with Gao et al. [31] who showed increased regional agreement by DSC from 0.7 to 0.74 by adding feature analysis of the edema region. Both regional agreement by DSC and quantitative bias as %LVM was improved by the addition of information on the infarct region from LGE images

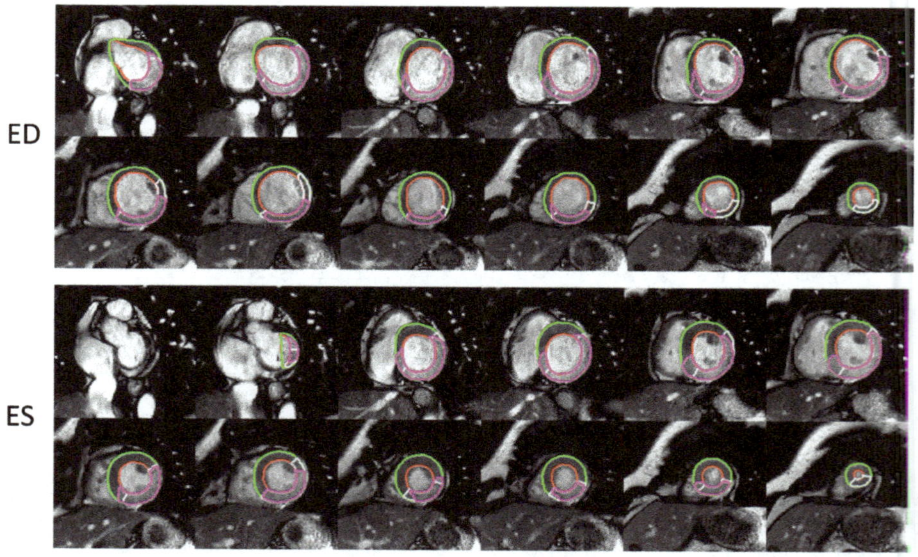

Fig. 3 Example of automatic segmentation and manual delineation of MaR in CE-SSFP. Typical MaR segmentation in all left ventricular short axis slice images from one patient in end-diastole (ED, top panel) and end systole(ES, bottom panel), for automatic segmentation by Segment MaR CE-SSFP, shown in white, and manual delineation, shown in purple. Endocardial borders are shown in red and epicardial border in green. For this patient MaR by manual segmentation was 44 %LVM and by automatic Segment MaR CE-SSFP 43 % LVM with a regional agreement DSC of 0.85

Table 3 Inter-observer variability analysis from subset $n = 15$ for manual delineation and automatic Segment MaR CE-SSFP segmentation compared to results for Segment MaR CE-SSFP against manual delineation

	MaR bias [% of LVM]	Regression *R*-value	DSC
Manual delineation vs. manual delineation	0 ± 3	0.93	0.92 ± 0.04
Segment MaR CE-SSFP vs. Segment MaR CE-SSFP	-1 ± 2	0.99	0.94 ± 0.03
Segment MaR CE-SSFP vs. manual delineation	2 ± 6	0.77	0.86 ± 0.05

MaR Myocardium at risk, *LVM* Left ventricular mass, *DSC* Dice similarity coefficient, *Segment MaR CE-SSFP* automatic segmentation proposed in this study, manual delineation performed by a reference and a second observer, automatic Segment MaR CE-SSFP performed by a reference and a second observer

which has not been implemented in previous studies. As for all automatic segmentation methods visual assessment and possibly manual corrections are needed and will probably influence the outliers seen after the fourth block of the algorithm and decrease the variability further.

Comparison to previous studies

Regional agreement to manual delineation was for Segment MaR CE-SSFP higher than for the automatic segmentation methods by Johnstone et al. [12] (DSC 0.50 ± 0.27) and Gao et al. [31] (DSC 0.74 ± 0.06), and higher respectively similar to inter-observer regional agreement of manual delineation in the same studies (DSC 0.72 ± 0.14 [12] and 0.85 ± 0.03 [31]). Regional agreement of interobserver variability bias of Segment MaR CE-SSFP was comparable to inter-observer variability of manual delineation found in this study and similar to inter-observer variability previously found in CE-SSFP (2 ± 4 %LVM [4] and 0 ± 6 %LVM [17]), and in T2-weighted imaging (-2 ± 5 %LVM [11] and 5 ± 5

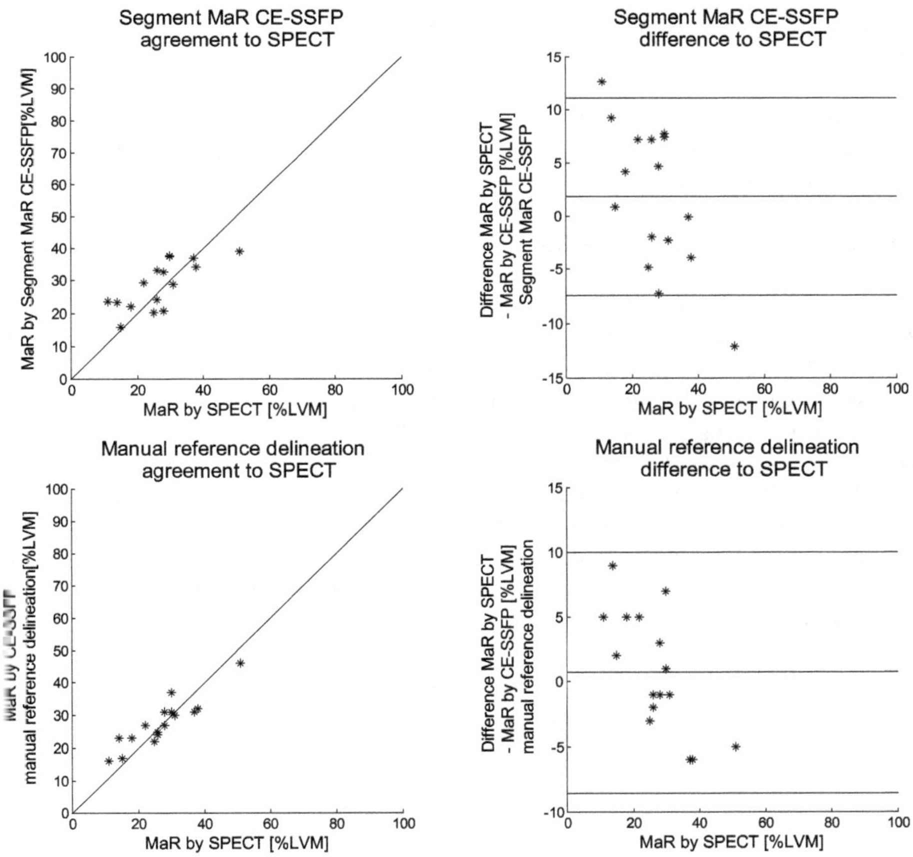

Fig. 4 Correlation and bias against SPECT for automatic segmentation and manual delineation in CE-SSFP. Correlation of MaR as % of LVM (left column) and Bland-Altman plot of MaR bias as % of LVM (right column) against SPECT for automatic segmentation algorithm Segment MaR CE-SSFP (top row) and manual reference delineation (bottom row). The line of identity is shown as a solid line for all correlations plots and mean bias (solid line) and mean ± two standard deviations (dashed line) is shown for all Bland-Altman plots. Correlation and Bland-Altman plots for manual delineation in CE-SSFP against SPECT (bottom row) are adopted from Sorenson et al. [4]

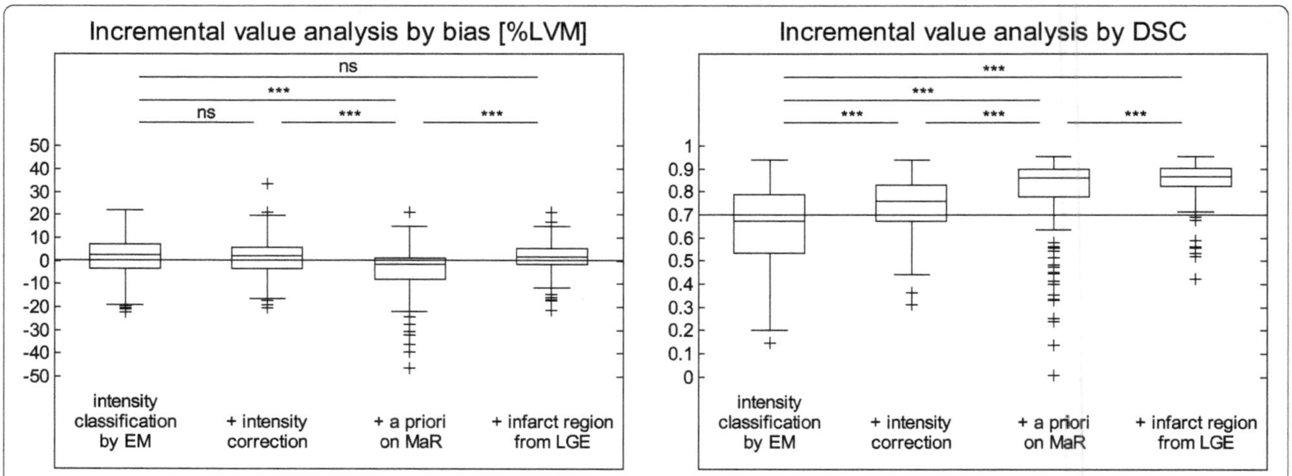

Fig. 5 Analysis of incremental value of blocks in the automatic segmentation algorithm. Incremental value of each block in the automatic segmentation algorithm analyzed by bias to manual delineation as %LVM, left panel and by regional agreement as Dice similarity coefficient DSC (right panel). Bias and DSC was calculated with segmentation based on only intensity classification by Expectation Maximization and calculated after the addition of the processing blocks of intensity correction, a priori on myocardium at risk (MaR) and infarct region from late gadolinium enhancement (LGE). For each block of the algorithm the upper limit of the box indicate upper quartile, middle line indicate median, lower limit of box indicate lower quartile, whiskers indicate minimum and maximum points within 1.5 interquartile range and points (+) indicate outliers. Bias zero is shown as dotted black line in the left panel, DSC above of 0.7 indicates good regional agreement [30], and is shown as dotted black line in the right panel. Two sided paired t-test was performed for each block in comparison to previous block and first block, ns: non significant, ***: $p < 0.0001$

%LVM [17]). Bias of Segment MaR CE-SSFP to SPECT was low and comparable to the results from the validation study of CE-SSFP with manual delineation (0 ± 5 %LVM [4]). Bias was lower and regional agreement was higher for Segment MaR CE-SSFP than for the threshold methods of 2SD, FWHM and Otsu.

Recently McAlindon et al. [21] showed that manual delineation in T2-weighted images was superior to simple threshold methods (2, 3 and 5 SD from remote, FWHM and Otsu) with manual corrections regarding accuracy and variability of intra-observer, inter-observer and test-retest. Khan et al. [22] also showed that using simple threshold methods with manual corrections for inclusion of hypoenhancement and exclusion of artifacts did not significantly reduce time for analysis compared to manual delineation. Automatic segmentation methods are desirable to increase accuracy, decrease subjectivity

Table 4 Analysis of incremental value of each block in the automatic *Segment MaR CE-SSFP* algorithm ($n = 183$)

	MaR bias [% of LVM]	Regression *R*-value	DSC
Intensity classification by EM	2 ± 8	0.60	0.65 ± 0.18
+ intensity correction[a]	2 ± 8	0.63	0.74 ± 0.12
+ a priori on MaR	-4 ± 10	0.62	0.81 ± 0.16
+ infarct region from LGE	1 ± 6	0.83	0.85 ± 0.08

EM Expectation Maximization, *MaR* Myocardium at risk, *LGE* late gadolinium enhancement, *LVM* Left ventricular mass, *DSC* Dice similarity coefficient, [a]applied in 127/183 patients

and reduce time for analysis. Using simple threshold methods for MaR quantification in T2-weighted images seems to achieve neither and might be explained by the regional agreement seen in T2-weighted images (DSC 0.69 ± 0.14, 0.46 ± 0.14 and 0.68 ± 0.10 for 2SD, FWHM and Otsu respectively) [11] and in CE-SSFP images of this study the regional agreement for simple threshold methods was even lower. The regional agreement of the Segment MaR CE-SSFP was however similar to that of the original Segment MaR in T2-weighted images (DSC 0.85 ± 0.07) [11].

Segment MaR CE-SSFP was designed to include hypoenhancement and exclude artifacts and thereby has a greater potential to reduce time for analysis, and with a low bias to manual delineation by expert readers and a regional agreement and bias to manual delineation comparable to inter-observer of manual delineation Segment MaR CE-SSFP shows potential to increase accuracy and reduce subjectivity.

Limitations

Limitations to the study are that test-retest scans were not performed and the effect of and time required for possible manual corrections following automatic segmentation was not evaluated. Contrast enhanced SSFP are not yet widely used for assessment of MaR but has been shown to be more robust than T2-weighted imaging in multi-center, multi-vendor studies [8] and can easily be implemented by acquiring cine SSFP images approximately 5 min after gadolinium injection.

Conclusion

This study has presented an automatic algorithm, Segment MaR CE-SSFP for quantification of MaR in CE-SSFP images based on four processing blocks, Expectation Maximization, surface coil intensity correction, *a priori* regional criteria and incorporation of infarct region from LGE images. Low bias and variability, strong correlation and high regional agreement was shown against manual delineation in CE-SSFP images from multi-center, multi-vendor randomized clinical trials. Bias and variability was comparable to inter-observer variability of manual delineation and inter-observer variability was decreased by use of the Segment MaR CE-SSFP algorithm.

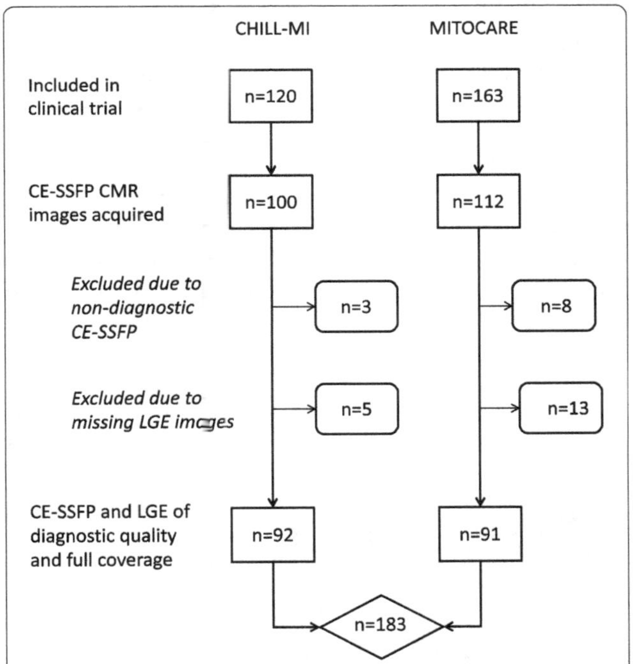

Fig. 6 Model of maximal extent for perfusion territory of each culprit artery. Bulls-eye representation of maximal extent model for the perfusion territories of left anterior descending artery (LAD), left circumflex artery (LCx), right coronary artery (RCA), and left main artery (LM). Models for LAD, LCX and RCA were defined in consensus by three experienced observers in an extended 17- segment AHA model and models for LM were defined from the models of LAD, LCX and RCA. The 17-segment model is extended to three slices in each of the basal, mid-ventricular and apical zones and 24 sectors in each slice. Black sectors are included in the maximal extent model. The septal part of the left ventricle is represented in the left of the bulls-eye plot, the lateral part in the right, anterior part in the top, inferior part in the bottom, the apical slices in the center and the basal slices in the outer part of the bulls-eye plot

Ethics approval and consent to participate

All three studies [4, 6, 7] from which patients were included were approved by the institutional review boards/ethics committees, and all patients provided written informed consent. No specific ethics approval or informed consent was needed for the development of the new automatic algorithm in the current study.

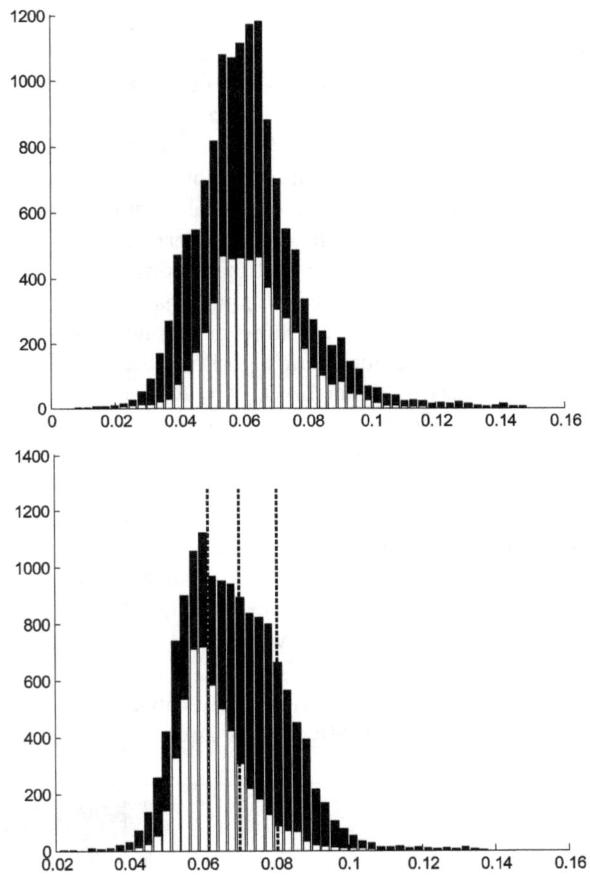

Fig. 7 Surface coil intensity correction. Histogram of myocardial intensities within the myocardium before intensity correction (top panel) and after intensity correction (bottom panel), represented in black for culprit region and white for remote region. After intensity correction a decreased standard deviation of remote region is obtained and the mean intensity of the culprit region is higher than remote region. Myocardial intensities as after intensity correction (bottom panel) are used as input to the EM-algorithm with remote region and culprit region as initial classification and dashed blue lines indicating the constraints. Intensities below the 50th percentile of the remote region are kept classified as normal myocardium through the iterations of the EM-algorithm (lower dashed blue line). Intensities above the 75th percentile of the intensities within the culprit region are kept classified as MaR through the iterations of the EM-algorithm (upper dashed blue line). Dashed red line indicates the resulting cut off 0.5 of the Bayesian probability of MaR resulting from the EM-algorithm after intensity correction

Availability of data and materials
The new automatic algorithm is freely available for research purposes and can be downloaded from http://segment.heiberg.se.

Appendix 1

Detailed description of the automatic segmentation method

The automatic segmentation Segment MaR CE-SSFP was developed for segmentation of MaR in CE-SSFP based on ideas from the algorithm developed for T2-weighted images [12]. The use of Expectation Maximization (EM) algorithm [21] for classification of myocardial intensities [12] was improved with modified constraints and surface coil intensity correction. For definition of the MaR region the implementation of *a priori* regional criteria [12] was improved and utilization of information on infarct region from LGE images was added. Maximal extent models for the perfusion territory of the culprit artery [12] were used to define the remote region and the culprit region based on user input. Figure 6 shows the maximal extent models as defined in consensus by three experienced observers [12]. As input to the automatic algorithm, the user defines the culprit artery as either LAD, LCx, RCA or LM based on the overall appearance of the hyper enhanced region and defines right ventricular insertion points in CE-SSFP and LGE images, to define maximal extent model and how to rotate the model. The maximal extent model is used with the user input of culprit artery and LV rotation to define the remote myocardium for surface coil intensity correction and initialization of the EM-algorithm and to define a MaR region within the maximal perfusion territory.

Varying surface coil sensitivity may cause an intensity gradient through the CMR images and can in CE-SSFP cause a larger variability in the myocardium than the contrast between MaR and normal myocardium and hence a surface coil correction needs to be applied before the EM-algorithm. A second order intensity correction is applied to account for a gradient proportional to the squared distance to the surface coil. The correction is calculated based on the intensity in the remote myocardium and blood pool with papillaries excluded from the blood pool by using a simple unconstrained EM-algorithm. The intensity correction should result in a reduced intensity variability in the remote myocardium and a mean intensity in the culprit region higher than in the remote region, otherwise the correction is not applied. If the mean intensity in the remote myocardium is higher than in the culprit region both before and after the intensity correction, no correction is applied and the user is notified with a warning on low image quality. Figure 7 shows the intensity histogram before and after intensity correction for the remote and culprit region.

For classification of pixel intensities as normal myocardium or MaR, a Bayesian probability is calculated by the use of a constrained EM-algorithm. The EM-algorithm [21] iteratively refines an initial classification to find the maximum likelihood estimate of the mean and standard deviation for the intensity distributions of normal myocardium and MaR. The initial classification is defined from the maximal extent model with all pixels in the remote region initially classified as normal myocardium and all pixels in the culprit region initially classified as MaR. The EM-algorithm was constrained to keep the initial classification of normal myocardium for pixels with intensity below the 50th percentile in the remote region, respectively, keeping classification of MaR for pixels with intensity above the 75th percentile in the culprit region. The Bayesian MaR probability is calculated

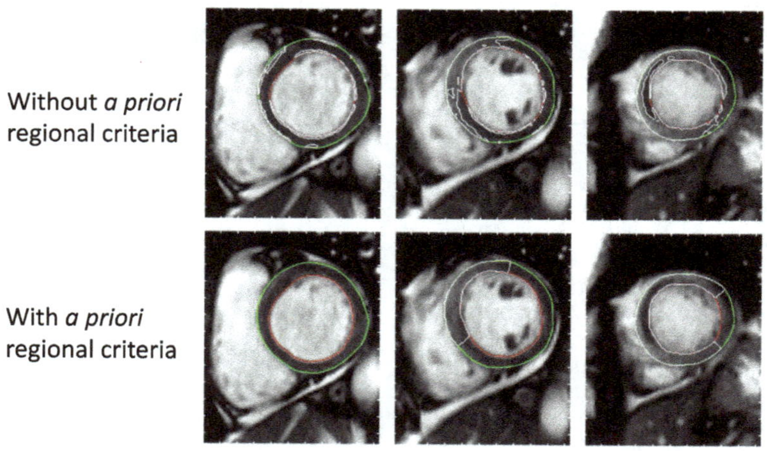

Fig. 8 Utilization of *a priori* information on extent and transmurality. Three short axis slice, basal, mid and apical with MaR segmentation, shown in white, based on only the Bayesian probability of MaR (top row) and with the addition of *a priori* regional criteria on extent and transmurality (bottom row)

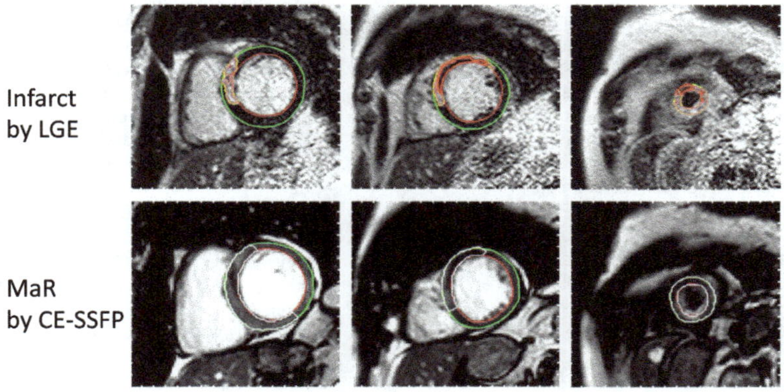

Fig. 9 Utilization of infarct segmentation from LGE. Three short axis slices, basal, midventricular and apcial, from LGE (top row) with infarct region in yellow, infarct core in pink and microvascular obstruction in red, and CE-SSFP (bottom row) with automatic segmentation by Segment MaR CE-SSFP after utilization of information on infarct region from LGE. The large region of hypoenhancement in CE-SSFP is included as MaR by utilizing the segmentation of infarct region

for each myocardial pixel as the intensity distribution of MaR divided by the sum of the intensity distributions of MaR and normal myocardium. The resulting Bayesian MaR probability cutoff 0.5 indicates higher probability of MaR and is shown in the histogram after intensity correction in Fig. 7.

The MaR region is defined as a connected region with high MaR probability which fullfills the *a priori* cirteria on transmurality and localization within the culprit artery's perfusion territory. The mean MaR probability is calculated for each sector in a bullseye representation with 24 sectors and 30 interpolated slices averaged over the time frames. Sectors with a mean MaR probability above 0.5 which are within the maximal extent and connected to its nearest neighboring sector within the slice or in an adjacent slice in a 4-neighbourhood constitute a region. If several connected regions are found the region with highest summed MaR probability is chosen. Gray scale morphological operations of opening and closing are applied to remove holes and small peninsulas in a 4-neighbourhood. Additionally holes within slices are removed to account for larger encapsulated regions of microvascular obstruction. Non-physiological extent in apical and basal slices is detected for LAD and LM as missing apical MaR sectors or false basal sectors and for LCx and RCA as false apical sectors. False and missing sectors was detected as extent larger than mean + 2 standard deviations respectively smaller than mean - 2 standard deviations of the extent in midventricular slices. If any non-physiological extent was detected and corrected for, then the user is notified to check correctness of MaR region in the basal or apical slices. Figure 8 shows one short axis slice with MaR segmentation before and after applying *a priori* regional criteria.

If LGE images with infarct segmentation are available the information on the infarct region can be used as part of the *a priori* regional criteria for definition of the MaR region. The infarct region is always a part of MaR but may due to hypoenhancment of microvascular obstruction not always be detected as MaR by the EM-algorithm. From the LGE images with delineation of the infarct, either by manual delineation or automatic segmentation [9], and right ventricular insertion points the infarct region, represented as a sector-wise bullseye, is used to define the MaR region. For each sector the fraction of infarct is calculated and the MaR region is defined from sectors with either the infarct fraction above 0.5 or mean MaR probability above 0.5. Figure 9 shows a short axis slice of a CE-SSFP image with a distinct region of microvascular obstruction which can be determined as MaR region by the use of the infarct segmentation from the LGE images.

From the bulls eye representation of the MaR region a MaR segmentation is defined in the short axis slices for each time frame and MaR is expressed as %LVM averaged over end-diastole and end-systole.

Abbreviations

%LVM: Percent of left ventricular mass; CE-SSFP: Contrast enhanced SSFP; DSC: Dice similarity coefficient; EM: Expectation maximization; FWHM: Full width half maximum; LAD: Left anterior descending artery; LCx: Left circumflex artery; LGE: Late gadolinium enhancement; LM: Left main artery; MaR: Myocardium at risk; MI: Myocardial infarction; MSI: Myocardial salvage index; RCA: Right coronary artery; RCT: Randomized clinical trials; SPECT: Single photon emission computed tomography.

Competing interests

EH is the founder of Medviso AB, Lund, Sweden, which sells a commercial version of Segment. JT is employed by Medviso AB on a part-time basis. HA is a share-holder of Imacor AB, Lund, Sweden, which performs core lab analysis of CMR images. HA, HE and MC have been employed by Imacor AB on a part-time basis. The other authors declare that they have no competing interests.

Authors' contributions

JT contributed to the design of the study, developed and implemented the automatic segmentation algorithm, analyzed and interpreted results, and drafted the manuscript. MC and HE contributed to the design of the study and the automatic algorithm and performed manual delineations in the test set. AA contributed to the design of the study and the automatic algorithm and provided in depth CMR knowledge needed for algorithm development. JFD, SK, DA and DE were responsible for data collection in the multi-center studies. PS was responsible for data collection for validation against SPECT and performed manual delineations in the additional set. JP was responsible for data collection for validation against SPECT. HA contributed to the design of the automatic algorithm, performed manual delineations and conceived the study. EH contributed to the design of the automatic algorithm and conceived the study. All authors revised the manuscript, and have read and approved the final version of the manuscript.

Fundings

This study has been funded by the Swedish Research Council (2011-3916, 2012-4944, 2011-4078), The Swedish Heart and Lung Foundation, Swedish Medical Society, The Medical Faculty of Lund University, Sweden, and Region of Scania, Sweden. Funding for the CHILL-MI trial was received from Philips Healthcare. Funding for the MITOCARE trial was received from the European Commission within the 7th Framework Programme for RTD – Project MITO-CARE – Grant Agreement HEALTH-2010-261034.

Author details

[1]Department of Clinical Physiology, Skåne University Hospital in Lund, Lund University, Lund, Sweden. [2]Department of Biomedical Engineering, Faculty of Engineering, Lund University, Lund, Sweden. [3]Laboratory of Medical Informatics, School of Medicine, Aristotle University of Thessaloniki, Thessaloniki, Greece. [4]Department of Cardiology, Henri Mondor Hospital, Creteil, France. [5]Department of Cardiology, Lund University, Lund, Sweden. [6]Department of Medicine, Karolinska Institutet, Karolinska University Hospital, Stockholm, Sweden. [7]Department of Cardiology B, Oslo, University Hospital Ullevål and Faculty of Medicine, University of Oslo, Oslo, Norway.

References

1. Engblom H, et al. Sample size in clinical cardioprotection trials using myocardial salvage index, infarct size or biochemical markers as endpoint. J Am Heart Assoc. 2016. In Press.
2. Kim RJ, et al. Relationship of MRI delayed contrast enhancement to irreversible injury, infarct age, and contractile function. Circulation. 1999;100(19):1992–2002.
3. Aletras AH, et al. Retrospective determination of the area at risk for reperfused acute myocardial infarction with T2-weighted cardiac magnetic resonance imaging: histopathological and displacement encoding with stimulated echoes (DENSE) functional validations. Circulation. 2006;113(15):1865–70.
4. Sorensson P, et al. Assessment of myocardium at risk with contrast enhanced steady-state free precession cine cardiovascular magnetic resonance compared to single-photon emission computed tomography. J Cardiovasc Magn Reson. 2010;12(1):25.
5. Carlsson M, et al. Myocardium at risk after acute infarction in humans on cardiac magnetic resonance: quantitative assessment during follow-up and validation with single-photon emission computed tomography. JACC Cardiovasc Imaging. 2009;2(5):569–76.
6. Erlinge D, et al. Rapid endovascular catheter core cooling combined with cold saline as an adjunct to percutaneous coronary intervention for the treatment of acute myocardial infarction. The CHILL-MI trial: a randomized controlled study of the use of central venous catheter core cooling combined with cold saline as an adjunct to percutaneous coronary intervention for the treatment of acute myocardial infarction. J Am Coll Cardiol. 2014;63(18):1857–65.
7. Atar D, et al. Effect of intravenous TRO40303 as an adjunct to primary percutaneous coronary intervention for acute ST-elevation myocardial infarction: MITOCARE study results. Eur Heart J. 2015;36(2):112–9.
8. Nordlund D, et al. Multi-vendor, multicentre comparison of contrast-enhanced SSFP and T2-STIR CMR for determining myocardium at risk in ST-elevation myocardial infarction. Eur Heart J Cardiovasc Imaging. 2016. doi:10.1093/ehjci/jew027.
9. Heiberg E, et al. Automated quantification of myocardial infarction from MR images by accounting for partial volume effects: animal, phantom, and human study. Radiology. 2008;246(2):581–8.
10. Amado LC, et al. Accurate and objective infarct sizing by contrast-enhanced magnetic resonance imaging in a canine myocardial infarction model. J Am Coll Cardiol. 2004;44(12):2383–9.
11. Sjogren J, et al. Semi-automatic segmentation of myocardium at risk in T2-weighted cardiovascular magnetic resonance. J Cardiovasc Magn Reson. 2012;14:10.
12. Johnstone R.I, et al. Assessment of tissue edema in patients with acute myocardial infarction by computer-assisted quantification of triple inversion recovery prepared MRI of the myocardium. Magn Reson Med. 2011;66(2): 564-73.
13. Atar D, Abitbol JL, Arheden H, Berdeaux A, Bonnet JL, Carlsson M, Clemmensen P, Cuvier V, Danchin N, Dubois-Randé JL, Engblom H, Erlinge D, Firat H, Eggert Jensen S, Halvorsen S, Hansen HS, Heiberg E, Larsen AI, Le Corvoisier P, Longlade P, Nordrehaug JE, Perez C, Pruss R, Sonou G, Schaller S, Tuseth V, Vicaut E. Rationale and design of the 'MITOCARE' Study: a phase II, multicenter, randomized, double-blind, placebo-controlled study to assess the safety and efficacy of TRO40303 for the reduction of reperfusion injury in patients undergoing percutaneous coronary intervention for acute myocardial infarction. Cardiology. 2012;123(4):201-7.
14. Simonetti OP, et al. An improved MR imaging technique for the visualization of myocardial infarction. Radiology. 2001;218(1):215–23.
15. Heiberg E, et al. Design and validation of Segment–freely available software for cardiovascular image analysis. BMC Med Imaging. 2010;10:1.
16. Beek AM, Nijveldt R, van Rossum AC. Intramyocardial hemorrhage and microvascular obstruction after primary percutaneous coronary intervention. Int J Cardiovasc Imaging. 2010;26(1):49–55.
17. Ubachs JF, et al. Myocardium at risk by magnetic resonance imaging: head-to-head comparison of T2-weighted imaging and contrast-enhanced steady-state free precession. Eur Heart J Cardiovasc Imaging. 2012;13(12):1008–15.
18. Ugander M, et al. Quantification of myocardium at risk in myocardial perfusion SPECT by co-registration and fusion with delayed contrast-enhanced magnetic resonance imaging–an experimental ex vivo study. Clin Physiol Funct Imaging. 2012;32(1):33–8.
19. Soneson H, et al. An improved method for automatic segmentation of the left ventricle in myocardial perfusion SPECT. J Nucl Med. 2009; 50(2):205–13.
20. Dempster AP, Laird NM, Rubin DB. Maximum likelihood from incomplete data via em algorithm. J R Stat Soc B-Methodol. 1977;39(1):1–38.
21. McAlindon E, et al. Quantification of infarct size and myocardium at risk: evaluation of different techniques and its implications. Eur Heart J Cardiovasc Imaging. 2015;16(7):738-46.
22. Khan JN, et al. Comparison of semi-automated methods to quantify infarct size and area at risk by cardiovascular magnetic resonance imaging at 1.5T and 3.0T field strengths. BMC Res Notes. 2015;8(1):1007.
23. Friedrich MG, et al. The salvaged area at risk in reperfused acute myocardial infarction as visualized by cardiovascular magnetic resonance. J Am Coll Cardiol. 2008;51(16):1581–7.
24. Wright J, et al. Quantification of myocardial area at risk with T2-weighted CMR: comparison with contrast-enhanced CMR and coronary angiography. JACC Cardiovasc Imaging. 2009;2(7):825–31.
25. Tilak GS, et al. In vivo T2-weighted magnetic resonance imaging can accurately determine the ischemic area at risk for 2-day-old nonreperfused myocardial infarction. Invest Radiol. 2008;43(1):7–15.
26. Burchell T, et al. Comparing analysis methods for quantification of myocardial oedema in patients following reperfused ST-elevation MI. J Cardiovasc Magn Reson. 2011;13 Suppl 1:M11.
27. Hsu LY, et al. Quantitative myocardial infarction on delayed enhancement MRI. Part I: Animal validation of an automated feature analysis and

combined thresholding infarct sizing algorithm. J Magn Reson Imaging. 2006;23(3):298–308.
28. Otsu N. Threshold selection method from gray-level histograms. IEEE Trans Syst Man Cybern. 1979;9(1):62–6.
29. Dice LR. Measures of the amount of ecologic association between species. Ecology. 1945;26(3):297–302.
30. Zijdenbos AP, et al. Morphometric Analysis of white-matter lesions in Mr-Images - method and validation. IEEE Trans Med Imaging. 1994;13(4):716–24.
31. Gao H, et al. Highly automatic quantification of myocardial oedema in patients with acute myocardial infarction using bright blood T2-weighted CMR. J Cardiovasc Magn Reson. 2013;15:28.
32. Aletras AH, et al. ACUT2E TSE-SSFP: a hybrid method for T2-weighted imaging of edema in the heart. Magn Reson Med. 2008;59(2):229–35.

19

Evaluation of quantitative parameters of dynamic contrast-enhanced magnetic resonance imaging in qualitative diagnosis of hepatic masses

Jingjing Chen[1], Youjiao Si[2], Kaikai Zhao[3], Xianglong Shi[1], Weiqun Bi[1], Shi-en Liu[1] and Hui Hua[4*]

Abstract

Background: To explore the value of parameters of multiphase dynamic contrast-enhanced magnetic resonance imaging (MDCE-MRI) in the qualitative diagnosis of hepatic masses.

Methods: Eighty patients with hepatic masses were retrospectively analyzed. All the patients underwent MDCE-MRI at 3.0 T MR before treatment. Mean enhancement time (MET), positive enhancement integral (PEI), a maximum slope of increase (MSI), and a maximum slope of decrease (MSD) were measured.

Results: There were significant differences between benign and malignant hepatic masses with respect to MET, PEI, and MSI values. The PEI and MSI values between hemangiomas, hepatocellular carcinomas (HCCs), cholangiocarcinomas, and metastatic tumors had significant differences. The MSD value between metastatic tumors, HCCs, and hemangiomas were significantly different. The area under the curve (AUC) values of the receiver operator characteristic curves for MET, PEI, and MSI were 0.70, 0.72, and 0.80, respectively. The specificity of MET, PEI, and MSI were all 77%, and the sensitivities of MSI was the highest, of which was 82.40%. Logistic regression analysis showed the regression equation to be $P = 1/[1 + e^{0.008 \times 1 + 0.007 \times 2-6.707}]$, and taking the Youden index maximum points as a diagnostic point was 0.2946.

Conclusion: Some parameters of MDCE-MRI have significant roles in differentiating hepatic masses.

Keywords: Hepatic tumor, Magnetic resonance imaging, Hemangioma, Hepatocellular carcinoma, Cholangiocarcinoma, Metastatic tumor

Background

There are numerous causes of solid hepatic masses, both benign and malignant. It is important to make a correct diagnosis, especially when the potential for therapy exists. While most of these lesions present as solitary masses, multiple lesions may be seen in patients with hemangiomas, hepatocellular carcinomas (HCCs), cholangiocarcinomas, and metastatic tumors. The detectability of hepatic tumors is rising in China with advances in detection of tumor biomarkers and imaging technology [1]. However, the positive predictive value of alpha-fetoprotein (AFP) in the diagnosis of primary liver cancer is only 67.8–74.4% [2]. Although biopsy and histopathologic verification are mandatory for the definitive diagnosis of hepatic masses, those cannot be regarded as ideal diagnostic methods as invasive procedures.

Recently, an increasing interest has been preferred to diagnosing hepatic masses non-invasively. Although magnetic resonance imaging (MRI) has high soft tissue resolution, its routine sequences are not satisfied in the diagnosis of hepatic masses which have the similar imaging appearances on both T1WI and T2WI in most hepatic masses [3–6]. In the last decade, molecular and functional methods of MRI, such as dynamic contrast-enhanced MRI, diffusion-weighted MRI, perfusion-weighted MRI, diffusion tensor imaging, and MR

* Correspondence: henysci@sina.com
[4]Department of Thyroid Surgery, The Affiliated Hospital of Qingdao University, No. 16 Jiangsu Road, Qingdao 266000, Shandong Province, China
Full list of author information is available at the end of the article

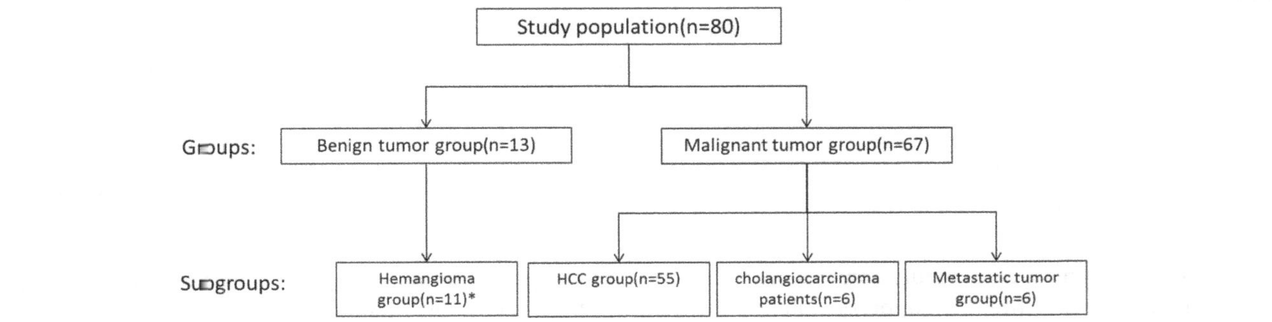

Fig. 1 Flow diagram of enrolled patients. *There were only two patients suffering from focal nodular hyperplasia, which was not included in statistics

spectroscopy have been investigated to improve the diagnostic capability of MRI.

Dynamic-enhanced CT and MR scanning technology can effectively reflect tumor neovascularization, But MR soft tissue resolution is much higher than that of CT. The organizational structure and hemodynamics are different in different hepatic lesions, resulting in varying dynamic contrast-enhanced MRI manifestations. So, MRI will play more important roles in the qualitative diagnosis of hepatic masses, especially on multiphase dynamic contrast-enhanced MRI (MDCE-MRI) [7].

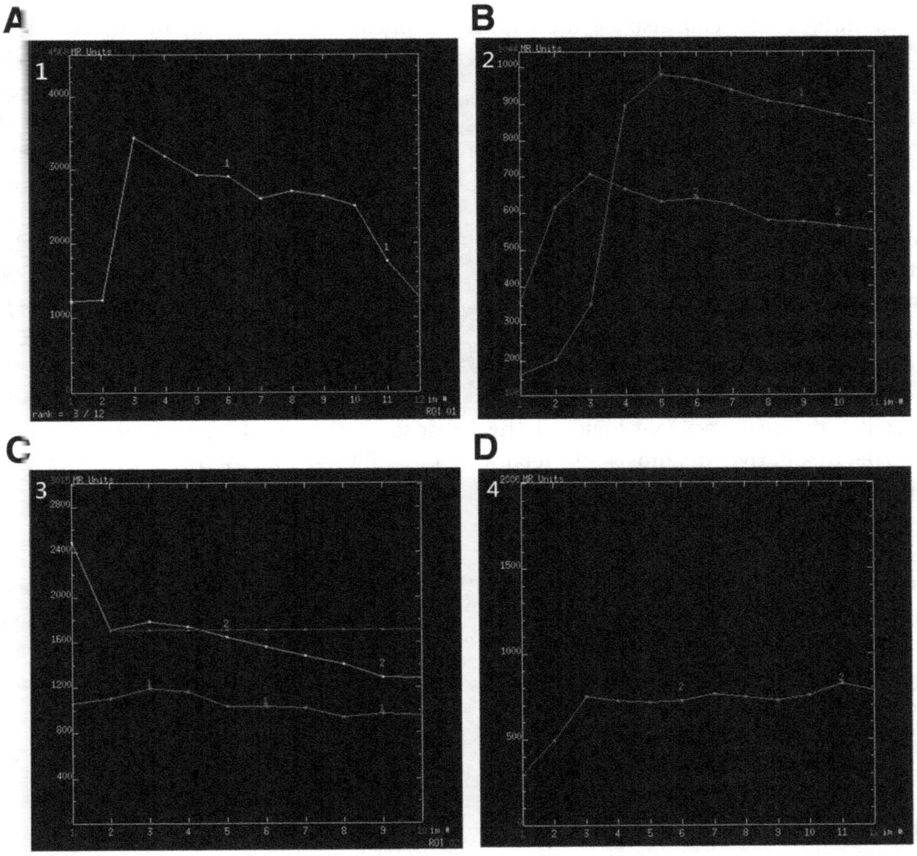

Fig. 2 The enhancement curves of the lesions. **a**: Male, 59 years old, High-differentiation HCC with rapid increase and rapid Decrease; **b**: Female, 40 years old, Hemangioma (Curve 1 is the enhancement curve of the lesion with rapid increase and slow decrease, and Curve 2 is the enhancement curve of normal liver tissue); **c**: Male, 51 years old, HCC (Curve 1 is the enhancement curve of the lesion with a slow increase and slow decrease, and Curve 2 is the enhancement curve of the abdominal aorta); **d**: Male, 63 years old, Cholangiocarcinoma (The enhancement curve of the lesion has a slow increase after no apparent decline)

Table 1 Comparison of each parameter value between benign and malignant hepatic tumors [M(QL~Qu)]

Group	MET*	PEI	MSI	MSD
Benign tumor	596.06 (516.01~596.06)	256.95 (36.50~421.59)	283.47 (162.12~437.08)	88.09 (77.13~153.69)
Malignant tumor	506.94 (478.48~591.06)	32.24 (3.34~99.07)	91.13 (50.95~150.53)	121.09 (80.94~161.74)
T value	2.53	2.77	3.76	1.02
P value	0.012	0.006	0.001	0.309

Remarks: Wilcoxon test,* Unit: s

Liver acceleration volume acquisition (LAVA) is a fast 3D volumetric T1-weighted fat-suppressed imaging technology [8], which depends on the design idea of GE high-density target coils that improve the acquisition speed by parallel acquisition techniques and achieving higher time resolution with the premise of ensuring enough spatial resolution within and between the levels. LAVA automatically uses K space-filling technology and piecewise special technology, which greatly shortens the scan time and obtains good fat suppression. Compared to the previous abdominal multi-period dynamic-enhanced scanning technology, the speed and resolution of LAVA can be improved by 25%, and the scanning range can also be increased by 25%. Clearly, LAVA improves the ability to display minimal change, and is widely used in abdominal lesions. The fine structure of liver lesions can be shown by LAVA involving the different morphology, growth mode, and dynamic enhanced features. Meanwhile, LAVA can also help to make a differential diagnosis of various pathologic types of tumors.

In this present study, we applied LAVA technology to eighty patients with hepatic masses to perform multiphase dynamic contrast-enhanced examinations in an effort to explore the diagnostic value of some quantitative and semi-quantitative parameters of MDCE-MRI in hepatic masses, and to provide a theoretical basis for the qualitative diagnosis of hepatic masses using non-invasive MRI.

Methods

Patient population and grouping

Between 2011 and 2014, a total of 80 patients (62 males and 18 females) with pathologically-confirmed hepatic masses by surgery or biopsy were scanned by MRI prior to surgery or biopsy. The mean age of the patients was 54 years (range, 26~78 years). The MR examination and diagnostic time interval were all within 30 days. None of the patients received anti-tumor therapy before MR examination and surgery. Informed consent was obtained from each patient prior to the MRI examination. The study was approved by the local ethics committee. Eighty cases were divided into 2 groups (benign and malignant tumor) according to pathologic results, and then, subdivided into 4 groups (hemangioma, HCC, cholangiocarcinoma, and metastatic tumor groups) further. Only two patients were suffering from focal nodular hyperplasia, which was not included in statistics (Fig. 1).

MRI

All the examinations were performed in GE Signa HDx 3.0 T clinical MRI system using an eight-channel phased array body coil. Gadolinium-diethylene triamine pentaacetic acid (Gd-DTPA) acted as a contrast agent in a concentration of 0.5 mmol/ml. All of the patients fasted for 12 h before the examination in the morning. During the examination the patients were asked to maintain eupnea and avoid abdominal breathing. The following MRI sequences were obtained: (1) axial fast spin echo (FSE) T2-weighted imaging (T2WI) sequence: Repetition Time (TR) 8000 ms, Echo Time (TE) 90 ms, slice thickness 6.0 mm, slice gap 2.0 mm, Matrix 256 × 192. (2) axial fast spin echo (FSE) T1-weighted imaging (T1WI) sequence: TR 150 ms, TE 2.0 ms slice thickness 6.0 mm, slice gap 2.0 mm, Matrix 256 × 192. (3) Multiphase dynamic contrast enhanced MRI: Applying liver acquisition with volume acceleration (LAVA) technologic, TE 1.16 ms; TR 2.52 ms; slice thickness 5.0 mm, slice gap 0 mm, scanning time 120 s, Matrix256x192. During contrast scan, a high-pressure injector was used at a dose of 0.2 mmol/kg of body weight and an injection rate of 3 ~ 4 ml/s following by 20 ml of physiologic saline in the same velocity.

Images analysis

After data acquisition, all of the images were transferred to the AW4.3 workstation and analyzed by Functool analysis software. ROI was drawn in the maximum cross-section of the lesion in a relatively uniform signal

Table 2 Comparison of the curve types between benign and malignant tumors (case)

Group	Curve types			
	I	II	III	IV
Benign tumor	0	10	0	3
Malignant tumor	31	9	5	22
P value	< 0.001			

Remark: Fisher exact probability test

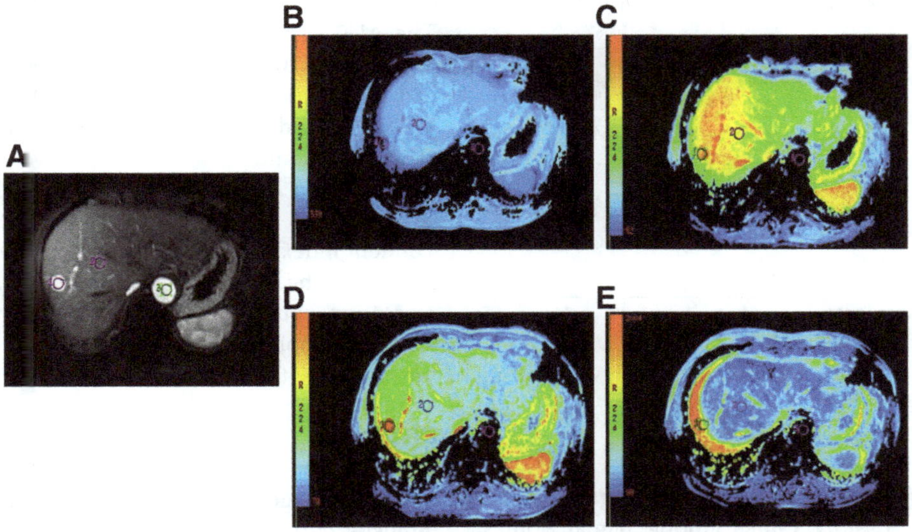

Fig. 3 Imaging from a patient of male, 59 years old with high differentiation HCC. Figs. **a-e** represent dynamic contrast-enhanced magnetic resonance imaging and the pseudo-color images of MET, PET, MSI, and MSD, respectively

intensity excluding the vessels, hemorrhage, necrosis, and cystic degeneration. Each measurement of the ROI was repeated by 3 times for statistical analysis. The Mean enhancement time (MET), positive enhancement integral (PEI), a maximum slope of increase (MSI), and a maximum slope of decrease (MSD) values and the curve types of ROIs were calculated and shown by Functool analysis software. The curve types of ROIs were divided into the following 4 categories: I, increase rapidly and decrease rapidly; II: increase rapidly and decrease slowly; III: increase slowly and decrease slowly; and IV, rise slowly after no apparent decline (Fig. 2a-d).

Data analysis

The statistical software package SPSS 20.0 (SPSS Inc., Chicago, IL, USA) was used for data analysis. We performed normal testing and homogeneity of variance testing for MET, PEI, MSI, and MSD values in the benign and malignant tumor groups, such as hemangioma, HCC, cholangiocarcinoma, and metastatic tumor groups. The Student *t*-test was used for comparison of each parameter value between benign and malignant hepatic tumors. Nonparametric analyses including the Kruskal-Wallis test and Wilcoxon-Mann-Whitney U test using the Bonferroni correction were performed on data of parameter values among four groups, and Fisher exact probability test was used in the analysis of the curve types among the four groups. Receiver Operator Characteristic (ROC) curves were evaluated to compare every parameter value in the differential diagnoses of hepatic tumors. The area under the curve (AUC) reflects the accuracy of diagnostic testing, in which the value of AUC in 50 ~ 70, 70% ~ 90%, and > 90% corresponding to low, medium, and higher the accuracy of diagnostic testing respectively. Logistic regression analysis was used to obtain the regression eq. A P value < 0.05 was considered statistically significant.

Results

Comparison of benign and malignant hepatic tumors

The MET, PEI, and MSI values were significantly lower in the malignant hepatic tumor group than that in the benign tumor group (Table 1). Different lesions had different curve types, with benign tumors presenting

Table 3 Comparison of each parameter value among four groups [M(QL~Qu)]

Group	MET*	PEI	MSI	MSD
HCC	528.14 (476.25~592.40)	20.51 (2.94~83.35)	83.93 (49.51~133.41)	131.65 (90.51~182.63)
Metastatic tumor	507.59 (505.30~534.64)	52.91 (31.89~114.30)	84.76 (49.37~130.52)	44.76 (42.49~57.24)
Cholangiocarcinoma	502.84 (491.57~546.42)	97.35 (47.92~183.20)	166.13 (128.10~233.93)	129.57 (105.80~147.67)
Hemangioma	536.35 (505.30~596.06)	353.89 (133.10~517.43)	340.72 (265.70~633.86)	88.09 (80.84~217.85)
F value	0.99	14.69	24.40	15.92
P value	0.803	0.002	< 0.001	0.001

Remark: Kruskal-Wallis test

Table 4 Comparison of the curve types among the four groups (case)

Group	Curve types			
	I	II	III	IV
HCC	31	7	4	13
Metastatic tumor	0	1	1	4
Cholangiocarcinoma	0	1	0	5
Hemangioma	0	10	0	1
P value	< 0.001			

Remark: Fisher exact probability test

with type II and malignant tumors mainly presenting with type I (Table 2).

Comparison between malignant hepatic tumors

The PEI, MSI and MSD values among hemangiomas, HCCs, cholangiocarcinomas, and metastatic tumors had significant differences (Fig. 3a-e and Table 3). HCCs mainly presented with type I, metastatic tumors, and cholangiocarcinomas mainly presented with type IV, and hemangiomas mainly presented with type II (Table 4).

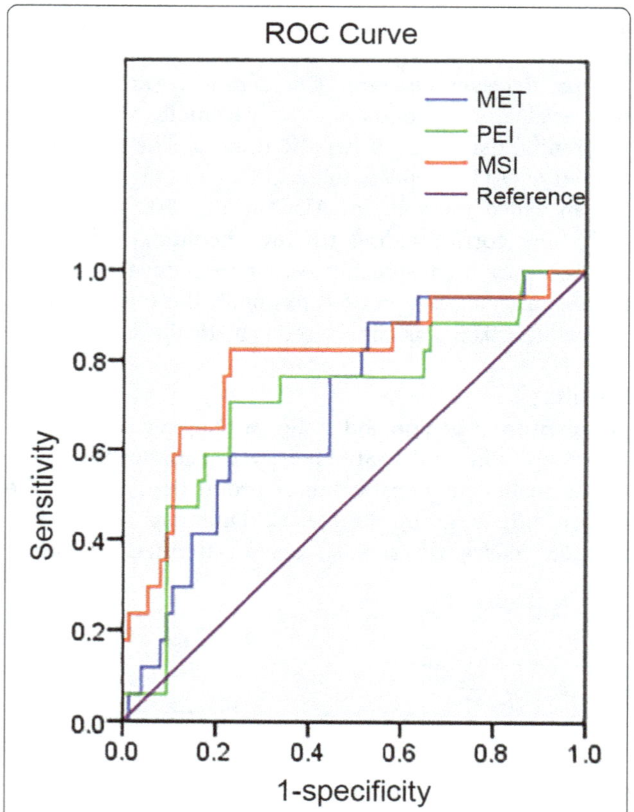

Fig. 4 ROC curves for MET, PEI, and MSI. Abbreviations: MET: Mean enhancement time; PEI: positive enhancement integral; MSI: a maximum slope of increase

Diagnosis of malignant hepatic tumor

The AUC values of the ROC curves for MET, PEI, and MSI were 0.70, 0.72, and 0.80 respectively, all of which had diagnostic significances (Fig. 4). The specificity of MET, PEI, and MSI were all 77%, and the sensitivity was 58.80, 70.60, and 82.40% retrospectively (Table 5). Logistic regression analysis showed the regression equation to be $P = 1/[1 + e^{0.008 \times 1 + 0.007 \times 2 - 6.707}]$, and taking the Youden index (sensitivity + specificity − 1) maximum points as the diagnostic point was 0.2946. When the regression equation calculated value was less than the diagnostic point, it is more likely to be a malignant tumor (Table 6).

Discussion

In this present study, we found that MDCE-MRI showed different characteristics of enhancement by a time-signal intensity curve, the various parameters in assessing the degree of tumor neovascularization non-invasively. These parameters can be used for the quantitative analysis of diseases. The MET reflects the average pass time, the PEI relates to the relative blood volume, the MSI represents the microcirculatory blood flow, and the MSD reflects the blood supply of the tumor velocity [9, 10]. The mean values of MET, PEI, and MSI for benign tumors were higher than malignant tumors, and the difference was statistically significant. When the thresholds were 592.13, 120.11, and 156.97 respectively, the diagnostic specificity of these parameters were 77%, and the sensitivities were 58.80, 70.60, and 82.40% respectively. A large proportion of benign tumors is hemangiomas and the pathology of hemangiomas is mainly composed of abnormal dilatation of hepatic sinusoids. Although the MSD of benign tumors was less than malignant tumors, the difference was not statistically significant. Based on the literature, many factors can affect the enhancement type of the tumor, such as the density and permeability of the tumor vessels and extracellular diffusion space [11, 12]. We compared each parameter value among the four groups of tumors and found that the PEI and MSI values between hemangiomas, HCCs, cholangiocarcinomas, and metastatic tumors had significant differences. The MSD values between metastatic tumors and HCCs also had significant differences. Furthermore, the MET, PEI, and MSI values of hemangiomas were all higher than other tumors.

These results may have a relationship to the pathology of hemangiomas, HCCs, cholangiocarcinomas, and metastatic tumors [13–16]. The pathology of hemangiomas is composed of abnormal dilatation of hepatic sinusoids; however, HCCs develop in multistage processes with an increase in the degree of malignancy as the

Table 5 ROC curve analysis of each parameter

Parameter	AUC	Standard error	*P* value	95% Confidence interval	Threshold value	Sensitivity (%)	Specificity (%)
MET	0.70	0.07	0.01	0.57~0.83	592.13	58.8	77
PEI	0.72	0.07	0.01	0.57~0.86	120.11	70.6	77
MSI	0.8	0.07	0.00	0.66~0.92	156.97	82.4	77

Remark: Fisher exact probability test

greater the blood supply in the hepatic artery. Cholangiocarcinomas are hypovascular tumors with increased fiber composition. According to the varied origin of cholangiocarcinomas, the blood supply of metastatic tumors is different and the rate of growth is usually rapid, thus the center of the tumor is prone to be liquefaction necrosis. Therefore, blood flow in hemangiomas is higher than other liver diseases.

Some research have suggested that parameters which are obtained from MDCE-MRI are highly related to tumor angiogenesis [17]. Because different lesions have different hemodynamic metabolic characteristics, the enhancement curve types were varied, which reflects the blood supply of tissues and vascular permeability state. Combined with the enhancement type curve of this study, we divided the curve type into the four categories. We found that there was a significant difference between benign and malignant tumors, as well as among each four groups. Benign tumors present with type II and malignant tumors mainly present with type I. HCCs mainly present with type I metastatic tumors and cholangiocarcinomas mainly present with type IV, and hemangiomas mainly present with type II, all of which are consistent with reports in the literature [18, 19]. This result reflects the pathologic changes of each lesion. The histologic characteristics of HCCs reflect the liver arterial blood supply, the histologic characteristics of cholangiocarcinomas reflect the hypovascular tumor containing more fibers, which results in slow contrast agent diffusion between the blood vessels and fibrous tissues. The pathologic features of hemangiomas reflect abnormal dilatation of hepatic sinusoids and the enhanced feature of metastasis depends on the blood supply of the primary tumor.

In addition, we adopted parameters that were significantly different between benign and malignant tumors and performed logistic regression analysis. We obtained the regression eq. ($P = 1/[1 + e^{0.008 \times 1 + 0.007 \times 2 - 6.707}]$) and took the Youden index maximum points as the diagnostic point, which was 0.2946. When the regression equation calculated value was less than the diagnostic point, the tumor was malignant.

Due to the small sample size, there are several limitations in the article, such as, it is not possible to characterise all metastases into a single group. There is no discussion of dysplastic nodules versus HCC. And HCCs accounted for a larger proportion of the tumors in the current study. For benign tumors, hemangiomas accounted for a larger proportion. There is no mention of differences between cirrhotic and normal background livers. The main focus of the discussion is on haemangiomas, which are almost always easy to diagnose. We will increase sample size for further research.

Table 6 Results of logistic regression analysis

Covariant	Regression coefficient	Standard error	*P* value
X1	0.008	0.003	0.011
X2	0.007	0.002	0
X3	0	0.001	0.543
constant	−6.707	1.892	0

Remark: X1 present with MET, X2 present with MSI, X3 present with PEI

Conclusion

Parameters obtained from MDCE-MRI can reflect the hemodynamic characteristics of lesions, which has application value in differential diagnoses of hepatic masses. A larger study is needed to validate the findings.

Abbreviations

AFP: alpha-fetoprotein; Gd-DTPA: Gadolinium-diethylene triamine pentaacetic acid; HCCs: hemangiomas, hepatocellular carcinomas; LAVA: Liver acceleration volume acquisition; MDCE-MRI: multiphase dynamic contrast-enhanced MRI; MRI: magnetic resonance imaging

Acknowledgements

Not applicable.

Funding

This work was supported by grants from the Shandong Province Science and Technology Development Projects (2011YD18034).

Authors' contributions

JJC, XLS and WQB carried out the studies, participated in collecting data, and drafted the manuscript. SEL and HH performed the statistical analysis and participated in its design. YJS and KKZ helped to draft the manuscript. All authors read and approved the final manuscript.

Consent for publication

Not applicable.

Competing interests

The authors declare that they have no competing interests.

Author details

[1]Department of Radiology, The Affiliated Hospital of Qingdao University, Qingdao 266000, Shandong Province, China. [2]Department of Radiology, Yantai Affiliated Hospital of Binzhou Medical University, Yantai 264100, Shandong Province, China. [3]Department of Oncology, Yantai Affiliated Hospital of Binzhou Medical University, Yantai 264100, Shandong Province, China. [4]Department of Thyroid Surgery, The Affiliated Hospital of Qingdao University, No. 16 Jiangsu Road, Qingdao 266000, Shandong Province, China.

References

1. Zhou X, Luo Y, Peng YL, Cai W, Lu Q, Lin L, Sha XX, Li YZ, Zhu M. Hepatic perfusion disorder associated with focal liver lesions: contrast-enhanced US patterns--correlation study with contrast-enhanced CT. Radiology. 2011;260:274–81.
2. Song P, Feng X, Inagaki Y, Song T, Zhang K, Wang Z, Zheng S, Ma K, Li Q, Kong D, et al. Clinical utility of simultaneous measurement of alpha-fetoprotein and des-gamma-carboxy prothrombin for diagnosis of patients with hepatocellular carcinoma in China: a multi-center case-controlled study of 1,153 subjects. Bioscience trends. 2014;8:266–73.
3. McGlynn KA, London WT. Epidemiology and natural history of hepatocellular carcinoma. Best Pract Res Clin Gastroenterol. 2005;19:3–23.
4. Lee VS, Lavelle MT, Rofsky NM, Laub G, Thomasson DM, Krinsky GA, Weinreb JC. Hepatic MR imaging with a dynamic contrast-enhanced isotropic volumetric interpolated breath-hold examination: feasibility, reproducibility, and technical quality. Radiology. 2000;215:365–72.
5. Semelka RC, Shoenut JP, Kroeker MA, Greenberg HM, Simm FC, Minuk GY, Kroeker RM, Micflikier AB. Focal liver disease: comparison of dynamic contrast-enhanced CT and T2-weighted fat-suppressed, FLASH, and dynamic gadolinium-enhanced MR imaging at 1.5 T. Radiology 1992;184: 687–694.
6. Isozaki T, Numata K, Kiba T, Hara K, Morimoto M, Sakaguchi T, Sekihara H, Kubota T, Shimada H, Morizane T, et al. Differential diagnosis of hepatic tumors by using contrast enhancement patterns at US. Radiology. 2003;229:798–805.
7. Kim MJ, Kim JH, Chung JJ, Park MS, Lim JS, Oh YT. Focal hepatic lesions: detection and characterization with combination gadolinium- and superparamagnetic iron oxide-enhanced MR imaging. Radiology. 2003;228:719–26.
8. Mostardi PM, Glockner JF, Young PM, Riederer SJ. Contrast-enhanced MR angiography of the abdomen with highly accelerated acquisition techniques. Radiology. 2011;261:587–97.
9. Kudo M, Tomita S, Tochio H, Kashida H, Hirasa M, Todo A. Hepatic focal nodular hyperplasia: specific findings at dynamic contrast-enhanced US with carbon dioxide microbubbles. Radiology. 1991;179:377–82.
10. Masselli G, Picarelli A, Di Tola M, Libanori V, Donato G, Polettini E, Piermattei A, Palumbo P, Pittalis A, Saponara A, et al. Celiac disease: evaluation with dynamic contrast-enhanced MR imaging. Radiology. 2010;256:783–90.
11. Ito K, Fujita T, Shimizu A, Koike S, Sasaki K, Matsunaga N, Hibino S, Yuhara M. Multiarterial phase dynamic MRI of small early enhancing hepatic lesions in cirrhosis or chronic hepatitis: differentiating between hypervascular hepatocellular carcinomas and pseudolesions. AJR Am J Roentgenol. 2004;183:699–705.
12. Sun HY, Lee JM, Shin CI, Lee DH, Moon SK, Kim KW, Han JK, Choi BI. Gadoxetic acid-enhanced magnetic resonance imaging for differentiating small hepatocellular carcinomas (< or =2 cm in diameter) from arterial enhancing pseudolesions: special emphasis on hepatobiliary phase imaging. Investig Radiol. 2010;45:96–103.
13. Glazer GM, Aisen AM, Francis IR, Gyves JW, Lande I, Adler DD. Hepatic cavernous hemangioma: magnetic resonance imaging. Work in progress Radiology. 1985;155:417–20.
14. Koh TS, Thng CH, Lee PS, Hartono S, Rumpel H, Goh BC, Bisdas S. Hepatic metastases: in vivo assessment of perfusion parameters at dynamic contrast-enhanced MR imaging with dual-input two-compartment tracer kinetics model. Radiology. 2008;249:307–20.
15. Jeong MG, Yu JS, Kim KW. Hepatic cavernous hemangioma: temporal peritumoral enhancement during multiphase dynamic MR imaging. Radiology. 2000;216:692–7.
16. Shimizu A, Ito K, Koike S, Fujita T, Shimizu K, Matsunaga N. Cirrhosis or chronic hepatitis: evaluation of small (<or=2-cm) early-enhancing hepatic lesions with serial contrast-enhanced dynamic MR imaging. Radiology. 2003;226:550–5.
17. Elsayes KM, Narra VR, Yin Y, Mukundan G, Lammle M, Brown JJ. Focal hepatic lesions: diagnostic value of enhancement pattern approach with contrast-enhanced 3D gradient-echo MR imaging. Radiographics. 2005;25:1299–320.
18. Lutz AM, Willmann JK, Goepfert K, Marincek B, Weishaupt D. Hepatocellular carcinoma in cirrhosis: enhancement patterns at dynamic gadolinium- and superparamagnetic iron oxide-enhanced T1-weighted MR imaging. Radiology. 2005;237:520–8.
19. Burns PN, Wilson SR. Focal liver masses: enhancement patterns on contrast-enhanced images--concordance of US scans with CT scans and MR images. Radiology. 2007;242:162–74.

A case report in cardiovascular magnetic resonance: the contrast agent matters in amyloid

Marianna Fontana[1,2], Thomas A. Treibel[2,3], Ana Martinez-Naharro[1], Stefania Rosmini[3], Raymond Y. Kwong[4], Julian D. Gillmore[1], Philip N. Hawkins[1] and James C. Moon[2,3*]

Abstract

Background: Cardiac amyloidosis is a progressive but underdiagnosed and underappreciated cause of heart failure. In the last few years, cardiovascular magnetic resonance (CMR) has become the gold standard for non invasive diagnosis of cardiac amyloidosis with the characteristic subendocardial late gadolinium enhancement.

Case presentation: We describe a case of a patient who, in the process of aligning protocols for a trial between different centers, had a paired study with two different contrast agents, Dotarem® and MultiHance®. MultiHance® surprisingly failed to demonstrate the characteristic imaging pattern, showing only non specific late gadolinium enhancement at the inferior right ventricular insertion point and different myocardial extracellular volume fraction compared to the one obtained with Dotarem®. MultiHance® is used by many centres, because its partial blood protein binding is a strength for MR angiography, but late gadolinium enhancement, particularly non-ischemic, appears to be compromised.

Conclusions: This case report suggests that contrast agents should be selected with caution, especially with new therapies lining up for amyloid and CMR being used as exploratory end point in clinical trials.

Keywords: Case report, Amyloidosis, CMR, Contrast

Background

In the last decade cardiovascular magnetic resonance (CMR) has grown dramatically and in amyloidosis has become the gold standard for non invasive diagnosis of cardiac involvement with the characteristic subendocardial late gadolinium enhancement (LGE) [1]. The number of new referrals for cardiac amyloidosis has significantly increased in the last few years, with the diagnosis being based on CMR and the characteristic LGE. New contrast agents favoured for their high relaxivity related to blood protein binding, [2] have become available but no one has ever tested the diagnostic performance of these new agents in infiltrative disease.

* Correspondence: j.moon@ucl.ac.uk
[2]Institute of Cardiovascular Science, University College London, London, UK
[3]Barts Heart Centre, West Smithfield, London EC1A 7BE, UK
Full list of author information is available at the end of the article

Case presentation

A 77-year old man presented with breathlessness and weight loss. Endoscopy and duodenal biopsy showed amyloid deposits, subtyped as transthyretin type (TTR). Investigations excluded a plasma cell dyscrasia, and showed atrial fibrillation on ECG (Fig. 1), and moderately increased wall thickness with moderate to severe diastolic dysfunction on echocardiography (Fig. 2, videos available as Additional files 1 and 2). TTR gene sequencing showed no mutation so the diagnosis was that of wild-type ATTR amyloidosis (senile systemic amyloidosis). Cardiac involvement, though likely, was not unequivocal as age/hypertension can confound.

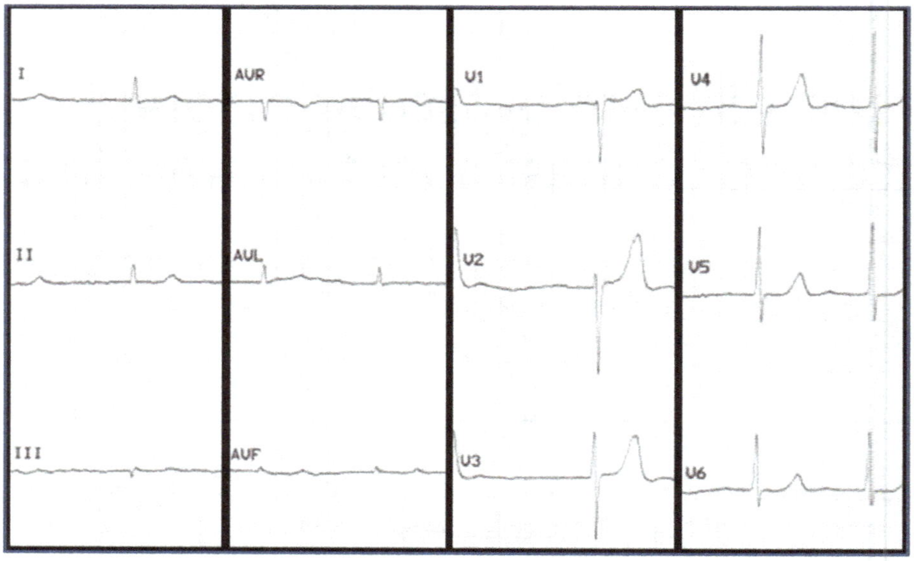

Fig. 1 Twelve lead ECG at presentation showing atrial fibrillation

Technetium-labelled bone scintigraphy and CMR were performed. Scintigraphy demonstrated grade 2 myocardial uptake, highly specific for cardiac amyloidosis. Cine CMR imaging supported the echocardiographic and scintigraphy findings. Tissue characterization showed clear amyloidosis with elevated native myocardial T1 (ShMOLLI, 1072 ms, normal 960 ms+/-30 ms) and, after contrast (Gadoterate meglumine, 0.1 mmol/kg, gadolinium-DOTA, Dotarem® Guerbet S.A. France), abnormal gadolinium kinetics on TI scout (nulling of the myocardium before the blood) and diffuse biventricular subendocardial LGE (Fig. 2) [1]. The extracellular volume fraction (ECV) at 15 min was 0.53.

Two weeks later, the CMR was repeated (same scanner and team with no changes in the patient regarding treatment or disease status) within the screening tests of a clinical trial, this time with a different contrast agent, gadobenate dimeglumine (0.1 mmol/kg, gadolinium-BOPTA, MultiHance®, Bracco, Milan, Italy). The cines and native T1 findings were the same (Fig. 3). The LGE however was markedly different – the subendocardial LGE so characteristic of amyloidosis was not visible, even with phase-sensitive inversion recovery (PSIR). There was just non-specific right ventricle insertion point LGE (Fig. 4). The ECV at 15 min obtained using Gd-BOPTA (MultiHance®) was now lower – 0.45 compared to 0.53 with gadolinium-DOTA (Dotarem®) (same acquisition time after contrast administration). This difference is higher than the expected variability of the technique. Prior publications demonstrate the ECV to

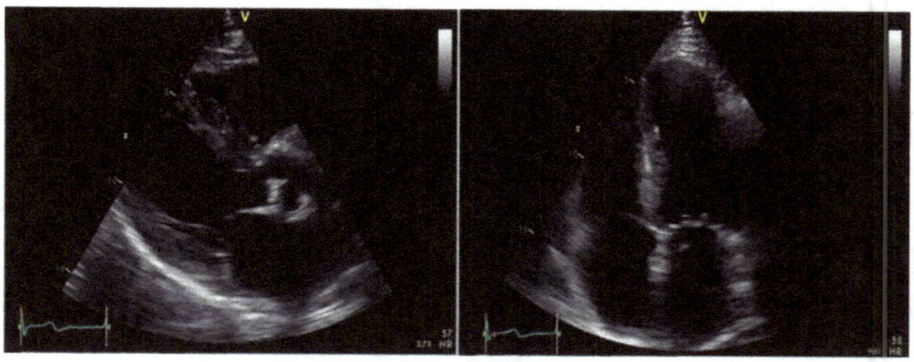

Fig. 2 Parasternal long axis (*left*) and apical four-chamber (*right*) views echocardiography images. Videos are available as Additional files 1 and 2

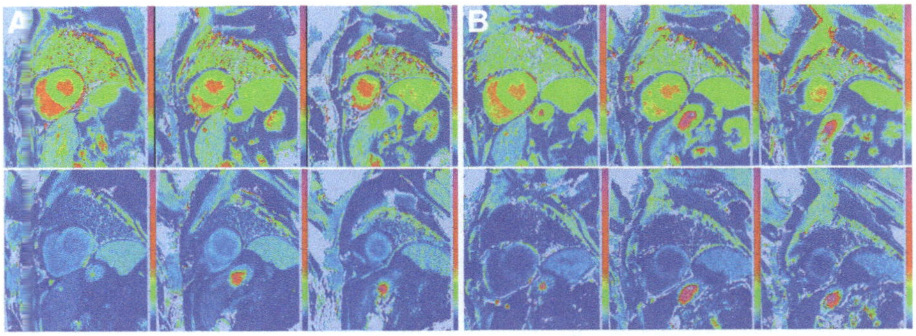

Fig. 3 Short axis ShMOLLI T1 mapping images pre-contrast (top) and post-contrast (bottom) with gadolinium-DOTA, Dotarem® (**a**) and with gadolinium-BOPTA, MultiHance® (**b**). Myocardial T1 post-contrast = 486 ms and blood T1 post-contrast =506 ms 15 min after gadolinium-DOTA, Dotarem®; and myocardial T1 post-contrast = 344 ms and blood T1 post-contrast = 287 ms 15 min after gadolinium-BOPTA, MultiHance®

be stable to a standard deviation of 0.02 (0.03 for amyloid); [3] here a 0.08 difference with contrast agent is recorded.

Discussion

Gd-BOPTA (MultiHance®) is an ionic linear chelate favoured for its high relaxivity related to blood protein binding, [2] which also makes it a partially "intra-vascular" contrast agent. Here, paired scanning performed serendipitously for a clinical trial failed to demonstrate the characteristic pattern of myocardial amyloidosis, and performed poorly compared to gadoterate meglumine. MultiHance® is widely used for CMR. This effect was unexpected – but theoretical concerns had been raised for ECV mapping with protein bound contrast agents [4]. Due to difference in relaxivity between the contrast agents, some Authors proposed the use of a lower dose of Gd-BOPTA for reaching similar T1 and ECV values. In this case the same dose was used for both contrasts and this could explain in part the differences observed. In this case, the use of MultiHance® did not affect the diagnosis, but reporting the MultiHance® CMR in isolation without the previous work-up by the National Amyloid Centre could have conceivably led to a misdiagnosis.

Conclusion

We suggest that protein bound agents for interstitial enhancement of non-ischaemic cardiomyopathy (myocardium, ECV measurement) should be used with caution whilst further work is undertaken as the diagnostic performance may not be the same as non-protein bound variants.

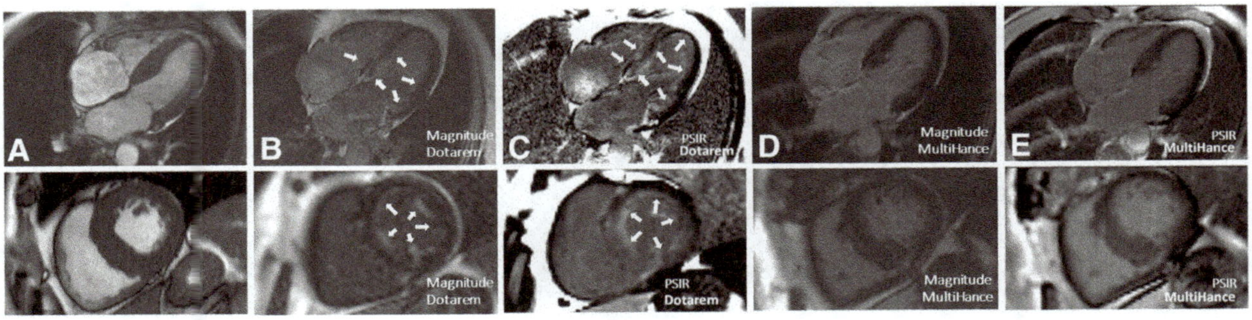

Fig. 4 CMR end-diastolic cine (**a**); late gadolinium images with Magnitude-FLASH (**b**) and late gadolinium images with PSIR-FLASH (**c**) after gadolinium-DOTA, Dotarem® showing the classic amyloid global, subendocardial late gadolinium enhancement pattern; late gadolinium images with Magnitude-FLASH (**d**) and late gadolinium images with PSIR-FLASH (**e**) after gadolinium-BOPTA MultiHance®, showing no features of amyloid

Abbreviations
CMR: Cardiovascular magnetic resonance; ECG: Electrocardiogram; ECV: Extracellular volume; Gd: Gadolinium; LGE: Late gadolinium enhancement; PSIR: Phase Sensitive Inversion Recovery; ShMOLLI: Shortened Modified Look-Locker Inversion recovery; TTR: Transthyretin type

Acknowledgments
Not applicable.

Funding
No funding.

Authors' contributions
MF and JCM have made substantial contributions to conception and design of the case, have been involved in drafting the manuscript and revising it critically for important intellectual content and have given final approval of the version to be published. TAT, AMN, RYK, JDG and PNH have made substantial contributions to conception and design of the case, have been involved in revising the manuscript critically for important intellectual content and have given final approval of the version to be published. All authors read and approved the final manuscript.

Competing interests
The authors declare that they have no competing interests.

Consent for publication
Written informed consent was obtained from the patient for publication of this Case report and any accompanying images. A copy of the written consent is available for review by the Editor-in-Chief of this journal.
The authors do hereby declare that all illustrations and figures in the manuscript are entirely original and do not require reprint permission.

Author details
[1]National Amyloidosis Centre, University College London, Royal Free Hospital, London, UK. [2]Institute of Cardiovascular Science, University College London, London, UK. [3]Barts Heart Centre, West Smithfield, London EC1A 7BE, UK. [4]Non-Invasive Cardiac Imaging, Cardiovascular Medicine Division, Brigham and Women's Hospital, Harvard Medical School, Boston, MA, USA.

References
1. Maceira AM, Joshi J, Prasad SK, Moon JC, Perugini E, Harding I, Sheppard MN, Poole-Wilson PA, Hawkins PN, Pennell DJ. Cardiovascular magnetic resonance in cardiac amyloidosis. Circulation. 2005;111(2):186–93.
2. Pintaske J, Martirosian P, Graf H, Erb G, Lodemann KP, Claussen CD, Schick F. Relaxivity of Gadopentetate Dimeglumine (Magnevist), Gadobutrol (Gadovist), and Gadobenate Dimeglumine (MultiHance) in human blood plasma at 0.2, 1.5, and 3 Tesla. Investig Radiol. 2006;41(3):213–21.
3. Fontana M, White SK, Banypersad SM, Sado DM, Maestrini V, Flett AS, Piechnik SK, Neubauer S, Roberts N, Moon JC. Comparison of T1 mapping techniques for ECV quantification. Histological validation and reproducibility of ShMOLLI versus multibreath-hold T1 quantification equilibrium contrast CMR. J Cardiovasc Magn Reson. 2012;14:88.
4. Moon JC, Messroghli DR, Kellman P, Piechnik SK, Robson MD, Ugander M, Gatehouse PD, Arai AE, Friedrich MG, Neubauer S, et al. Myocardial T1 mapping and extracellular volume quantification: a Society for Cardiovascular Magnetic Resonance (SCMR) and CMR Working Group of the European Society of Cardiology consensus statement. J Cardiovasc Magn Reson. 2013;15:92.

21

Importance of correctly interpreting magnetic resonance imaging to diagnose posterior reversible encephalopathy syndrome associated with HELLP syndrome

Syuichi Tetsuka[1*] and Hiroaki Nonaka[2]

Abstract

Background: Severe haemolysis, elevated liver enzyme levels, and low platelet count (HELLP) syndrome in pregnancy are possible underlying trigger factors for posterior reversible encephalopathy syndrome (PRES). Magnetic resonance imaging (MRI) shows diffuse signal abnormalities involving the subcortical white matter in the parieto-occipital lobes. Although the diagnosis of RPES was clearly established by the distinctive reversibility of clinical and radiological abnormalities, it is difficult to distinguish from differential diagnosis. Thus, it is important to correctly interpret MRI.

Case presentation: We describe a case of HELLP syndrome with PRES. A 38-year-old pregnant woman was admitted to our hospital as an emergency case with a complaint of upper abdominal pain and headache at 29 weeks of pregnancy and the development of HELLP syndrome. An emergency caesarean section was immediately performed. After the operation, the patient received intravenous corticosteroids, and her blood pressure was controlled. Thereafter, she showed an altered mental status. MRI showed hypersignal intense lesions in the cortical and subcortical white matter in the occipital lobes, basal ganglia and callosal splenium in both the fluid-attenuated inversion recovery (FLAIR) sequence and apparent diffusion coefficient (ADC), but these lesions were not recognized in diffusion-weighted imaging (DWI). These images were suggestive of PRES. The patient was kept in the hospital and received the appropriate treatment, after which the patient's level of consciousness improved and all laboratory tests and imaging examinations returned normal.

Conclusion: The MRI findings were useful for the prompt diagnosis of PRES, characterized by hypersignals in FLAIR and ADC, but not in DWI. Additionally, there was an "atypical" MRI appearance of basal ganglial and callosal splenial involvement in this case, which may mistakenly lead clinicians to diagnose other aetiologies than typical PRES. It is considered that vasogenic oedema is the main pathology of PRES according to the MRI image findings. MRI is the gold standard for diagnosing PRES because it can provide information about cerebral involvement earlier than CT; further, it can be a useful tool in the differential diagnosis. This technique facilitated the prompt diagnosis and treatment of the said patient, ultimately resulting in a good outcome.

Keywords: HELLP syndrome, Posterior reversible encephalopathy syndrome, Magnetic resonance imaging

* Correspondence: syuichi@jichi.ac.jp
[1]Department of Neurology, Hospital of Yuki, 9629-1, Yuki, Yuki-City, Ibaraki 307-0001, Japan
Full list of author information is available at the end of the article

Background

Haemolysis, elevated liver enzymes, and low platelet count (HELLP) syndrome is a complication of severe forms of pre-eclampsia that compromises the blood system with haemolysis, hepatic lesions, and low platelet counts and can cause a lethal condition with a high mortality rate of up to 25% [1]. Along with maternal death, HELLP syndrome is associated with the development of focal neurological complications, including seizure, ischaemic and haemorrhagic strokes, cerebral venous thrombosis, eclampsia, cerebral artery dissection, encephalitis, and posterior reversible encephalopathy syndrome (PRES).

PRES is a clinical condition characterized by temporary neurological symptoms such as acute headache, altered mental status, vision loss, and coma. The prognosis of PRES is good when an appropriate treatment is received; symptoms generally improve in approximately 3–8 days, and imaging abnormalities disappear within a few weeks. However, 5%–12% of such cases can assume a negative course with irreversible brain damage culminating in persistent severe neurological deficit or death [2, 3]. Early diagnosis and prompt treatment of PRES are essential to avoid irreversible neurological deficits. The neuroradiographic findings of PRES by magnetic resonance imaging (MRI) are symmetrical subcortical white matter or cortical oedema in the occipital and parietal lobes, brain stem, basal ganglia, frontal lobes, and cerebellum [4, 5]. The typical manifestations of PRES are MRI abnormalities that occur primarily in the subcortical white matter and often extend to the cortical surface, sparing the deep white matter in the classic posterior parietal or occipital lobe region most consistently. The "atypical" findings of basal ganglial and callosal splenial involvement on MRI may mistakenly lead clinicians to diagnose other aetiologies, such as stroke, hypoxic-ischaemic injury, or an overdose of pain medication (e.g., opioids). Intravenous contrast administration is not indicated to diagnose PRES because contrast enhancement is reported to have a variable incidence [6]. Thus, plain MRI is essential in the diagnosis of PRES. We report a case of PRES that showed atypical findings of basal ganglial and callosal splenial involvement on MRI in the setting of severe HELLP syndrome that improved without sequelae because of prompt diagnosis and treatment.

Case presentation

A 38-year-old primigravid reported for a pregnancy screening after her normal gestation period of 28 weeks without hypertension and a normal blood and urine test. She had not experienced any problems during her pregnancy until then. However, later, she was admitted to our hospital of International University of Health and Welfare as an emergency case with a complaint of upper abdominal pain and headache at 29 weeks of pregnancy. On arrival, her Glasgow Coma Scale (GCS) was E4V5M6. Her blood pressure at admission was 200/100 mmHg. Her blood biochemistry showed hypertransaminasemia with aspartate aminotransferase (AST) at 821 IU/L, elevated lactate dehydrogenase (LDH) at 1895 IU/L, and a low platelet count at $4.3 \times 10^5/\mu L$. The patient's serum bilirubin level was 1.7 mg/dl. Glucose, creatinine (Cr), and serum electrolytes were normal. According to HELLP syndrome for the diagnostic criteria (Table 1) [7], she was diagnosed with pregnancy–HELLP syndrome and was immediately scheduled for an emergency caesarean section. The new-born male weighed 975 g with an Apgar score of 7 at the first minute and 8 at the fifth minute. After the operation, the patient was administered intravenous corticosteroids, and nifedipine was continued to maintain her blood pressure below approximately 150/90 mmHg. Gabexate mesilate and anti-thrombin III were also infused to treat intravascular coagulation, which is often observed in patients with HELLP syndrome.

On the second postoperative day, she was assessed by a neurologist. She was conscious but very drowsy and could move her limbs and follow simple orders, and her GCS was E3V4M5. However, she occasionally presented with delirium, which is characterized by a fluctuating mental status. A brain MRI was immediately performed because of her drowsy and confused state on the neurological examination. MRI showed hypersignal intense lesions in the cortical and subcortical white matter in the occipital lobes, basal ganglia and callosal splenium in both the fluid-attenuated inversion recovery (FLAIR) sequence (Fig. 1a) and apparent diffusion coefficient (ADC) (Fig. 1b), but these lesions were not recognized in diffusion-weighted imaging (DWI) (Fig. 1c). DWI was normal. These images were suggestive of PRES. The aforementioned treatment was continued. On biochemical analysis, it was observed that the liver function improved (AST 59 IU/L, LDH 932 IU/L); however, renal impairment deteriorated further (Cr 4.27 mg/dl). In addition, her urine volume decreased to approximately

Table 1 The diagnostic criteria and classification of HELLP syndrome [7]

Class 1: requires severe thrombocytopenia (platelets ≤50,000/μl), evidence of hepatic dysfunction (AST [aspartate aminotransferase] and/or ALT [alanine aminotransferase] ≥70 IU/l), and evidence suggestive of hemolysis (total serum LDH [lactate dehydrogenase] ≥600 IU/l).
Class 2: requires similar criteria except thrombocytopenia is moderate (>50,000 to ≤100,000/μl).
Class 3: includes patients with mild thrombocytopenia (platelets >100,000 but ≤150,000/μl), mild hepatic dysfunction (AST and/or ALT ≥40 IU/l), and hemolysis (total serum LDH ≥600 IU/L).

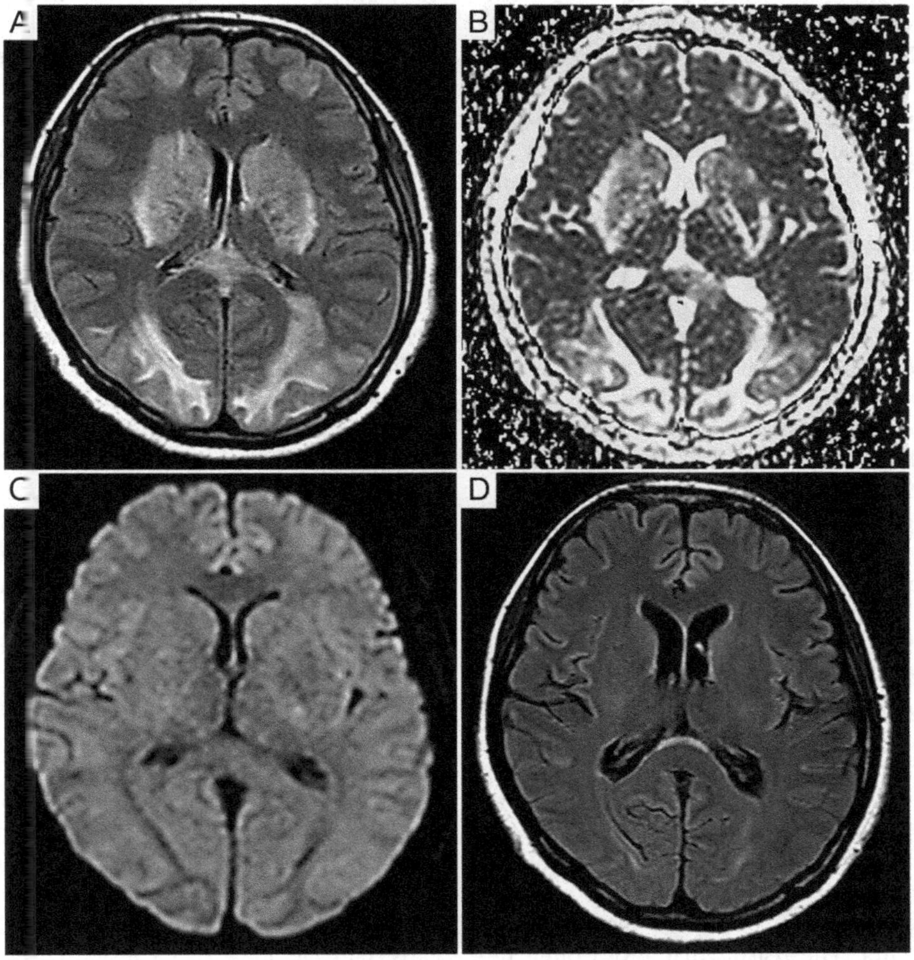

Fig. 1 MRI showed hypersignal intense lesions in the cortical and subcortical white matter in the occipital lobes, basal ganglia and callosal splenium in both the fluid-attenuated inversion recovery (FLAIR) sequence (**a**) and apparent diffusion coefficient (ADC) (**b**), but these lesions were not recognized in diffusion-weighted imaging (DWI) (**c**). (**b**) The follow-up brain MRI, performed 2 weeks later, showed complete resolution of the lesions

400 ml/day. Subsequently, she received haemodialysis 4 times starting on the 5th postoperative day.

Subsequently, patient's level of consciousness improved, and her renal functional also gradually improved. A complete resolution of the lesions (Fig. 1d) was observed on the follow-up brain MRI performed in 2 weeks after caesarean section. The patient was kept in the hospital for 21 days, and throughout this period, all laboratory tests and imaging examinations returned to normal. The patient was then released, and outpatient follow-up was continued.

Discussion

We present a case of HELLP syndrome that occurred during pregnancy associated with clinical and neuroradiological findings consistent with PRES. The major complications in such cases are eclampsia, haematologic (intravascular disseminated coagulation) and cardiopulmonary (pulmonary oedema and acute cardiac insufficiency) events, and neurological alterations (cerebral bleeding, hypoxic–ischaemic encephalopathy, eclampsia). When HELLP syndrome complicates eclampsia, the maternal and perinatal death rates increase with delayed diagnosis or inappropriate treatment, accounting for the poor overall prognosis [8]. Early treatment reduces both maternal and perinatal complications. Headache, altered consciousness, seizures, and visual symptoms, including cortical blindness, are frequent clinical findings associated with PRES.

PRES is predominantly characterized by reversible brain oedema affecting the occipital and posterior parietal regions and is usually described in association with hypertensive encephalopathy, eclampsia, and renal failure [4, 5]. A mild elevation in blood pressure may occur with PRES, even in patients without hypertension [4, 9].

We hypothesize that because blood pressure has a tendency to increase during pregnancy, a physiological state connected to PRES may be involved in the development of this case. However, PRES commonly occurs in patients with eclampsia. Cerebral vasospasm is the proposed aetiology of eclampsia, although the patient did not show eclampsia, which suggests that vasogenic oedema of the brain plays a major pathophysiological role in most patients with PRES. However, PRES is not always reversible. McKinney et al. [10] reported that DWI abnormalities were found in a minority (15–20%), which later studies have shown to potentially lead to neurologic sequelae and encephalomalacia. The lack of DWI abnormalities in this patient solidified the diagnosis of PRES. However, this patient had basal ganglial abnormalities, which could confound the diagnosis described in 10–15% of the patients in the aforementioned study [10]. Considering these factors, this PRES case was relatively rare.

Vasogenic oedema due to cerebrovascular autoregulatory dysfunction results in the leakage of fluid into the interstitium. It was considered that vasogenic oedema is the main pathology of PRES by MRI imaging findings. Endogenous-exogenous factors injure the endothelial cells in the brain blood vessels in PRES. Furthermore, ischaemia due to vasospasm accelerates endothelial injury. If there is an increase in blood pressure due to whole-body vasospasm and hypertension, even if it is slight, it is considered that the autoregulatory capacity of the blood–brain barrier and cerebral blood flow collapses immediately. Therefore, it is presumed that vasogenic oedema easily occurs. The reason that PRES often develops with an increase in blood pressure is thought to involve an increase in blood pressure accompanying vasospasm and injury of vascular endothelial cells, including ischaemia. More recent evidence suggests that endothelial injury is a more likely cause, as many (up to 50%) PRES patients do not have elevated BP. However, BP and other factors certainly contribute. Additionally, the fact that DWI is positive suggests that cytotoxic oedema can coexist or occur superimposed in a minority and that vasogenic oedema is just one component of the injury. It has become clear that perhaps hypoperfusion or hyperperfusion alone are inadequate explanations for the manifestations of PRES. A more novel theory is that of a systemic toxicity, perhaps with increased leukocyte trafficking, which results in endothelial dysfunction. Hypoperfusion and vasoconstriction may lead to hypoxia with the upregulation of vascular endothelial growth factor; as a result, endothelial permeability increases. This process may be modulated by changes in blood pressure, with increased autoregulatory vasoconstriction in response to increases in blood pressure. In summary, 1) severe hypertension leads to failed auto-regulation, subsequent hyperperfusion, and endothelial injury/vasogenic oedema; and 2) vasoconstriction and hypoperfusion lead to brain ischaemia and subsequent vasogenic oedema [11, 12]. This is important when considering the MRI findings of PRES. Both vasogenic and cytotoxic oedema show signal hyperintensity on FLAIR. However, DWI only shows markedly high density for cytotoxic oedema. In addition, ADC maps only display the diffusion component and are hyperintense in PRES, in contrast to being hypointense in cytotoxic oedema that causes ischaemia (cerebral infraction) (Table 2). Such MRI findings were also recognized in this case. In addition, there are characteristic differences on brain lesions, indicating abnormal MRI imaging between PRES patients unrelated to pregnancy and those with HELLP syndrome. Although abnormal findings on MRI are almost always located only in the occipital and parietal lobe in most patients with non-associated PRES [13], many studies since then have shown that "atypical" variants abound [14], but the constellation of findings on imaging along with clinical features suggest PRES.

However, in HELLP syndrome, lesions are frequency observed in the brain stem, basal ganglia and thalamus, which are arterially supplied by small end arteries with little collateral circulation [15]. Based on these results, thrombotic microangiopathy in HELLP syndrome may result in higher incidence of those lesion [16]. However, FLIAR-MRI abnormalities in the occipital lobe, basal ganglia and callosal splenium were recognized in this case (Fig. 1a). This is a relatively rare case. Although the reversibility of vasogenic oedema in PRES is typical, early damage may also cause ischaemia [8]. PRES is usually considered a reversible condition if it is promptly diagnosed and properly treated. However, a delayed or incorrect diagnosis may lead to irreversible damage [17]. The differential diagnosis of PRES caused by stroke, cerebral venous thrombosis, encephalitis, and metabolic and demyelinating disorders may be difficult in pregnancy and puerperium [4]. In addition, given presence of basal ganglial and callosal lesions visualized on the MRI in this case (Fig. 1a), the differential diagnosis should be expanded to include hypoxic-ischaemic injury, or overdose of pain medication (e.g., opioids). The mistreatment of vasogenic oedema associated with PRES because ischaemic changes due to acute stroke might result in the

Table 2 Characteristics of PRES on MRI

Image conditions (MRI)	Vasogenic oedema	Cytotoxic oedema	PRES	Cerebral infraction (Acute stage)
FLAIR	↑	↑	↑	N, then ↑
DWI	N	↑	N	N, then ↑
ADC	↑	↓	↑	↓

N normal, *PRES* posterior reversible encephalopathy syndrome; ↑, hyperintense signal; ↓, hypointense signal

stopping of prompt antihypertensive treatment. In contrast, the appropriate and rapid lowering of blood pressure in patients with PRES is essential to avoid any permanent brain injury, and PRES is reversible when early diagnosis is established and appropriate treatment is started without delay [18]. However, prospective studies are warranted to establish predictors of fatality in patients with PRES [19]. Therefore, MRI plays an important role in the prompt diagnosis of PRES.

In this case, corticosteroids were promptly used for the treatment of HELLP syndrome, and this treatment is considered to slow disease progression and prevent new major maternal morbidity [20]. Corticosteroids should reduce vasogenic oedema. Thus, aggressively used potent glucocorticoids are recommended for the management of patients considered to have HELLP syndrome [6]. Although there are only a few reports in the literature on the use of steroids in patients with PRES [21], corticosteroids might have been effective for PRES in this case.

Conclusion

In this article, we report and highlight a rare association between severe HELLP syndrome and PRES. MRI findings were useful for the prompt diagnosis of PRES, which is characterized by hypersignals in FLAIR and ADC, but not in DWI. Additionally, the "atypical" MRI appearance of basal ganglial and callosal splenial involvement, as demonstrated in this case, may mistakenly lead clinicians to diagnose other aetiologies compared to typical PRES. It is considered that vasogenic oedema is the main pathology of PRES according to MRI image findings. This technique facilitated prompt diagnosis and treatment, resulting in a good outcome. We believe that clinicians should be aware of this neurological syndrome because prompt diagnosis and treatment may result in complete resolution.

Abbreviations

ADC: Apparent diffusion coefficient; AST: Aspartate aminotransferase; Cr: Creatinine; DWI: Diffusion-weighted image; FLAIR: Fluid-attenuated inversion recovery; GCS: Glasgow coma scale; HELLP: Haemolysis, elevated liver enzymes, and low platelet count; LDH: Lactate dehydrogenase; MRI: Magnetic resonance imaging; PRES: Posterior reversible encephalopathy syndrome

Acknowledgements

The authors would like to thank American Journal Experts (http://bit.ly/AJE_BS) for the English language review.

Funding

This case report was not founded by any grant or company.

Authors' contributions

Study concept and design: ST. Acquisition of data: HN. Analysis and interpretation of data: ST and HN. Drafting of the manuscript: ST. Critical revision of the manuscript for important intellectual content: All authors. Both authors read and approved the final manuscript.

Competing interests

The authors declare that they have no conflicts of interest.

Consent for publication

Written informed consent was obtained from the patient for publication of this case report and any accompanying images.

Author details

[1]Department of Neurology, Hospital of Yuki, 9629-1, Yuki, Yuki-City, Ibaraki 307-0001, Japan. [2]Obstetrics & Gynecology, Hospital of International University of Health and Welfare, 537-3, Iguchi, Nasushiobara, Tochigi 329-2763, Japan.

References

1. Ellison J, Sattar N, Greer I. HELLP syndrome: mechanisms and management. Hosp Med. 1999;60:243–9.
2. Singhal AB, Kimberly WT, Schaefer PW, Hedley-Whyte ET. Case records of the Massachusetts general hospital. case 8–2009. A 36-year-old woman with headache, hypertension, and seizure 2 weeks post partum. N Engl J Med. 2009;360:1126–37.
3. Fugate JE, Wijdicks EF, Parisi JE, Kallmes DF, Cloft HJ, Flemming KD, et al. Fulminant postpartum cerebral vasoconstriction syndrome. Arch Neurol. 2012;69:111–7.
4. Hinchey J, Chaves C, Appignani B, Breen J, Pao L, Wang A, et al. A reversible posterior leukoencephalopathy syndrome. N Engl J Med. 1996;334:494–500.
5. Garg RK. Posterior leukoencephalopathy syndrome. Postgrad Med J. 2001;77:24–8.
6. Karia SJ, Rykken JB, McKinney ZJ, Zhang L, McKinney AM. Utility and significance of gadolinium-based contrast enhancement in posterior reversible encephalopathy syndrome. AJNR Am J Neuroradiol. 2016;37:415–22.
7. Martin Jr JN, Rose CH, Briery CM. Understanding and managing HELLP syndrome: the integral role of aggressive glucocorticoids for mother and child. Am J Obstet Gynecol. 2006;195:914–34. Review.
8. Norwitz ER, Hsu CD, Repke JT. Acute complications of preeclampsia. Clin Obstet Gynecol. 2002;45:308–29.
9. Kastrup O, Maschke M, Wanke I, Diener HC. Posterior reversible encephalopathy syndrome due to severe hypercalcemia. J Neurol. 2002;249: 1563–6.
10. McKinney AM, Short J, Truwit CL, McKinney ZJ, Kozak OS, SantaCruz KS, et al. Posterior reversible encephalopathy syndrome: incidence of atypical regions of involvement and imaging findings. AJR Am J Roentgenol. 2007;189:904–12.
11. Rykken JB, McKinney AM. Posterior reversible encephalopathy syndrome. Semin Ultrasound CT MR. 2014;35:118–35.
12. Bartynski WS. Posterior reversible encephalopathy syndrome, part 2: controversies surrounding pathophysiology of vasogenic edema. AJNR Am J Neuroradiol. 2008;29:1043–9.
13. Bartynski WS, Boardman JF. Distinct imaging patterns and lesion distribution in posterior reversible encephalopathy syndrome. AJNR Am J Neuroradiol. 2007;28:1320–7.
14. McKinney AM, Jagadeesan BD, Truwit CL. Central-variant posterior reversible encephalopathy syndrome: brainstem or basal ganglia involvement lacking cortical or subcortical cerebral edema. AJR Am J Roentgenol. 2013;201:631–8.
15. Negro A, Zuccoli G, Regolisti G, Mastrangeli S, Rossi E. Reversible posterior leukoencephalopathy associated with postpartum HELLP syndrome. Eur J Intern Med. 2005;16:291–3.

16. Fakhouri F. Pregnancy-related thrombotic microangiopathies: clues from complement biology. Transfus Apher Sci. 2016;54:199–202.
17. Antunes NL, Small TN, George D, Boulad F, Lis E. Posterior leukoencephalopathy syndrome may not be reversible. Pediatr Neurol. 1999;20:241–3.
18. Cozzolino M, Bianchi C, Mariani G, Marchi L, Fambrini M, Mecacci F. Therapy and differential diagnosis of posterior reversible encephalopathy syndrome (PRES) during pregnancy and postpartum. Arch Gynecol Obstet. 2015;292:1217–23.
19. Siebert E, Bohner G, Liebig T, Endres M, Liman TG. Factors associated with fatal outcome in posterior reversible encephalopathy syndrome: a retrospective analysis of the Berlin PRES study. J Neurol. 2016;4:1–6.
20. Martin Jr JN, Owens MY, Keiser SD, Parrish MR, Tam Tam KB, Brewer JM, et al. Standardized Mississippi protocol treatment of 190 patients with HELLP syndrome: slowing disease progression and preventing new major maternal morbidity. Hypertens Pregnancy. 2012;31:79–90.
21. Roth C, Ferbert A. The posterior reversible encephalopathy syndrome: what's certain, what's new? Pract Neurol. 2011;11:136–44.

22

Cardiovascular magnetic resonance in the evaluation of heart valve disease

G. S. Gulsin*, A. Singh and G. P. McCann

Abstract

Background: Over the last 25 years, cardiovascular magnetic resonance imaging (CMR) has emerged as an alternative to echocardiography for assessment of valvular heart disease (VHD). Although echo remains the first-line imaging modality for the assessment of patients with VHD, CMR can now provide a comprehensive assessment in many instances. Using a combination of techniques, CMR provides information on valve anatomy and enables quantitative analysis of the severity of the valve lesion.

Main text: In this review, the fundamentals of CMR in assessment of VHD are described, together with its strengths and weaknesses. We detail the utility of CMR for studying all aspects of VHD, including valve anatomy, flow quantification as well as ventricular volumes and function. The optimisation of CMR for evaluating the commonest valve lesions (aortic stenosis, aortic regurgitation, mitral regurgitation, mitral stenosis) as well as in right-sided VHD and prosthetic valves is summarised. The focus of this review is to enable the reader to optimise the use of CMR in his or her own evaluation of heart valve lesions in clinical practice.

Conclusions: CMR can be used for the comprehensive evaluation of VHD. This exciting, non-invasive imaging modality is likely to have increasing utility in the clinical evaluation of patients with VHD.

Background

Over the last 25 years, CMR has emerged as an alternative to echocardiography for assessment of valvular heart disease (VHD). Although echocardiography remains the first-line imaging modality for the assessment of patients with VHD, CMR can now provide a comprehensive assessment in many instances. This is especially true in patients with poor acoustic windows and where echocardiography is limited by operator dependence.

Using a combination of techniques, CMR provides information on valve anatomy and enables quantitative analysis of the severity of the valve lesion. CMR allows unparalleled evaluation of the consequences of valve disease on the relevant ventricle and on the anatomy of surrounding structures. Tissue characterisation, particularly with late gadolinium enhanced (LGE) also provides additional information regarding myocardial infarction or fibrosis, which may be clinically relevant in patients with VHD. The relative strengths and weaknesses of CMR in the evaluation of VHD are listed in Table 1, below.

* Correspondence: Gaurav.gulsin@nhs.net
Department of Cardiovascular Sciences, University of Leicester and the NIHR Biomedical Research Centre Glenfield Hospital, Groby Road, Leicester, UK

In this article, we review the role of CMR in the evaluation of VHD, with emphasis on clinical applications of CMR techniques. In particular, we focus on the four key left-sided valve pathologies: aortic stenosis (AS), aortic regurgitation (AR), mitral stenosis (MS) and mitral regurgitation (MR). We also highlight the role of CMR in the assessment of other, rarer valve lesions.

General principles

CMR pulse sequences for evaluation of valvular heart disease

Several CMR radiofrequency pulse sequences are used in the assessment of VHD. The pulse sequences have utility in different circumstances applicable to VHD (Table 2).

Heart valve anatomy

The complete valve anatomy can be visualised by CMR, including the valve leaflets, chordae tendinae and papillary muscles. CMR can also identify the presence of valve masses, such as vegetations, thrombi and tumours, highlighting their attachment site and mobility [1, 2].

Table 1 The strengths and weakness of CMR in the evaluation of VHD

CMR strengths	CMR weaknesses
Unlimited windows	Regurgitant jet visualisation inferior to echocardiography
Excellent image quality	Low through-plane spatial resolution
Flow quantification	Low(er) temporal resolution
Gold standard imaging modality for left and right ventricle assessment	Averages of multiple R-R intervals
Multi-parametric comprehensive assessment (LGE, T1 mapping, ischaemia)	Peak velocities can be underestimated
	Flow quantification can be prone to errors

The steady-state free precession (SSFP) pulse sequence is the most widely used for assessment of valve morphology and function [3]. To visualise each valve throughout systole and diastole, image acquisition is gated to the ECG over several cardiac cycles. Each slice can be obtained within a single breath hold lasting only 5-8 s. SSFP sequences are favoured for their high contrast between blood pool and surrounding structures, together with a high signal-to-noise ratio. SSFP can be used to produce 2D cine images of all four heart valves in any prescribed plane, with multiple phases throughout the cardiac cycle. This allows all four valves to be imaged irrespective of challenging thoracic or cardiac anatomy and is particularly useful for right-sided heart valves, which are often difficult to study with echocardiography. Furthermore, planimetry enables direct measurement of valve orifice area for stenotic valves.

Several limitations of CMR assessment of valve anatomy exist. Foremost is the relatively large slice thickness (typically 5-8 mm) of CMR cine images. Thin structures as cardiac valves (which are usually 1-2 mm thick) are therefore susceptible to partial volume effects. Careful planning of imaging slices perpendicular to the valve enhance assessment and in plane resolution will typically be in the order of 1.0–1.5 mm if a matrix of 256 is used and the field of view is 260mm x 390mm. Thinner slice thickness (4–5 mm) can improve the accuracy of evaluation but at the expense of reduced signal to noise ratio. This is particularly important for measurement of valve orifice area, where positioning of the slice image at the valve tips is vital to avoid error in planimetry. Such errors can be avoided by imaging across the valve area with multiple parallel slices to determine the position closest to the valve tips (Fig. 1).

Table 2 CMR pulse sequences with utility in the evaluation of VHD [4]

CMR pulse sequence	Utility in VHD
Steady-state free precession	Valve anatomy and motion Ventricular volumes and function Turbulent blood flow jet visualisation
Gradient echo	Valve anatomy and motion Turbulent blood flow jet visualisation Prosthetic valve assessment
Phase contrast	Flow velocity Forward and reverse volumes
Turbo spin echo	Evaluation of valve masses
Segmented inversion recovery gradient echo	Evaluation of valve masses

Flow

SSFP and gradient echo cine images provide visualisation of turbulent flow jets across stenosed or regurgitant valves. These are seen as signal voids and occur due to spin-dephasing in moving protons. A visual assessment of the site and direction of stenotic or regurgitant flow, similar to that with colour flow echo Doppler, can be made prior to further evaluation of the valve lesion. In this regard SSFP is less sensitive than gradient echo in depicting regurgitant jets. In gradient echo sequences the sensitivity for detecting spin-dephasing is a function of the echo time, i.e. the longer the echo time, the larger and more pronounced the jet [4].

Flow velocity can be directly quantified by CMR using through-plane phase contrast velocity mapping. Phase-contrast pulse sequences are based on the property that protons moving within a magnetic field gradient acquire a shift in the phase of their rotational spin compared with stationary protons. The magnitude of this shift is proportional to velocity. The net phase of moving protons is proportional to the velocity of blood and can be displayed as a phase map, where different velocities are represented by different signal intensities. Flow in the direction of the phase-encoding appears white whereas flow in the opposite direction appears black. Stationary objects (i.e. those with a phase-shift of zero) appear grey.

Velocity mapping generates two sets of images: 1) magnitude images, which delineate the anatomy of the vessel(s) being studied and their surrounding structures, and 2) phase velocity maps, where the velocities within each pixel are encoded (Fig. 2). The region of interest is traced on these images for each frame of the cardiac cycle. Flow volume (cm^3/s) is calculated by multiplying the velocity within each pixel (cm/s) by the area (cm^2) and a flow-time graph can be generated over one cardiac cycle (Fig. 3).

CMR 2D phase-contrast flow measurements can be performed with free-breathing or breath-held techniques.

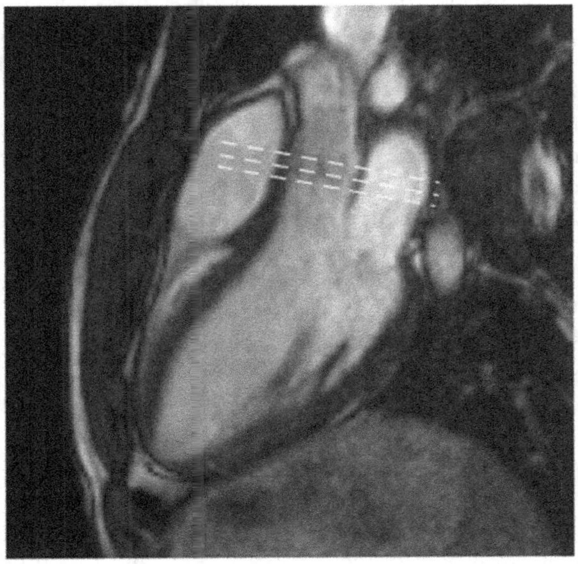

Fig. 1 SSFP cine three-chamber image of the normal aortic valve. Dashed lines indicate location of multiple parallel slices that should be used to avoid errors in planimetry. Source: University Hospitals of Leicester NHS Trust

Breath-held acquisitions are shorter, but may not account for the physiological effects of breathing on cardiac filling. Breath holding may also prove difficult in patients with dyspnoea. Free-breathing techniques have a longer sampling time and require temporal averaging of flow measurements, but may better account for physiological effects of breath holding. Because phase-contrast flow mapping relies on ECG gating to average flow information over multiple cardiac cycles, it is prone to errors in patients with arrhythmias, where there are beat-to-beat flow variations. In such cases, real-time phase contrast flow imaging may be performed without ECG gating [5].

CMR flow measurements correlate strongly with Doppler and invasive in-vivo flow measurements [6–8]. However the temporal resolution of CMR flow measurement (25–45 ms) is lower than that of continuous wave Doppler echo (2 ms). For high flow velocities of short duration, there is the risk that CMR flow measurement may underestimate peak velocity. Nevertheless the temporal resolution of CMR is sufficient for most flow measurements.

A key limitation of clinical flow acquisition is the occurrence of positive or negative phase offset errors, which occur due to local non-compensated eddy currents. Phase offset errors can lead to considerable miscalculations in flow quantification. Even small velocity offset errors can lead to sizeable flow quantification errors, because flow volume is calculated by integrating velocities across the cross-sectional area of the vessel over the entire cardiac cycle [9]. Velocity offset errors can be minimised by ensuring that the vessel of interest is positioned into the isocenter plane for flow imaging. Post-acquisition offset correction methods may also improve the reliability of flow quantification. In routine practice, clinicians should be aware of potential inaccuracies in flow quantification and aim to internally validate flow measurement in the aorta versus LV stroke volumes in patients without mitral regurgitation. Alternatively, scanning a stationary gel phantom with identical flow acquisitions as a baseline reference for zero velocity is proposed as a measure to tackle phase offset correction [10].

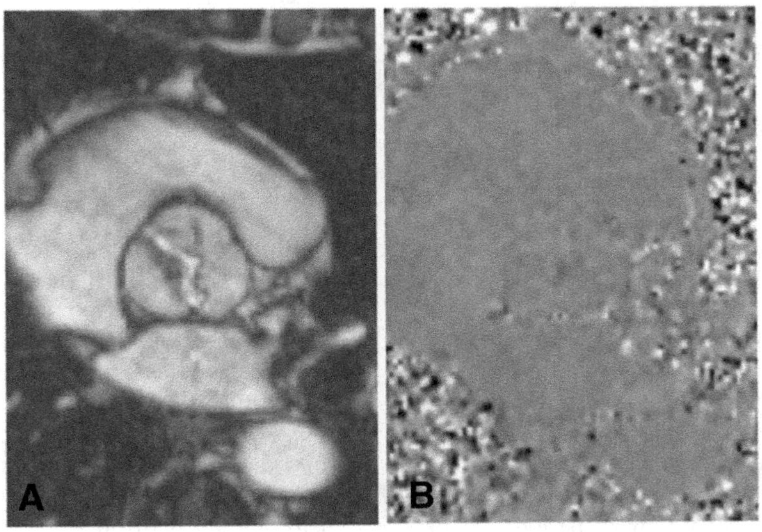

Fig. 2 a magnitude and **b** phase images generated by CMR flow velocity mapping in a patient with a type 1 bicuspid aortic valve. The magnitude image provides visualisation of the valve anatomy and the phase map is used to calculate velocity within each pixel. Source: University Hospitals of Leicester NHS Trust

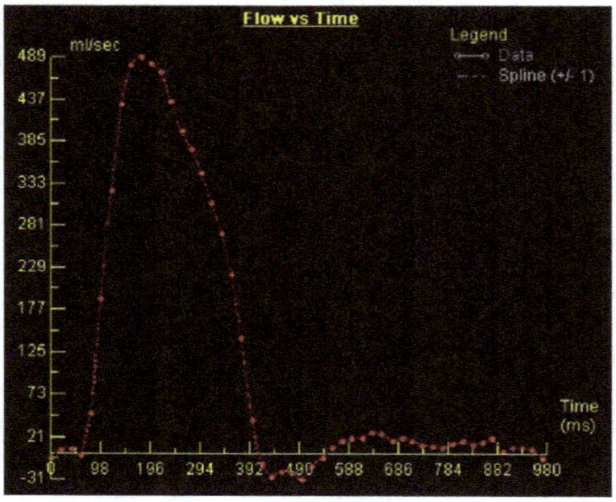

Fig. 3 A normal ascending aortic flow-time graph generated by CMR through-plane phase-contrast velocity mapping. Source: University Hospitals of Leicester NHS Trust

Ventricular volumes and function

CMR is the gold-standard imaging modality for evaluation of left and right ventricular volumes, mass and function [11]. Accurate assessment of the consequence of a valve lesion on the relevant ventricle is imperative in establishing the timing for intervention. Following acquisition of the localiser images, cine imaging is acquired, using the SSFP pulse sequence, in the two-, three- and four- chamber views. The long-axis views are then used to plan a full "stack" of short-axis slices, the first being planned at the mitral valve annulus, perpendicular to the inter-ventricular septum, with a slice every 10 mm, until full coverage of the left ventricle (LV) is achieved (Fig. 4). For quantification, LV epicardial and endocardial contours are drawn at end-diastole and end-systole (Fig. 5), allowing calculation of LV end-diastolic volume (LVEDV), LV end-systolic volume (LVESV), stroke volume (SV), LV ejection fraction (LVEF) and LV mass (LVM) [12].

Aortic stenosis (AS)

AS is the commonest valve disease requiring surgery in the developed world. Up to 3% of individuals aged ≥75 years are affected by AS, most commonly occurring due to calcific degeneration of the aortic valve [13, 14]. Other causes of AS include a congenital bicuspid aortic valve or rheumatic valve disease [14]. Calcific AS advances from a prolonged asymptomatic period with progressive narrowing of the aortic valve orifice. There is a corresponding increase in the pressure gradient across the aortic valve with associated LV pressure overload and LV hypertrophy. Subsequent onset of symptoms – typically angina, heart failure and syncope – portends a poor prognosis without intervention, with death usually occurring within 5 years [15]. Most patients with asymptomatic disease are recommended to undergo periodic monitoring to assess severity and adverse ventricular remodelling [16].

Application of CMR in the evaluation of AS includes anatomical assessment of the aorta and aortic valve, quantification of LV volumes, mass and function, and calculation of stenotic jet velocity [3]. The three standard measures used to establish the severity of AS are valve area, peak velocity and pressure gradient (Table 3) [4].

Cine imaging and determination of aortic valve area

CMR imaging in AS begins with standard three-chamber and coronal SSFP cine views, which provide a visual assessment of the aortic valve, LV, and LV outflow tract structure and function. All AS results in calcification of the aortic valve, which appears as signal void on CMR (Fig. 6).

More detailed aortic valve anatomy is achieved by through-plane SSFP imaging. Planimetry of the orifice should be precisely at the level of the valve tips, which is defined as the minimum area on any slice. Multiple, thin (4–5 mm) slices parallel to the valve should be acquired and we tend to use 0 slice gap, or even half moves of the positioning slice so that there is overlap (2–3 mm) between consecutive slices. This will enable direct planimetry of the valve orifice during systole (Fig. 7). This is the preferred method for grading severity. This method correlates well with aortic valve areas measured by cardiac catheterisation, trans-thoracic and trans-oesophageal echo, and direct measurement of autopsy specimens [17, 18]. Planimetry, however, can be suboptimal in cases of heavily calcified aortic valves due to signal void and stenotic jet turbulence [4]. A spoiled gradient echo pulse sequence can be used as an alternative and is recommended at 3 T as there is less flow artefact compared to SSFP [19].

Quantification by flow mapping

Trans-valvular velocity is measured by velocity mapping, as described above. It is important that the correct slice position is identified for flow measurement, to maximise the accuracy of assessment. Initially in-plane velocity mapping in the LV outflow tract enables the identification of the area of maximal velocity, usually situated just beyond the valve tips in systole. Through-plane velocity mapping perpendicular to this identified area of maximal velocity is then performed, from which peak velocity is measured. Velocity encoding (VENC) is set manually on the phase contrast sequence and must be adjusted to avoid aliasing. Aliasing appears in the centre of the flow

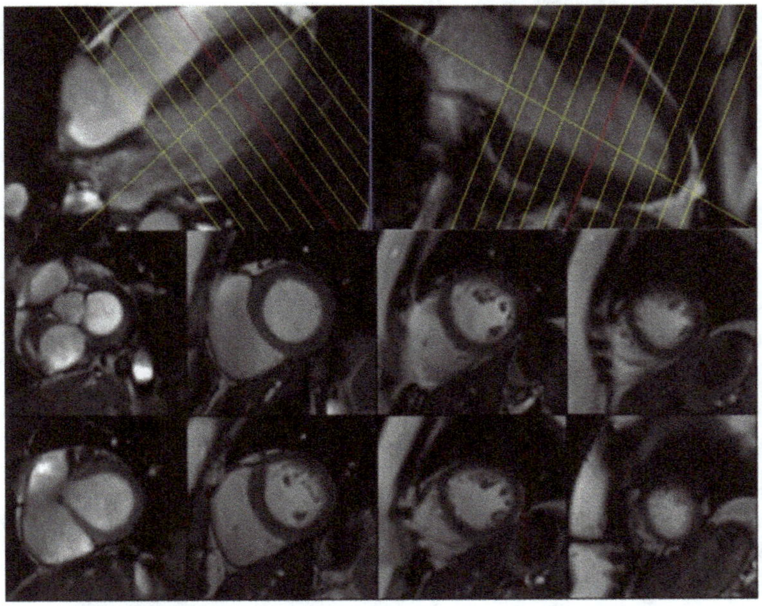

Fig. 4 An example of the planning used for the short-axis SSFP cine stack shown on 4- chamber and 2-chamber slices (top panel), with examples of some short-axis slices (bottom panel). Source: University Hospitals of Leicester NHS Trust

area, as the opposite colour to forward flow. We tend to gauge the required VENC based on how stenotic the valve appears on cine imaging and usually a value of 2.5-4 m/s is chosen. Although some vendors have built-in adjustments of VENC for aliasing, the sequence should be repeated with a higher VENC if there is significant aliasing (>1-2 pixels). Any velocity > 4 m/s should be considered as severe AS unless there is severe combined aortic regurgitation (AR), which increases stroke volume and flow across the valve.

Peak velocity in AS measured by CMR has been validated against continuous-wave Doppler echocardiography and there is a tendency for CMR to underestimate peak velocity [4]. This is the result of partial-volume effects within the vena contracta of very high velocity jets, as well as artefacts generated from turbulent jets as already described [3, 4]. However, CMR is advantageous in cases where correct echo beam alignment through the stenotic jet is difficult.

Aorta imaging

Another benefit of CMR is the ability to characterise the aortic anatomy, which may be affected by post-stenotic aortic root dilatation, and can influence subsequent surgical management. This is especially important in those with a bicuspid aortic valve, where there is particular susceptibility to aortic root dilatation and an association with aortic coarctation. Recent 4D flow studies have suggested that abnormal helical and chaotic flow patterns associated with bicuspid aortic valve disease are likely to

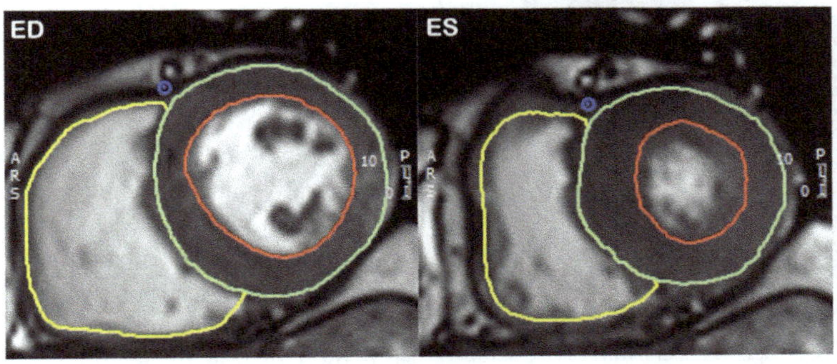

Fig. 5 An example of epicardial (green), endocardial (red) and right ventricular (yellow) contours at end-diastole (ED) and end-systole (ES). Source: University Hospitals of Leicester NHS Trust

Table 3 AHA/ACC recommendations for classification of valve severity [56]

	Aortic sclerosis	Mild	Moderate	Severe
Aortic jet velocity (m/s)	≤2.5	2.6-2.9	3.0-4.0	>4.0
Mean gradient (mmHg)	–	<20	20-40	>40
AVA (cm^2)	–	>1.5	1.0-1.5	<1.0

be the cause of aortic dilatation, rather than an inherited aortopathy [20, 21].

In patients being considered for aortic valve intervention it is essential that aortic annulus measurements are given. This helps guide size of prosthesis and is particularly important for transcutaneous valve insertion [22].

Tissue characterisation

Tissue characterisation by LGE enables the identification of replacement fibrosis in subjects with AS. Over one quarter of patients with AS demonstrate areas of LGE, which correlates with disease severity and is an independent predictor of mortality [23, 24]. When LGE is evident in AS, the typical pattern is one of a patchy mid-wall distribution. The regions of hyperenhancement represent areas of focal fibrosis, but more diffuse myocardial fibrosis may be underestimated by LGE [25]. Markers of diffuse myocardial fibrosis, such as extracellular volume fraction (ECV) and native T1 relaxation times, are also increased in AS and progress with disease severity [26, 27]. Several studies are currently in progress assessing whether multiparametric CMR can predict symptom development and recently, indexed ECV has been shown to be more strongly associated with mortality than LV mass index in AS [28].

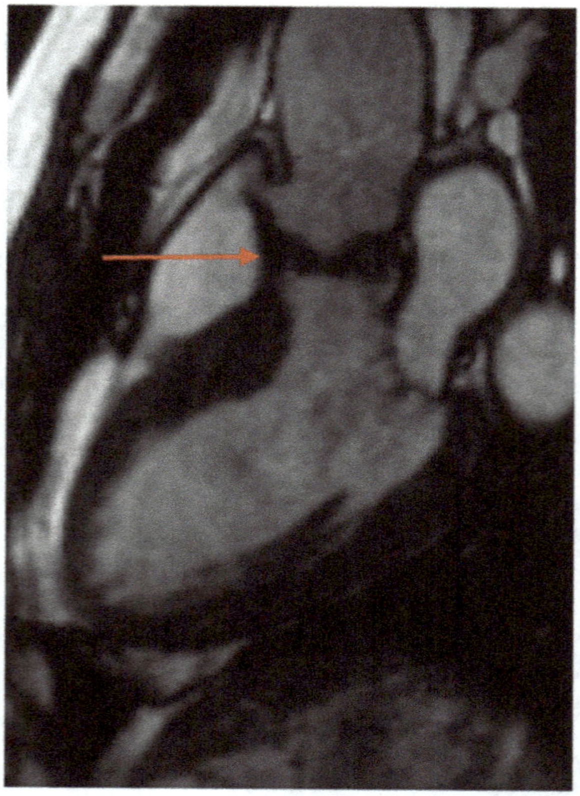

Fig. 6 Three-chamber SSFP cine image of patient with calcific aortic stenosis. Calcification of the aortic valve (arrow) results in signal void on SSFP images. Source: University Hospitals of Leicester NHS Trust

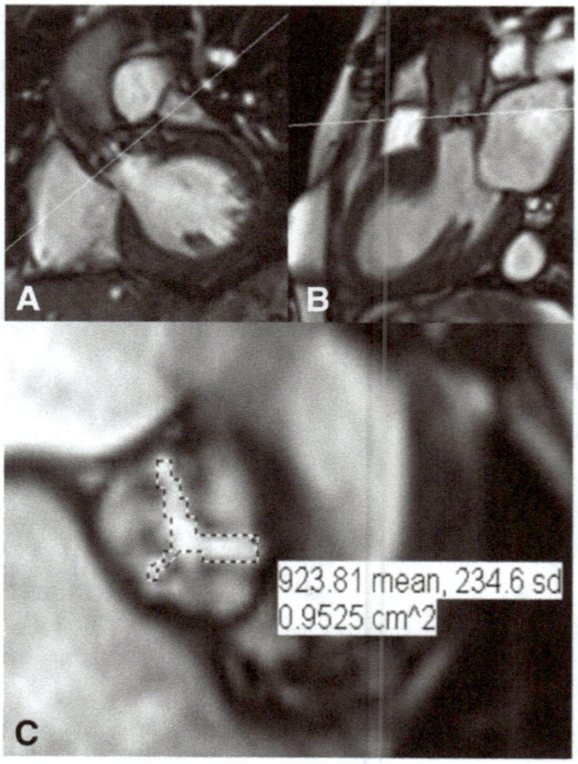

Fig. 7 CMR-derived AV area by 2D planimetry. SSFP cine sequences of (**a**) the LV outflow tract and (**b**) three-chamber with LV outflow tract showing restricted AV leaflets and a stenotic jet. The perpendicular white lines indicate the slice position used for planimetry. (**c**) Direct planimetry of the AV orifice during systole. The calculated aortic valve area (0.95cm^2 indicates severe AS). Source: University Hospitals of Leicester NHS Trust

Aortic regurgitation (AR)

Several disease processes can lead to the development of aortic regurgitation (AR). The commonest of these are degenerative and bicuspid aortic valves, although endocarditis of the aortic valve or diseases of the aortic root causing functional dilatation (e.g. hypertension, aortic dissection and Marfan syndrome) may also cause AR [29]. CMR evaluation of AR is advantageous owing to the high degree of accuracy for assessment of LV volumes and function as well as the capability for determining aortic regurgitant volumes [3, 29]. As with AS,

Table 4 ESC guidelines on grading the severity of AR by echocardiography [57]

	Mild	Moderate	Severe
Qualitative			
Aortic valve morphology	Normal/abnormal	Normal/ abnormal	Abnormal/flail/large coaptation defect.
Colour flow AR jet width	Small in central jets	Intermediate	Large in central jets, variable in eccentric jets
Continuous wave signal of AR jet	Incomplete/faint	Dense	Dense
Diastolic flow reversal in descending aorta	Brief, protodiastolic flow reversal	Intermediate	Holodiastolic flow reversal (end-diastolic velocity > 20 cm/s)
Semi-quantitative			
Vena contracta width (mm)	<3	Intermediate	>6
Pressure half-time (ms)	>500	Intermediate	<200
Quantitative			
Effective regurgitant orifice area (mm^2)	<10	10-29	≥30
Regurgitant volume (mL)	<30	30-59	≥60

periodic monitoring of AR is recommended [30]. Echocardiographic guidelines for grading the severity of AR are shown in Table 4.

Cine imaging

A similar approach to AS is used for CMR imaging in AR. This begins with the standard visual assessment of the aortic valve, LV, and LV outflow tract structure and function using SSFP cine sequences (Fig. 8a). The impact of AR on the LV is assessed with accurate LV volume and function quantification by CMR. Serial measurements can be performed with high reproducibility and provide useful information regarding disease progression. In a multi-centre observational study LV EDV >246 mL predicted those patients who developed a class I guideline indication for surgery [31].

Valve morphology (e.g. bicuspid/tricuspid) and aortic root anatomy are of particular interest in patients with AR. Planimetry of the valve orifice should be acquired as for AS (Fig. 5b). The regurgitant orifice area may be measured directly by planimetry. It should be noted that calculation of the regurgitant jet area or length are not reliable indices of disease severity and are therefore not usually performed [4]. Assessment of the aortic root anatomy can aid in the identification of the cause of AR as well as determining the requirement for aortic root repair/replacement alongside AVR.

Calculation of AR severity

Phase-contrast velocity mapping is used to calculate forward and reverse flow per cardiac cycle. Positioning of the imaging slice is important to ensure accurate assessment [32]. In AR the imaging slice is usually positioned at the level of sinotubular junction allowing direct measurement of the trans-valvular forward and regurgitant volumes. However, others advocate measurement at the valve tips or annulus and a recent paper in normal subjects showed that stroke volume measured at the annulus was more closely associated with LV stroke volume than flow measured at the sino-tubular junction. We

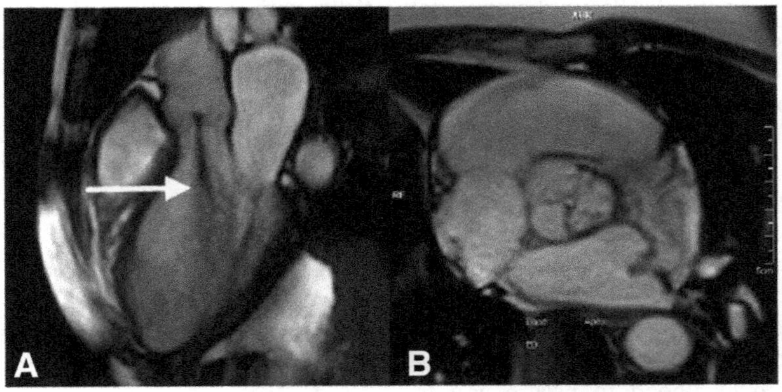

Fig. 8 SSFP cine three-chamber image showing aortic regurgitation. **a** The central regurgitant jet (arrow) is visible as signal void on SSFP sequences. **b** Visualisation of the central AV regurgitant orifice by direct planimetry. Source: University Hospitals of Leicester NHS Trust

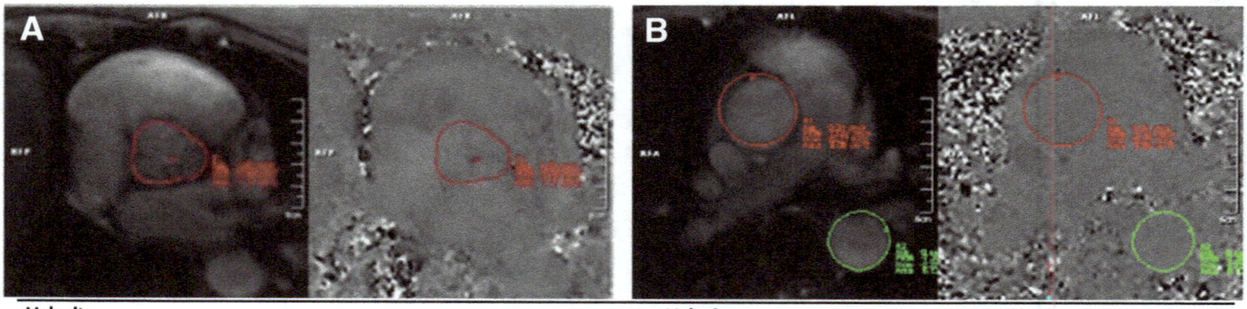

Velocity:		Velocity:	
Peak velocity	321.02 cm/sec	Peak velocity	207.54 cm/sec
Average Velocity	6.19 cm/sec	Average Velocity	6.12 cm/sec
Flow:		**Flow:**	
Forward volume	50.40 mL	Forward volume	69.91 mL
Reverse volume	6.03mL	Reverse volume	15.67 mL

Fig. 9 Phase contrast velocity mapping in aortic regurgitation. Aortic flow has been measured at (**a**) aortic level and (**b**) pulmonary artery level. Note the difference in forward and reverse volumes generated by velocity mapping at the different sites. At (**a**) the aortic level the regurgitant fraction is 12% compared with 23% at (**b**) the PA level, which reflects lower calculated stroke volumes if flow is calculated at aortic level. Source: University Hospitals of Leicester NHS Trust

have seen multiple cases where the stroke volume was lower at the annulus and we suggest that flow is measured at the annulus, sino-tubular junction and pulmonary artery bifurcation (Fig. 9) [33].

For inexperienced centres, we recommend that aorta flow is routinely measured in patients between contrast administration and late gadolinium enhanced image acquisition. This allows centres to obtain a good 'feel' for how accurate aorta flow measurement is against LV stroke volume.

Regurgitant volume is simply the difference between LV stroke volume from the LV measurements and forward aortic volume. From these the regurgitant fraction is calculated (regurgitant volume/forward volume × 100) [3]. Although there is a moderate correlation between regurgitant volumes measured by echocardiography and CMR, the limits of agreement are wide but observer variability is significantly lower with CMR, suggesting this may be the preferred method of assessment [34]. Flow mapping alone can be used to calculate severity of AR and flow reversal can be directly quantified with this technique. Alternatively the regurgitant volume can be calculated by cine assessment and comparison of LV and right ventricle (RV) stroke volumes. The difference in ventricular stroke volumes represents the regurgitant volume, assuming no other valve disease is present [3, 4].

Regurgitant fraction is an independent predictor of outcome in patients with AR, and a regurgitant fraction of >33% has been shown to predict the likelihood of requiring surgery within nine years [31]. A combination of LV EDV and regurgitant fraction are proposed as powerful discriminators for the likelihood to progression to surgery but randomised trials are required to demonstrate clinical benefit [31].

Mitral stenosis (MS)

Rheumatic heart disease is by far the commonest cause of MS, accounting for over 95% of cases [35]. As a consequence the prevalence of MS has fallen with the decline of rheumatic fever in the developed world [36]. Rarer causes include carcinoid, Fabry's disease, mucopolysaccharidoses, Whipple's disease, rheumatoid arthritis, gout and congenital mitral stenosis [37]. Over one-third of patients with rheumatic mitral valve disease have involvement of other valves, most commonly the aortic valve [35]. This should be considered as part of the CMR evaluation of MS. Severity of MS by echo is graded predominantly by valve area, although mean gradient and pulmonary artery pressure are also useful markers of severity (Table 5) [38].

Standard assessment of MS begins with the standard SSFP cine views, followed by mitral valve (MV) planimetry and MV flow velocities. The two-chamber, four-chamber and LVOT views are of particular interest initially, with visualisation of the signal void generated by the stenotic jet (Fig. 10a). The impact of MS on the left atrium is easily quantified by these images. MV planimetry may be performed in a manner similar to the AV (Fig. 10b). An imaging plane close to the MV tips should be acquired during diastole. Multiple, thin (4-5 mm)

Table 5 Echocardiographic parameters for determining the severity of MS [38]

	Mild	Moderate	Severe
Valve area (cm^2)	>1.5	1.0–1.5	<1.0
Mean gradient (mmHg)	<5	5-10	>10
Pulmonary artery pressure (mmHg)	<30	30-50	>50

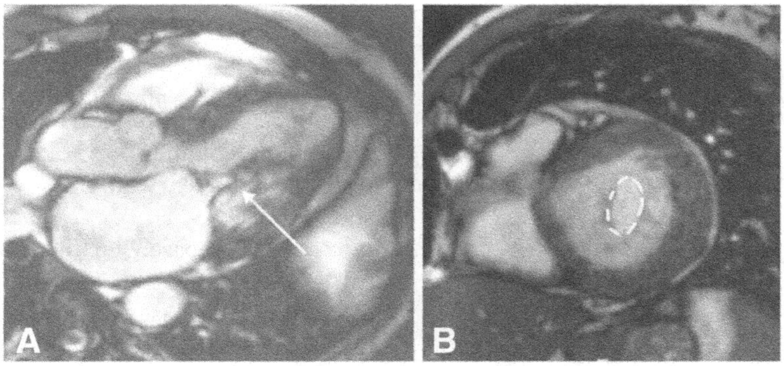

Fig. 10 CMR evaluation of MS. **a** SSFP cine images enable visualisation of the stenotic jet in MS (arrow). **b** Planimetry of the mitral valve (dashed line) to calculate valve orifice area should be performed in diastole. Source: University Hospitals of Leicester NHS Trust

slices should be imaged parallel to the mitral annulus to ensure accuracy.

Mitral diastolic inflow velocities performed with Doppler echocardiography correlate well with CMR-derived values [39, 40]. Mitral flow velocities curves are acquired by phase-contrast velocity mapping in the same plane as used for planimetry of the MV (Fig. 11). In patients with atrial fibrillation, however, the accuracy of flow measurements by CMR is limited [41]

Mitral regurgitation (MR)

MR is broken down in to primary and secondary causes. In primary MR there is disease affecting the mitral valve (MV) leaflets or the MV apparatus. In secondary (or functional) MR, the MV is normal and regurgitation results from annular or ventricular dilatation, which causes reduced or absent leaflet coaptation [42]. In patients with severe MR undergoing surgical intervention, the commonest causes are mitral valve prolapse, ischaemic MR, rheumatic heart disease and endocarditis [43]. Guidelines for grading severity of MR are shown in Table 6.

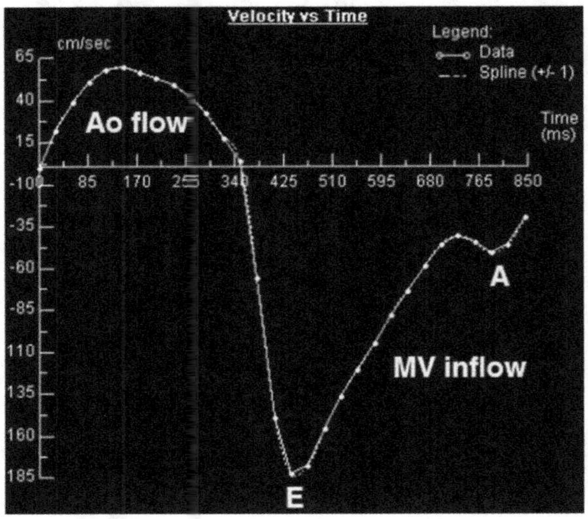

Fig. 11 Flow-time curve generated by CMR phase-contrast velocity mapping across the mitral valve (MV) in a patient with MS. Aortic (Ao) and mitral valve (MV) flow are shown. E and A waves are labelled at their respective peaks. The E deceleration time is prolonged, indicating mitral stenosis. Source: University Hospitals of Leicester NHS Trust

The unlimited imaging planes available through CMR are advantageous for evaluation of the complex MV anatomy. Quantification of regurgitation alongside LV volumes and function remain the major benefits of CMR in the assessment of MR. A visual assessment of the signal void created by the regurgitant jet can give an initial impression of the severity of MR, with wider jets indicative of more severe disease, particularly in the presence of a core area of high signal within the jet. However quantification should be carried out as described below.

Cine imaging in MR

A useful approach to assessment of the MV leaflet anatomy is to image the valve in three planes according to the coaptation of the individual scallops (i.e. A1P1, A2P2 and A3P3) (Fig. 12). This will enable the identification of the site of regurgitation or prolapse. A basal short axis slice through the MV commissure can be used to plan subsequent imaging planes. SSFP cine image slices through each of the three scallops can then be acquired. Direct planimetry though the mitral annulus may also be performed to enable measurement of the regurgitant orifice area [3]. A regurgitant orifice of $\geq 40mm^2$ portends a poor prognosis in patients with MR and has been proposed as an indication for surgical intervention [44]. Alternative imaging can be performed by a stack of axial slices or perpendicular to the four-chamber view.

Quantification of MR

Two methods for quantification of MR are possible by CMR: direct and indirect. The preferred method is

Table 6 ACC/AHA guidelines for grading severity of MR [30]

	Mild	Moderate	Severe
Qualitative			
Angiographic grade	1+	2+	3-4+
Colour Doppler jet area	Small, central jet (<4cm^2 or <20% LA area)	Signs of MR greater than mild present, but no criteria for severe MR.	Vena contracta width greater than 0.7 cm with large central MR jet (area < 40% of LA area) or with a wall-impinging jet of any size, swirling in LA.
Doppler vena contracta width (cm)	<0.3	0.3-0.69	≥0.7
Quantitative (cardiac catheterisation or echo)			
Regurgitant volume (ml)	<30	30-59	≥60
Regurgitant fraction (%)	<30	30-49	≥50
Regurgitant orifice area (cm^2)	<0.2	0.2-0.39	≥0.4
Additional essential criteria			
LA size			Enlarged
LV size			Enlarged

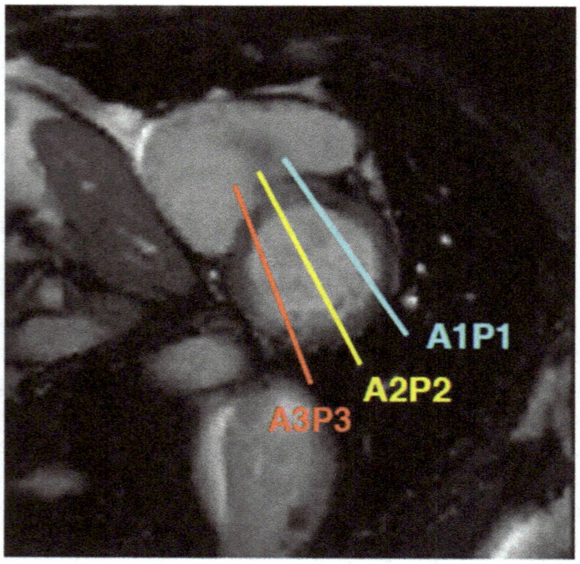

Fig. 12 Suggested imaging planes for visualisation of MV leaflets, according to the coaptation of the individual scallops. Slice position is planned from the basal short axis image (bottom left panel). Cine sequences are then acquired perpendicular to the mitral commissure corresponding to each of the three scallops, denoted by the coloured lines and respective coloured text. Source: University Hospitals of Leicester NHS Trust

indirect quantification, which enables calculation of MR volume by subtracting aortic forward flow (by phase-velocity mapping, as described above, or pulmonary flow) from the LV stroke volume. MR regurgitant fraction is calculated similar to that for the aortic valve: regurgitant volume/LV stroke volume × 100. Alternatively the difference in stroke volume between the LV and RV can be used to calculate the MR volume, although this is based on the assumption that no other valve lesion is present. For direct quantification of MR, through-plane phase-contrast velocity mapping may be undertaken, with care being taken to ensure the imaging plane is perpendicular to the regurgitant jet on the atrial side of the valve (Fig. 13). Direct quantification is made challenging by the highly mobile nature of the MV and the often eccentric jets of MR [3]. Nevertheless there is good agreement for MR quantification between the direct and indirect methods, although the indirect method is preferred in patients with variable heart rates where phase-contrast mapping may be prone to errors [41].

Indirect quantification of MR by CMR correlates only modestly with echocardiography but has markedly lower inter- and intra-observer variability [34, 45]. Moreover, emerging data show that there is marked discrepancy in

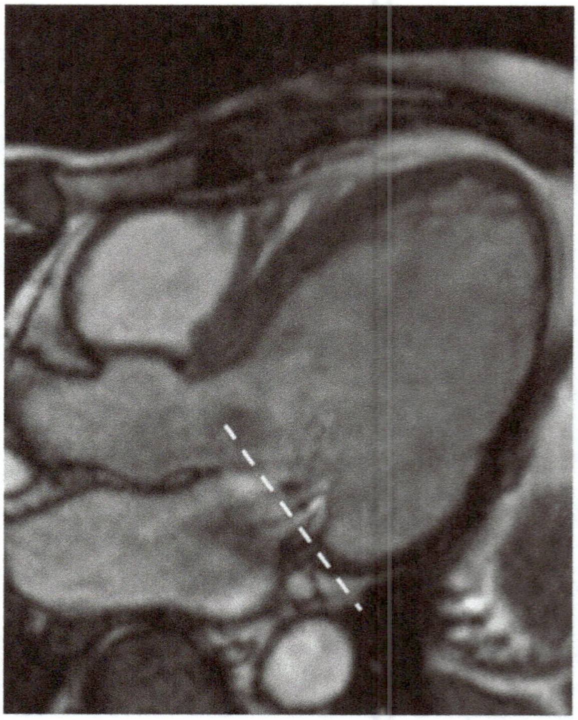

Fig. 13 Three-chamber SSFP cine image in subject with ischaemic MR. Dashed line indicates the slice position used for through-plane phase-contrast velocity mapping. Care should be taken that this is located perpendicular to the regurgitant jet. Source: University Hospitals of Leicester NHS Trust

the severity of MR assessment using echocardiography and CMR [46]. Whilst these findings do not prove that CMR is superior to echo, the fact that reductions in LV volumes following MV surgery were closely related to regurgitant volumes measured on CMR but not echocardiography do suggest that CMR is preferred method of quantification [46].

A regurgitant fraction of ≥40% is proposed as the threshold for surgery in asymptomatic MR [47]. However, there are no published data on cut-offs to predict outcome using CMR and there are no randomised trials comparing management of patients using CMR and echocardiography, so caution must be exercised in interpreting values in the meantime.

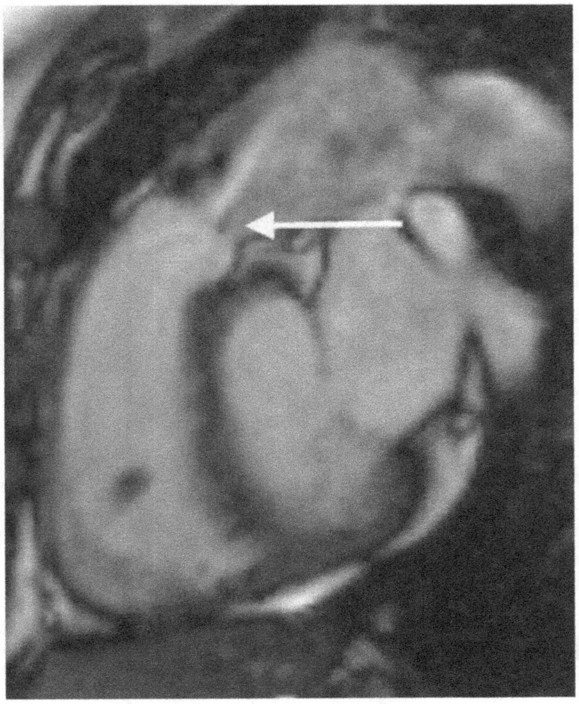

Fig. 14 SSFP RV outflow tract cine image in a subject with PS. Arrow indicates the location of the pulmonary valve, after which the stenotic jet is seen. Source: University Hospitals of Leicester NHS Trust

Right-sided heart valve disease

CMR is the gold-standard tool for quantification of RV volumes and function. Furthermore, CMR enables imaging of the pulmonary valve and RV outflow tract with precision not possible with 2D echo. The complex structure of the RV makes volumetric assessment by echo difficult. CMR is therefore the preferred modality for RV and pulmonary valve disease evaluation.

Pulmonary valve disease

Phase-contrast velocity mapping for quantification of pulmonary regurgitation (PR) has been validated against CMR derived LV and RV stroke volumes [48]. Assessment of PR by echo is only qualitative and comparison with CMR is therefore limited. As with AR, flow mapping alone can be used to calculate severity of PR and flow reversal can be directly quantified with this technique. Trivial PR is a common finding in normal subjects [49]. The occurrence of clinically significant PR is primarily the result of congenital cardiac disease – usually following surgical repair of tetralogy of Fallot [50]. Detailed CMR assessment of PR is therefore beyond the scope of this review. Pulmonary stenosis (PS) is easily visualised using CMR by acquiring SSFP cine views of the RV outflow tract (Fig. 14).

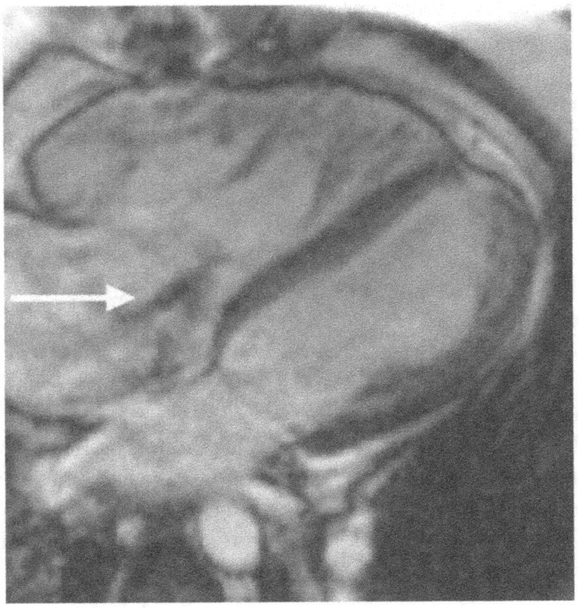

Fig. 15 SSFP four-chamber cine image in a subject with TR. The regurgitant jet (arrow) is seen as signal void on SSFP cine images. Source: University Hospitals of Leicester NHS Trust

Tricuspid valve disease

Assessment of the tricuspid valve (TV) by CMR is performed in a manner similar to that of the MV, and axial cuts may be particularly useful. Tricuspid regurgitation (TR) is seen as signal void on SSFP cine images, best seen in the long axis slices (Fig. 15). For quantification of TR, an indirect method is preferred. Through-plane phase-contrast velocity mapping in the pulmonary artery is undertaken to calculate forward flow volumes. This is subtracted from the total RV stroke volume to provide a TR regurgitant volume [4]. Tricuspid stenosis is rare and not ordinarily assessed by CMR [3].

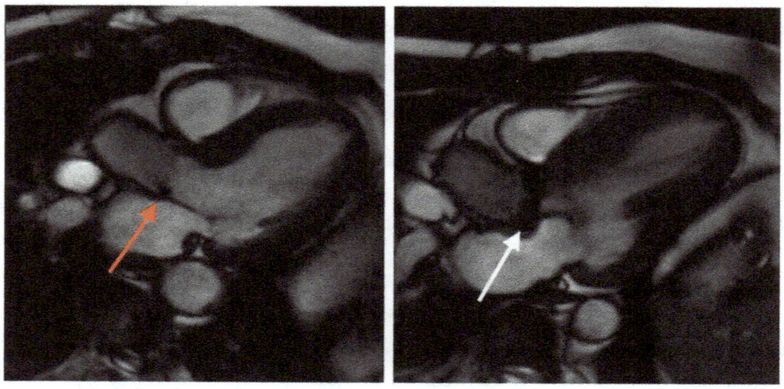

Fig. 16 SSFP three-chamber cine images in two subjects with prosthetic aortic valves. The degree of artefact is determined by the proportion of metal in the valve prosthesis. The red arrow points to a patient with a bioprosthetic AVR, with minimal artefact generated by the small metal component of the supporting structure of the valve. By comparison, a much greater degree of artefact is created by the metallic AVR (white arrow), which has larger metallic component. Source: University Hospitals of Leicester NHS Trust

Prosthetic heart valves

CMR is a safe technique for imaging patients with prosthetic heart valves. All prosthetic valves can be imaged safely at a field strength of 1.5 T and the vast majority at 3 T, although not all prostheses have been tested at 3 T [51]. In the event of concern the safety of any prosthesis can be checked using online resources.

The primary issue when imaging prosthetic valves is the occurrence of artefacts. SSFP cine sequences are highly susceptible to artefacts produced by ferromagnetic objects. The proportion of metal within the prosthetic valve therefore determines the degree of artefact (Fig. 16). This can vary from very little to large areas of artefact that obscure the surrounding anatomy [52, 53]. In the event of very severe artefacts with SSFP sequences, a spoiled gradient echo sequence can be used to acquire cine images. Gradient echo is less susceptible to artefacts from prosthetic valves, but this is at the expense of lower signal to noise [53].

Through-plane velocity mapping can be applied to prosthetic heart valves in the same way as for native valves. Varying degrees of signal voids occur above and below prosthetic valves. The imaging plane should be positioned downstream of the signal void artefact [3, 53]. Different valve types generate different flow patterns on phase-contrast imaging [3].

Finally, CMR is extremely valuable for assessing reverse ventricular remodelling following valve interventions, particularly when comparing different valve types as small numbers of patients are required to show statistically significant differences [54, 55].

Conclusions

CMR can be used for the comprehensive evaluation of VHD. The main strength of CMR lies in the highly accurate and reproducible assessment of ventricular volumes and function in patients with left- or right-sided valve disease. The ability to image in unlimited planes is particularly important in patients with right-sided valve disease, which is poorly evaluated by echo. The quantification of regurgitant volumes/fraction with CMR is a particularly promising area, and one which is established for pulmonary regurgitation following surgical correction of Fallot's. However further prospective studies, and ideally randomised controlled trials comparing MR and echocardiography, are required before the assessment of left sided valve lesions can be considered the clinical routine. The limitations of CMR should be borne in mind and CMR can never replace echo for use at the bedside or in the critically ill patient. Despite these shortcomings CMR is an exciting non-invasive imaging modality in patients with VHD and improvements in techniques and technologies are likely to enhance its utility in clinical practice.

Abbreviations

ACC: American College of Cardiology; AHA: American Heart Association; AR: Aortic regurgitation; AS: Aortic stenosis; CMR: Cardiac magnetic resonance imaging; ECV: Extracellular volume fraction; EDV: End-diastolic volume; EF: Ejection fraction; ESV: End-systolic volume; LGE: Late gadolinium enhancement; LV: Left ventricle; LVM: Left-ventricular mass; MR: Mitral regurgitation; MS: Mitral stenosis; MV: Mitral valve; PR: Pulmonary regurgitation; RV: Right ventricle; SSFP: Steady state free precession; SV: Stroke volume; TV: Tricuspid valve; VENC: Velocity encoding; VHD: Valvular heart disease

Acknowledgements
None.

Funding
None.

Authors' contributions
GSG and GPM conceived the idea for the manuscript. GSG and AS prepared the initial draft. GPM critically appraised the manuscript and ensured the accuracy of it's intellectual content. All authors read and approved the final manuscript.

Ethics approval and consent to participate
Acquisition of all clinical images was granted by subject verbal consent. The images in this review were obtained and accessed from the University Hospitals of Leicester Department of Cardiovascular Imaging local image bank. This is a repository of anonymised images accessible locally for educational purposes and no identifiable information is stored or available. Ethical approval for their use in publication was therefore deemed unnecessary. Permission for use and publication of images in the repository was granted by Prof. Gerry McCann, Head of Cardiovascular Imaging, University Hospitals of Leicester.

Consent for publication
Not applicable.

Competing interests
The authors declare that they have no competing interests.

References

1. Caduff JH, Hernandez RJ, Ludomirsky A. MR visualization of aortic valve vegetations. J Comput Assist Tomogr. 1996;20(4):613–5.
2. Wintersperger BJ, Becker CR, Gulbins H, Knez A, Bruening R, Heuck A, et al. Tumors of the cardiac valves: imaging findings in magnetic resonance imaging, electron beam computed tomography, and echocardiography. Eur Radiol. 2000;10(3):443–9.
3. Myerson SG. Heart valve disease: investigation by cardiovascular magnetic resonance. J Cardiovasc Magn Reson. 2012;14:7.
4. Cawley PJ, Maki JH, Otto CM. Cardiovascular magnetic resonance imaging for valvular heart disease: technique and validation. Circulation. 2009;119(3):468–78.
5. Andersson C, Kihlberg J, Ebbers T, Lindstrom L, Carlhall CJ, Engvall JE. Phase-contrast MRI volume flow–a comparison of breath held and navigator based acquisitions. BMC Med Imaging. 2016;16:26.
6. Hundley WG, Li HF, Hillis LD, Meshack BM, Lange RA, Willard JE, et al. Quantitation of cardiac output with velocity-encoded, phase-difference magnetic resonance imaging. Am J Cardiol. 1995;75(17):1250–5.
7. Chatzimavroudis GP, Oshinski JN, Franch RH, Walker PG, Yoganathan AP, Pettigrew RI. Evaluation of the precision of magnetic resonance phase velocity mapping for blood flow measurements. J Cardiovasc Magn Reson. 2001;3(1):11–9.
8. Van Rossum AC, Sprenger M, Visser FC, Peels KH, Valk J, Roos JP. An in vivo validation of quantitative blood flow imaging in arteries and veins using magnetic resonance phase-shift techniques. Eur Heart J. 1991;12(2):117–26.
9. Gatehouse PD, Rolf MP, Graves MJ, Hofman MB, Totman J, Werner B, et al. Flow measurement by cardiovascular magnetic resonance: a multi-centre multi-vendor study of background phase offset errors that can compromise the accuracy of derived regurgitant or shunt flow measurements. J Cardiovasc Magn Reson. 2010;12:5.
10. Chernobelsky A, Shubayev O, Comeau CR, Wolff SD. Baseline correction of phase contrast images improves quantification of blood flow in the great vessels. J Cardiovasc Magn Reson. 2007;9(4):681–5.
11. Grothues F, Smith GC Moon JC, Bellenger NG, Collins P, Klein HU, et al. Comparison of interstudy reproducibility of cardiovascular magnetic resonance with two-dimensional echocardiography in normal subjects and in patients with heart failure or left ventricular hypertrophy. Am J Cardiol. 2002;90(1):29–34.
12. Miller CA, Jordan P, Borg A, Argyle R, Clark D, Pearce K, et al. Quantification of left ventricular indices from SSFP cine imaging: impact of real-world variability in analysis methodology and utility of geometric modeling. J Magn Reson Imaging. 2013;37(5):1213–22.
13. Nkomo VT, Gardin JM, Skelton TN, Gottdiener JS, Scott CG, Enriquez-Sarano M. Burden of valvular heart diseases: a population-based study. Lancet. 2006;368(9540):1005–11.
14. Carabello BA. Clinical practice. Aortic stenosis N Engl J Med. 2002;346(9): 677–82.
15. Saikrishnan N, Kumar G, Sawaya FJ, Lerakis S, Yoganathan AP. Accurate assessment of aortic stenosis: a review of diagnostic modalities and hemodynamics. Circulation. 2014;129(2):244–53.
16. Nishimura RA, Otto CM, Bonow RO, Carabello BA, Erwin JP 3rd, Guyton RA, et al. 2014 AHA/ACC guideline for the management of patients with valvular heart disease: a report of the American College of Cardiology/ American Heart Association task force on practice guidelines. J Thorac Cardiovasc Surg. 2014;148(1):e1–e132.
17. Reant P, Lederlin M, Lafitte S, Serri K, Montaudon M, Corneloup O, et al. Absolute assessment of aortic valve stenosis by planimetry using cardiovascular magnetic resonance imaging: comparison with transesophageal echocardiography, transthoracic echocardiography, and cardiac catheterisation. Eur J Radiol. 2006;59(2):276–83.
18. Buchner S, Debl K, Schmid FX, Luchner A, Djavidani B. Cardiovascular magnetic resonance assessment of the aortic valve stenosis: an in vivo and ex vivo study. BMC Med Imaging. 2015;15:34.
19. Singh A, Ford I, Greenwood JP, Khan JN, Uddin A, Berry C, et al. Rationale and design of the PRognostic importance of MIcrovascular dysfunction in asymptomatic patients with aortic Stenosis (PRIMID-AS): a multicentre observational study with blinded investigations. BMJ Open. 2013;3(12):e004348.
20. Bissell MM, Hess AT, Biasiolli L, Glaze SJ, Loudon M, Pitcher A, et al. Aortic dilation in bicuspid aortic valve disease: flow pattern is a major contributor and differs with valve fusion type. Circ Cardiovasc Imaging. 2013;6(4):499–507.
21. Girdauskas E, Borger MA, Secknus MA, Girdauskas G, Kuntze T. Is aortopathy in bicuspid aortic valve disease a congenital defect or a result of abnormal hemodynamics? A critical reappraisal of a one-sided argument. Eur J Cardiothorac Surg. 2011;39(6):809–14.
22. Cavalcante JL, Schoenhagen P. Role of cross-sectional imaging for structural heart disease interventions. Cardiol Clin. 2013;31(3):467–78.
23. Debl K, Djavidani B, Buchner S, Lipke C, Nitz W, Feuerbach S, et al. Delayed hyperenhancement in magnetic resonance imaging of left ventricular hypertrophy caused by aortic stenosis and hypertrophic cardiomyopathy: visualisation of focal fibrosis. Heart. 2006;92(10):1447–51.
24. Dweck MR, Joshi S, Murigu T, Alpendurada F, Jabbour A, Melina G, et al. Midwall fibrosis is an independent predictor of mortality in patients with aortic stenosis. J Am Coll Cardiol. 2011;58(12):1271–9.
25. Nigri M, Azevedo CF, Rochitte CE, Schraibman V, Tarasoutchi F, Pommerantzeff PM, et al. Contrast-enhanced magnetic resonance imaging identifies focal regions of intramyocardial fibrosis in patients with severe aortic valve disease: correlation with quantitative histopathology. Am Heart J. 2009;157(2):361–8.
26. Bull S, White SK, Piechnik SK, Flett AS, Ferreira VM, Loudon M, et al. Human non-contrast T1 values and correlation with histology in diffuse fibrosis. Heart. 2013;99(13):932–7.
27. Hein S, Arnon E, Kostin S, Schonburg M, Elsasser A, Polyakova V, et al. Progression from compensated hypertrophy to failure in the pressure-overloaded human heart: structural deterioration and compensatory mechanisms. Circulation. 2003;107(7):984–91.
28. Chin CW, Everett RJ, Kwiecinski J, Vesey AT, Yeung E, Esson G, et al. Myocardial Fibrosis and Cardiac Decompensation in Aortic Stenosis. JACC Cardiovasc Imaging. 2016.
29. Everett RJ, Newby DE, Jabbour A, Fayad ZA, Dweck MR. The role of imaging in aortic valve disease. Curr Cardiovasc Imaging Rep. 2016;9:21.
30. Nishimura RA, Otto CM, Bonow RO, Carabello BA, Erwin JP 3rd, Guyton RA, et al. 2014 AHA/ACC guideline for the management of patients with valvular heart disease: executive summary: a report of the American College of Cardiology/American Heart Association task force on practice guidelines. J Am Coll Cardiol. 2014;63(22):2438–88.
31. Myerson SG, d'Arcy J, Mohiaddin R, Greenwood JP, Karamitsos TD, Francis JM, et al. Aortic regurgitation quantification using cardiovascular magnetic resonance: association with clinical outcome. Circulation. 2012;126(12):1452–60.
32. Chatzimavroudis GP, Oshinski JN, Franch RH, Pettigrew RI, Walker PG, Yoganathan AP. Quantification of the aortic regurgitant volume with

magnetic resonance phase velocity mapping: a clinical investigation of the importance of imaging slice location. J Heart Valve Dis. 1998;7(1):94–101.
33. Bertelsen L, Svendsen JH, Kober L, Haugan K, Hojberg S, Thomsen C, et al. Flow measurement at the aortic root - impact of location of through-plane phase contrast velocity mapping. J Cardiovasc Magn Reson. 2016;18(1):55.
34. Cawley PJ, Hamilton-Craig C, Owens DS, Krieger EV, Strugnell WE, Mitsumori L, et al. Prospective comparison of valve regurgitation quantitation by cardiac magnetic resonance imaging and transthoracic echocardiography. Circ Cardiovasc Imaging. 2013;6(1):48–57.
35. Horstkotte D, Niehues R, Strauer BE. Pathomorphological aspects, aetiology and natural history of acquired mitral valve stenosis. Eur Heart J. 1991; 12(Suppl B):55–60.
36. Carabello BA. Modern management of mitral stenosis. Circulation. 2005; 112(3):432–7.
37. Nishimura RA, Otto CM, Bonow RO, Carabello BA, Erwin JP 3rd, Guyton RA, et al. 2014 AHA/ACC guideline for the Management of Patients with Valvular Heart Disease: a report of the American College of Cardiology/ American Heart Association task force on practice guidelines. Circulation. 2014;129(23):e521–643.
38. Baumgartner H, Hung J, Bermejo J, Chambers JB, Evangelista A, Griffin BP, et al. Echocardiographic assessment of valve stenosis: EAE/ASE recommendations for clinical practice. J Am Soc Echocardiogr. 2009;22(1):1–23. quiz 101-2
39. Heidenreich PA, Steffens J, Fujita N, O'Sullivan M, Caputo GR, Foster E, et al. Evaluation of mitral stenosis with velocity-encoded cine-magnetic resonance imaging. Am J Cardiol. 1995;75(5):365–9.
40. Lin SJ, Brown PA, Watkins MP, Williams TA, Lehr KA, Liu W, et al. Quantification of stenotic mitral valve area with magnetic resonance imaging and comparison with Doppler ultrasound. J Am Coll Cardiol. 2004;44(1):133–7.
41. Myerson SG, Francis JM, Neubauer S. Direct and indirect quantification of mitral regurgitation with cardiovascular magnetic resonance, and the effect of heart rate variability. MAGMA. 2010;23(4):243–9.
42. Harb SC, Griffin BP. Mitral valve disease: a comprehensive review. Curr Cardiol Rep. 2017;19(8):73.
43. Enriquez-Sarano M, Akins CW, Vahanian A. Mitral regurgitation. Lancet. 2009; 373(9672):1382–94.
44. Enriquez-Sarano M, Avierinos JF, Messika-Zeitoun D, Detaint D, Capps M, Nkomo V, et al. Quantitative determinants of the outcome of asymptomatic mitral regurgitation. N Engl J Med. 2005;352(9):875–83.
45. Van De Heyning CM, Magne J, Pierard LA, Bruyere PJ, Davin L, De Maeyer C, et al. Assessment of left ventricular volumes and primary mitral regurgitation severity by 2D echocardiography and cardiovascular magnetic resonance. Cardiovasc Ultrasound. 2013;11:46.
46. Uretsky S, Gillam L, Lang R, Chaudhry FA, Argulian E, Supariwala A, et al. Discordance between echocardiography and MRI in the assessment of mitral regurgitation severity: a prospective multicenter trial. J Am Coll Cardiol. 2015;65(11):1078–88.
47. Myerson SG, d'Arcy J, Christiansen JP, Dobson LE, Mohiaddin R, Francis JM, et al. Determination of clinical outcome in mitral regurgitation with cardiovascular magnetic resonance quantification. Circulation. 2016;133(23):2287–96.
48. Rebergen SA, Chin JG, Ottenkamp J, van der Wall EE, de Roos A. Pulmonary regurgitation in the late postoperative follow-up of tetralogy of Fallot. Volumetric quantitation by nuclear magnetic resonance velocity mapping. Circulation. 1993;88(5 Pt 1):2257–66.
49. Klein AL, Burstow DJ, Tajik AJ, Zachariah PK, Taliercio CP, Taylor CL, et al. Age-related prevalence of valvular regurgitation in normal subjects: a comprehensive color flow examination of 118 volunteers. J Am Soc Echocardiogr. 1990;3(1):54–63.
50. Ammash NM, Dearani JA, Burkhart HM, Connolly HM. Pulmonary regurgitation after tetralogy of Fallot repair: clinical features, sequelae, and timing of pulmonary valve replacement. Congenit Heart Dis. 2007;2(6):386–403.
51. Shellock FG. MR imaging of metallic implants and materials: a compilation of the literature. AJR Am J Roentgenol. 1988;151(4):811–4.
52. Hasenkam JM, Ringgaard S, Houlind K, Botnar RM, Stodkilder-Jorgensen H, Boesiger P, et al. Prosthetic heart valve evaluation by magnetic resonance imaging. Eur J Cardiothorac Surg. 1991;16:300–5.
53. Cardiology ESo. MRI evaluation in patients with prosthetic valves: European Society of Cardiology; 2016 [Available from: http://www.escardio.org/Education/Practice-Tools/EACVI-toolboxes/Valvular-Imaging/Atlas-of-valvular-imaging/Prosthetic-valves/MRI-evaluation-in-patients-with-prosthetic-valves.
54. Sensky PR, Loubani M, Keal RP, Samani NJ, Sosnowski AW, Galinanes M. Does the type of prosthesis influence early left ventricular mass regression after aortic valve replacement? Assessment with magnetic resonance imaging. Am Heart J. 2003;146(4):E13.
55. Fairbairn TA, Steadman CD, Mather AN, Motwani M, Blackman DJ, Plein S, et al. Assessment of valve haemodynamics, reverse ventricular remodelling and myocardial fibrosis following transcatheter aortic valve implantation compared to surgical aortic valve replacement: a cardiovascular magnetic resonance study. Heart. 2013;99(16):1185–91.
56. American College of Cardiology/American Heart Association Task Force on Practice G, Society of Cardiovascular A, Society for Cardiovascular A, Interventions, Society of Thoracic S, Bonow RO, et al. ACC/AHA 2006 guidelines for the management of patients with valvular heart disease: a report of the American College of Cardiology/American Heart Association Task Force on Practice Guidelines (writing committee to revise the 1998 Guidelines for the Management of Patients With Valvular Heart Disease): developed in collaboration with the Society of Cardiovascular Anesthesiologists: endorsed by the Society for Cardiovascular Angiography and Interventions and the Society of Thoracic Surgeons. Circulation. 2006; 114(5):e84–231.
57. Lancellotti P, Moura L, Pierard LA, Agricola E, Popescu BA, Tribouilloy C, et al. European Association of Echocardiography recommendations for the assessment of valvular regurgitation. Part 2: mitral and tricuspid regurgitation (native valve disease). Eur J Echocardiogr. 2010;11(4):307–32.

Comparison of two different measurement methods in evaluating basilar atherosclerotic plaque using high-resolution MRI at 3 tesla

Luguang Chen, Qian Zhan, Wenjia Peng, Tao Song, Qi Liu and Jianping Lu*

Abstract

Background: To compare the Self-referenced and Referenced measurement methods in assessing basilar artery (BA) atherosclerotic plaque employing dark blood high-resolution MRI at 3 Tesla.

Methods: Forty patients with > 20% stenosis as identified by conventional MRA were recruited and evaluated on a 3 Tesla MRI system. The outer wall, inner wall and lumen areas of maximal lumen narrowing site and the outer wall and lumen areas of sites that were proximal and distal to the maximal lumen narrowing site were manually traced. Plaque area (PA), stenosis rate (SR) and percent plaque burden (PPB) were calculated using the Self-referenced and Referenced measurement methods, respectively. To assess intra-observer reproducibility, BA plaque was measured twice with a 2-week interval in between measurements.

Results: Thirty-seven patients were included in the final analysis. There were no significant differences in PA, SR and PPB measurements between the two methods. The intra-class coefficients and coefficient of variations (CV) ranged from 0.976 to 0.990 and from 3.73 to 5.61% for the Self-referenced method and ranged from 0.928 to 0.971 and from 4.64 to 9.95% for the Referenced method, respectively. Both methods are effective in the evaluation of BA plaque. However, the CVs of the Self-referenced method is lower than the Referenced measurement method. Moreover, Bland-Altman plots showed that the Self-referenced method has a narrower interval than the Referenced measurement method.

Conclusions: The Self-referenced method is better and more convenient for evaluating BA plaque, and it may serve as a promising method for evaluation of basilar atherosclerotic plaque.

Keywords: Basilar artery, Atherosclerosis, Magnetic resonance imaging

Background

Atherosclerosis is a disease that progresses slowly and silently over decades, and the slow progress offers a chance for diagnosis before symptoms occur [1, 2]. Intracranial atherosclerosis is the most common reason for mortality in Asian populations [3]. The basilar artery (BA) is one of the largest intracranial arteries and is located in the posterior cerebral circulation. Basilar atherosclerotic plaque usually occurs in patients with ischaemic stroke and transient ischaemic attack (TIA) [4]. Evaluation of morphologic characteristics of BA plaque (such as PA, plaque area; SR, stenosis rate and PPB, percent plaque burden) is important and may guide treatment decisions in the clinical setting.

The rapid development of magnetic resonance imaging technology, especially at 3 Tesla field strength, offers a significant improvement in the signal-to-noise ratio, vessel wall to lumen contrast-to-noise ratio and image quality compared to imaging at 1.5 Tesla [5]. Dark blood high-resolution magnetic resonance imaging (HRMRI) has been demonstrated as a non-invasive and useful technique for evaluating the vessel wall in in vivo atherosclerotic disease [1]. It has been used to assess

* Correspondence: cjr.lujianping@vip.163.com
Department of Radiology, Changhai Hospital of Shanghai, The Second Military Medical University, No.168 Changhai Road, Shanghai 200433, China

various major arteries in the whole body including the intracranial [6–10], carotid [11–15], coronary [16–18] and peripheral arteries [19–21] and the aorta [11, 22]. Accurate and fast assessment of the plaque burden and morphology of the basilar artery are paramount for determining treatment strategies for patients. Kim et al. used the maximal lumen narrowing (MLN) sites as the referenced sites to evaluate the degree of stenosis in basilar atherosclerotic plaque using HRMRI [23]. Previous studies have used the nearest plaque-free or minimally diseased segments proximal and distal to the MLN sites as the referenced sites to calculate morphologic parameters (herein referred to as the Referenced measurement method) [24–26]. In the present study, we have also employed the MLN sites as the referenced sites to compute the morphological parameters (herein referred to as the Self-referenced measurement method). Figure 1 shows the definitions of the Self-referenced and Referenced measurement methods and their calculation rules for assessing BA plaque. However, studies on the comparison of the Self-referenced and Referenced measurement methods in assessing basilar atherosclerotic plaque have been limited. We hypothesized that the Self-referenced measurement method is better than the Referenced measurement method in evaluating plaque morphologic characterization. To the best of our knowledge, no such studies have been reported yet except our group [27].

Therefore, the goal of this study was to compare the Self-referenced and Referenced measurement methods in assessing basilar atherosclerotic plaque employing dark blood HRMRI at 3 Tesla.

Methods

Subjects

This prospective study was approved by the Committee on Ethics of Biomedical Research, Changhai Hospital of Shanghai, and written informed consent was obtained from each patient. Forty patients with > 20% stenosis as identified by conventional contrast-enhanced magnetic resonance angiography were recruited during the period from January 2014 to July 2016. The inclusion criteria were listed as follows: 1) Patients who had ischaemic stroke or TIA in the basilar artery territory within one month; 2) Occurrence of an ischaemic event in a vascular area that lies outside of the stenotic basilar artery; and 3) More than two risk factors for cardiovascular disease (e.g., hypertension, diabetes, smoking and hypercholesterolemia). The following criteria were used to exclude patients: 1) the degree of stenosis of the basilar artery was normal, occluded or < 20%; 2) arteritis; 3) claustrophobia; and 4) poor image quality.

Magnetic resonance imaging

Cross-sectional imaging was performed on a 3 Tesla MRI system (MAGNETOM Skyra, Siemens medical solution, Erlangen, Germany) using a standard 20-channel phased-array head/neck coil, with a peak gradient strength of 45 mT/m and a slew rate of 200 $mTm^{-1} ms^{-1}$. Three-dimensional time-of-flight magnetic resonance angiography (3D TOF-MRA) images were used for HRMRI image positioning and obtained with repetition time/echo time (TR/TE) = 21/3.4 ms, field of view (FOV) = 180 × 200 mm^2, matrix = 330 × 384, thickness =

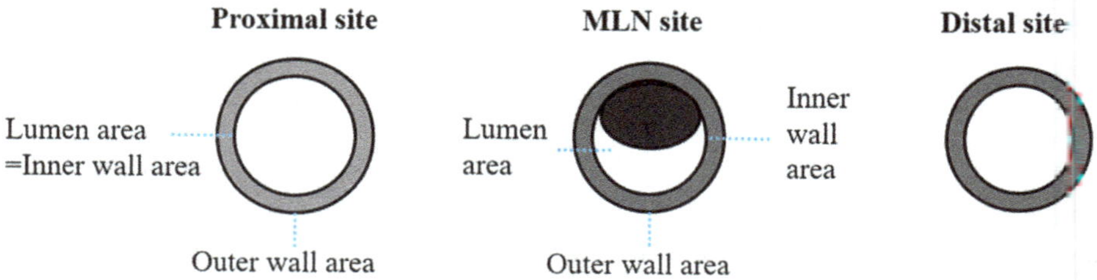

Self-referenced measurement method:
Plaque area = Inner area at MLN site – Lumen area at MLN site
Stenosis rate = Plaque area/Inner area at MLN site
Percent plaque burden = Plaque area/Outer wall area at MLN site

Referenced measurement method:
Outer wall area at reference site = average of the proximal and distal wall areas
Lumen area at reference site = average of the proximal and distal lumen areas
Wall area at reference site = Outer wall area at reference site – Lumen area at reference site
Wall area at MLN site = Outer wall area at MLN site – Lumen area at MLN site
Plaque area = Wall area at MLN site – Wall area at reference site
Stenosis rate = 1 – Lumen area at MLN site/Wall area at reference site
Percent plaque burden = Plaque area/Outer wall area at MLN site

Fig. 1 Definitions of the Self-referenced and Referenced measurement methods and their calculation rules for assessing BA plaque

0.7 mm, and average = 1, acquisition time (TA) = 4 min 40 s. The main parameters of two-dimensional T2-weighted turbo spin echo (T2W TSE) were TR/TE = 2890/46 ms, FOV = 100 × 100 mm^2, matrix = 256 × 256, thickness = 2 mm, Gap = 0.5 mm, echo train length = 20, and averages = 2, TA = 3 min 40 s. Fat saturation was applied to suppress signal from adjacent fatty tissues and improve identification of vessel wall boundaries. The black blood method with a regional saturation pulse of 60 mm thickness was employed to saturate the inflow arterial signal. The total scan time was approximately 8 min.

Image analysis

Two experienced radiologists with 5 and 6 years of experience in vessel wall imaging and who were blinded to the clinical information of each patient assessed the image quality by consensus using 4-scale scores (score 1, poor quality; score 2, adequate quality; score 3, good quality; score 4, excellent quality) [28]. Images with a score of 1 were excluded from the final analysis. Quantitative measurement was carried out on images with a score of ≥2. The outer wall, inner wall and lumen areas of the MLN site and the outer wall and lumen areas of the proximal and distal sites were manually traced using advanced image software (CMRTools, Cardiovascular Imaging Solutions London, UK; Fig. 2). The calculation of PA, SR and PPB using the Referenced measurement method was carried out as per a previous study [24], which used the nearest normal segments proximal and distal to the MLN sites as the reference to calculate the above parameters (Fig. 1). In brief, outer wall and lumen areas at the reference points were averages of the proximal and distal outer wall and lumen areas. Wall area was calculated by subtracting the lumen area from the outer wall area. The calculations for PA, SR and PPB were as follows: PA = wall area at MLN site – wall area at the reference site, SR = 1-lm area at MLN site/lumen area at the reference site, PPB = PA/outer wall area at MLN site. For the Self-referenced measurement method, the MLN site was used to as the reference. PA = inner wall area at MLN site - lumen area at MLN site, SR = PA/ inner wall area at MLN site, PPB = PA/outer wall area at MLN site (Fig. 1). The distance between proximal and distal reference locations was calculated and recorded (*distance* = *m* * Slice thickness + *(m - 1)* * Gap, *m* indicates the number of slices between both locations). To measure the intra-observer variability, BA plaque was measured twice at two different time points that were separated by a 2-week interval to avoid any recall bias.

Statistical analysis

All statistical analyses were performed using the SPSS software for Windows (version 16.0, SPSS Inc., Chicago, IL, USA) and MedCalc (version 13.0.0.0, MedCalc Software, Mariakerke, Belgium). A Kolmogorov-Smirnov test was used to test for normal distribution. Quantitative data were described as the means ± standard deviation. Qualitative data were expressed as count (percentage). Statistically significant differences between the Self-referenced and Referenced measurement methods and between the repeated measurements of PA, SR and PPB with both methods were assessed using a two-tailed paired t-test. The coefficient of variation (CV) was calculated by determining the standard deviation (SD) of the two paired measurements of T2W images and dividing the mean of those measurements. The intraclass correlation coefficient (ICC) with a two-way mixed model and single consistency type was determined and used to evaluate the agreement between the repeat measurements.

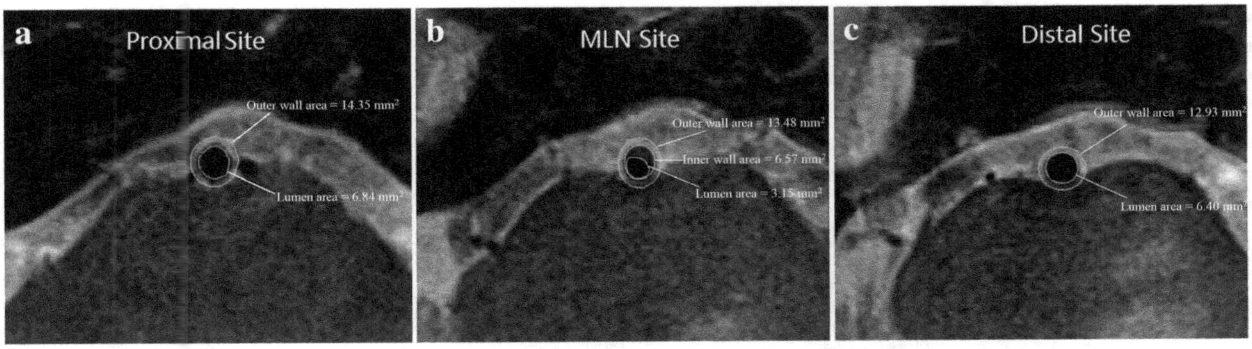

Fig. 2 Examples of outer wall areas, inner wall areas and lumen areas at the proximal sites (**a**), maximal lumen narrowing (MLN) sites (**b**) and distal sites (**c**) that were traced manually in a 53-year-old female patient with basilar atherosclerotic plaque. For the Self-referenced measurement method, the plaque area is 3.42 mm^2, stenosis rate is 0.521, and percent plaque burden is 0.254. For the Referenced measurement method, the outer wall area at the reference site is 13.64 mm^2, the lumen area at reference site is 6.62 mm^2, the wall area at the reference site is 7.02 mm^2, the wall area at the MLN site is 10.33 mm^2, the plaque area is 3.31 mm^2, the stenosis rate is 0.551, and the percent plaque burden is 0.246

Table 1 Patient demographics

Variable	$n = 37$
Male sex	28 (75.7%)
Age (years)	62.4 ± 10.1
Body mass index	24.4 ± 3.1
Hypertension	27 (73.0%)
Systolic pressure(mmHg)	159.0 ± 26.5
Diastolic pressure (mmHg)	94.8 ± 17.0
Diabetes mellitus	17 (45.9%)
Fasting blood-glucose (mg/dL)	8.3 ± 9.7
Hyperlipidaemia	19 (51.4%)
Total cholesterol (mmol/L)	4.08 ± 1.05
Triglyceride (mmol/L)	1.41 ± 0.53
High-density lipoprotein (mmol/L)	1.06 ± 0.19
Low density lipoprotein (mmol/L)	2.52 ± 0.95
Stenosis rate	0.69 ± 0.18
Apolipoprotein A1 (g/L)	1.14 ± 0.23
Apolipoprotein B (g/L)	0.83 ± 0.19
Smoking	16 (43.2%)

According to Shout and Fleiss [29], values of ICC < 0.4 represent poor agreement, 0.4 to 0.75 represent good agreement, and > 0.75 represent excellent agreement. Bland-Altman plots were also derived for those measurements [30] and bias and limits of agreement were calculated. A P-value of < 0.05 was considered as statistically significant.

Results

While all patients completed HRMRI examinations, three patients were excluded in the final analysis because of poor image quality. The scores of images quality were as follows: 2 in 5 patients, 3 in 21 patients and 4 in 11 patients. Thus, thirty-seven patients (28 males and 9 females, 47–79 years old, mean age = 62 years) were included in the study, and quantitative analysis was performed with their data. The patient demographics were presented in Table 1. The time interval between the stroke event and plaque imaging was also recorded, and the average time was 16.2 ± 8.2 days. The distances between proximal and distal reference locations were 11.12 ± 3.73 mm.

Comparison of self-referenced and referenced measurement methods

The results of the Self-referenced and Referenced measurement methods are presented in Table 2. PA determined by both measurement methods were 9.015 ± 4.916 mm^2 and 8.678 ± 4.634 mm^2, respectively. The SR values were 0.699 ± 0.172 and 0.688 ± 0.184 for the Self-referenced and Referenced methods, respectively. In addition, the PPB values of the two measurement methods were 0.375 ± 0.111 and 0.361 ± 0.117, respectively. The bias and limit of agreement measurements using Bland-Altman plots for the PA, SR and PPB were 0.336 (− 2.018, 2.690), 0.011 (− 0.072, 0.094) and 0.014 (− 0.083, 0.110) (Fig. 3), respectively. There were no statistically significant differences between the two methods in those measurements (p-values > 0.05).

Reproducibility of the self-referenced measurement method

The results for the Self-referenced measurement reproducibility analysis are presented in Table 3. Repeated measurements with the Self-referenced method were 8.954 ± 4.833 mm^2 and 9.071 ± 5.023 mm^2 for PA, 0.697 ± 0.173 and 0.695 ± 0.172 for SR, and 0.374 ± 0.112 and 0.372 ± 0.112 for PPB. No statistically significant differences were observed for those measurements (p-values > 0.05). The results indicate an excellent reproducibility for the repeated measurements, with the ICC and CV values ranging from 0.976 to 0.990 and 3.73 to 5.61%, respectively. Excellent agreement was also observed in the repeated measurement reproducibility analysis employing Bland-Altman plots (Fig. 4).

Reproducibility of the referenced measurement method

The results for the Referenced measurement reproducibility are presented in Table 4. The repeated measurements of the Referenced method were 8.569 ± 4.444 mm^2 and 8.783 ± 4.892 mm^2 for PA, 0.686 ± 0.185 and 0.684 ± 0.186 for SR, and 0.361 ± 0.112 and 0.361 ± 0.117 for PPB. No statistically significant differences were observed for those measurements (p-values > 0.05). The results indicate an excellent reproducibility for the repeated measurements, with the ICC and CV values

Table 2 Comparison of Self-referenced and Referenced measurement methods in assessing basilar plaque

	Self-referenced (Mean ± SD)	Referenced (Mean ± SD)	Bias	LoA	p
Plaque area (mm^2)	9.015 ± 4.916	8.678 ± 4.634	0.336	(−2.018, 2.690)	0.097
Stenosis rate	0.699 ± 0.172	0.688 ± 0.184	0.011	(−0.072, 0.094)	0.121
Percent plaque burden	0.375 ± 0.111	0.361 ± 0.117	0.014	(−0.083, 0.110)	0.761

SD Standard deviation, *LoA* Limit of Agreement

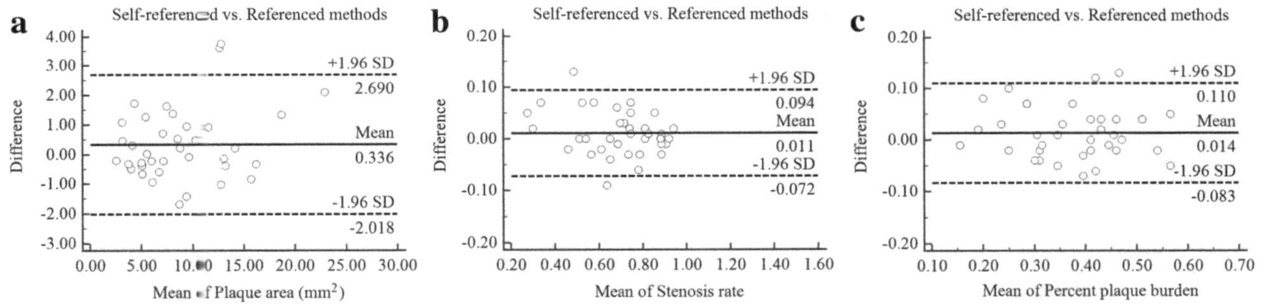

Fig. 3 Comparison of the Self-referenced and Referenced measurement methods for BA plaque using Bland-Altman plots, plaque area (**a**), stenosis rate (**b**) and percent plaque burden (**c**)

ranging from 0.928 to 0.971 and 4.64 to 9.87%, respectively. Excellent agreement was also observed in the repeated measurement reproducibility analysis employing Bland-Altman plots (Fig. 5).

Discussion

The present study evaluated the Self-referenced and Referenced measurement methods in assessing basilar atherosclerotic plaque employing dark blood HRMRI at 3 Tesla. The results show no significant differences between the Self-referenced and Referenced measurement. In addition, repeated measurements of PA, SR and PPB demonstrate excellent reproducibility in evaluating basilar atherosclerotic plaque.

This study employed Self-referenced and Referenced measurement methods to assess basilar atherosclerotic plaque and compared both techniques in evaluating morphologic parameters of the basilar artery. For the Self-referenced measurement method, the MLN site was used as the reference site to assess several parameters such as PA, SR and PPB. It is a simple and fast method to evaluate those parameters compared with the Referenced measurement method, in which both the nearest normal segments that are proximal and distal to the MLN site were used as the reference. Our data indicate that there were no significant difference between both methods in assessing the PA, SR and PPB of basilar plaque. In addition, only a small degree of bias was observed between the Self-referenced and Referenced measurement methods using Bland-Altman plots (Fig. 3). In addition, there was excellent reproducibility in the measurements of PA, SR and PPB by both methods, with ICC and CV values ranging from 0.941 to 0.990 and 3.73 to 9.87%, respectively. The reliability of these methods is of significant importance for the evaluation of basilar atherosclerotic plaque morphologic parameters. Briefly, the Self-referenced measurement method is a suitable alternative to the Referenced measurement method in quantifying basilar plaque morphology.

Dark blood HRMRI has been increasingly used to evaluate the morphology of basilar atherosclerotic plaque, as it offers good boundary outlines for the vessel-blood and the vessel-cerebral spine fluid borders [25, 31–33]. Kim et al. found that evaluation of stenosis associated with basilar atherosclerotic plaque using HRMRI is more accurate than evaluation using magnetic resonance angiography. The study involved a large sample size (219 patients) compared with other studies, and the Self-referenced measurement method was used to assess the degree of stenosis [23]. The discrepancy between HRMRI and magnetic resonance angiography was more obvious with mild stenosis, which shows that HRMRI is more sensitive for evaluating the early phase of intracranial atherosclerosis [23]. Ma et al. investigated the morphology of advanced basilar atherosclerotic plaque using the Referenced measurement method [26], Zhu et al. also used this method to assess the morphologic characteristics of atherosclerotic middle cerebral arteries using HRMRI at 3 Tesla [24] and Feng et al. explored arterial remodelling of basilar atherosclerosis in

Table 3 Reproducibility of Self-referenced measurement method in assessing basilar plaque

	Measurement 1 (Mean ± SD)	Measurement 2 (Mean ± SD)	ICC (95% CI)	CV (%)	*p*
Plaque area (mm^2)	8.954 ± 4.833	9.071 ± 5.023	0.990 (0.981–0.995)	5.61	0.329
Stenosis rate	0.697 ± 0.173	0.695 ± 0.172	0.977 (0.955–0.988)	3.73	0.759
Percent plaque burden	0.374 ± 0.112	0.372 ± 0.112	0.976 (0.954–0.988)	4.59	0.549

SD Standard deviation, *ICC* Intra-class coefficient, *CI* Confidence interval, *CV* Coefficient of variability

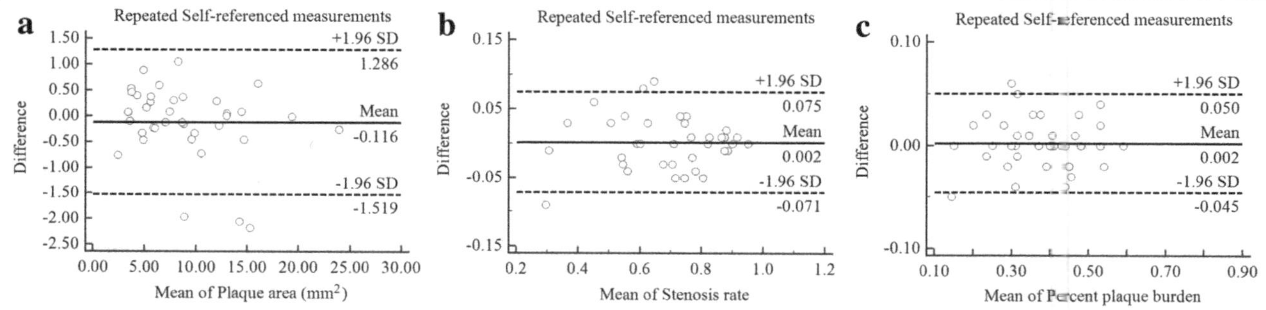

Fig. 4 Bland-Altman plots of reproducibility for the Self-referenced method, plaque area (**a**), stenosis rate (**b**) and percent plaque burden (**c**) of BA plaques were evaluated using the Self-referenced measurement method

pontine infarction [25]. However, sites that were proximal and distal to the MLN were first selected, and then PA, SR and PPB were evaluated using the Referenced measurement method in those studies. In contrast, the Self-referenced measurement method, only needed the MLN site to calculate those parameters. In short, the main differences between the Self-referenced measurement method and the Referenced measurement method are presented as follows: (1) Only one site (MLN) was used in Self-referenced measurement method, while three sites (proximal, MLN and distal) were needed in the Referenced measurement method. (2) For plaque area quantification, the former method is more simple and rapid, as there is no need to calculate the reference outer wall, lumen and wall areas, which are needed in the latter method. Therefore, the Self-referenced method is a simple and convenient method for assessing plaque morphologic characteristics compared with the Referenced method. Our comparison of the Self-referenced and Referenced measurement method in evaluating basilar atherosclerotic plaque morphology demonstrates an excellent agreement between both the methods in assessment of PA, SR and PPB parameters, which indicates that the Self-referenced measurement method can be used in the clinical setting.

Imaging modalities including transcranial doppler ultrasound, computed tomography angiography and magnetic resonance angiography have been used to assess intracranial atherosclerosis. However, while those imaging techniques offer an evaluation of the vascular lumen, they are incapable of providing vessel wall information [23]. More importantly, the vessel wall characteristics can help us better understand the pathophysiology of atherosclerosis, which has a significant effect on patient management [4]. Dark blood HRMRI can delicately delineate plaque presence and morphology and provide new insights into atherosclerotic burden [2]. To increase the black blood effect, saturation band, inversion recovery, motion-sensitized driven-equilibrium, and delay alternating with nutation for tailored excitation are the most commonly used techniques during the magnetization preparation phase [34–37]. Because of the inherent flow void effect of the TSE protocol and due to its simplicity and low specific absorption ratio properties, the saturation band was used to saturate the inflow blood signal when imaging basilar plaque. Black blood high-resolution T2W images were used to obtain quantitative measurements because of the good contrast that was obtained between the lumen and plaque, the vessel wall and cerebrospinal fluid compared to the other imaging protocols [38].

The present study has several limitations. First, the sample size is relatively small. Further studies with a larger sample size are needed to validate the present results. Second, the Self-referenced measurement method could not be directly used to calculate the remodelling patterns of basilar atherosclerotic plaque, such as positive and negative remodelling patterns. However, we can use the Referenced measurement method to calculate

Table 4 Reproducibility of Referenced measurement method in assessing basilar plaque

	Measurement 1 (Mean ± SD)	Measurement 2 (Mean ± SD)	ICC (95% CI)	CV (%)	*p*
Plaque area (mm^2)	8.569 ± 4.444	8.783 ± 4.892	0.971 (0.944–0.985)	9.87	0.289
Stenosis rate	0.686 ± 0.185	0.684 ± 0.186	0.970 (0.942–0.985)	4.64	0.774
Percent plaque burden	0.361 ± 0.112	0.361 ± 0.117	0.941 (0.887–0.969)	7.64	0.967

SD Standard deviation, *ICC* Intra-class coefficient, *CI* Confidence interval, *CV* Coefficient of variability

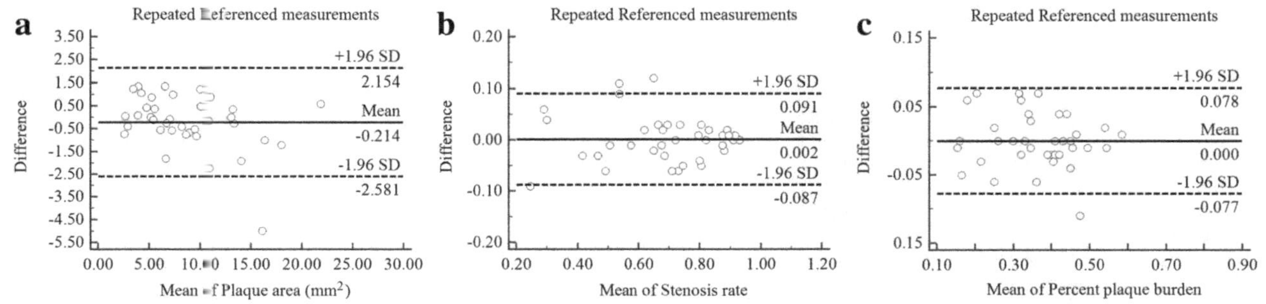

Fig. 5 Bland-Altman plots of reproducibility for the Referenced methods, plaque area (**a**), stenosis rate (**b**) and percent plaque burden (**c**) of BA plaques were evaluated using the Referenced measurement method

those patterns if needed. Lastly, the outer wall, inner wall and lumen boundaries on the T2W images were manually outlined to assess the PA, SR and PPB of basilar atherosclerotic plaque. An automatic plaque measurement tool is needed, as this may improve efficiency and reduce errors between the repeated measurements.

Conclusions

In conclusion, the Self-referenced and Referenced methods are slightly equivalent and both reliable, however, the former is quicker and easier and it may serve as a promising method for evaluation of basilar atherosclerotic plaque.

Abbreviations

3D TOF-MRA: Three-dimensional time-of-flight magnetic resonance angiography; BA: Basilar artery; CV: Coefficient of variation; FOV: Field of view; HRMRI: High-resolution magnetic resonance imaging; ICC: Intraclass correlation coefficient; MLN: Maximal lumen narrowing; PA: Plaque area; PPB: Percent plaque burden; SD: Standard deviation; SR: Stenosis rate; TA: Acquisition time; TIA: Transient ischaemic attack; TR/TE: Repetition time/echo time

Acknowledgements

Thanks for the International Society for Magnetic Resonance in Medicine (ISMRM) committee to accepted this work as a traditional poster in 2017 (https://www.ismrm.org/17TraditionalPoster.pdf, NO. 2456).

Funding

This work was supported by the national key clinical specialist construction programs of China (Grant Number N/A) and the National Natural Science Foundation of China (Grant Number 31470910, 31600755).

Authors' contributions

JL, and QL conceived of the present idea. LC and ZQ designed the study. Data acquisition was performed by LC. LC and WP performed the statistical analysis. TS, QZ and WP contributed to the data analysis and interpretation. LC was contributed to writing the manuscript. All the authors read and approved the final manuscript.

Consent for publication

Written informed consent was obtained from each patient to publish.

Competing interests

The authors declare that they have no conflict of interest.

References

1. El Aidi H, Mani V, Weinshelbaum KB, Aguiar SH, Taniguchi H, Postley JE, et al. Cross-sectional, prospective study of MRI reproducibility in the assessment of plaque burden of the carotid arteries and aorta. Nat Clin Pract Cardiovasc Med. 2009;6:219–28.
2. Dong L, Wang J, Yarnykh VL, Underhill HR, Neradilek MB, Polissar N, et al. Efficient flow suppressed MRI improves interscan reproducibility of carotid atherosclerosis plaque burden measurements. J Magn Reson Imaging. 2010; 32:452–8.
3. Suh DC, Lee SH, Kim KR, Park ST, Lim SM, Kim SJ, et al. Pattern of atherosclerotic carotid stenosis in Korean patients with stroke: different involvement of intracranial versus extracranial vessels. AJNR Am J Neuroradiol. 2003;24:239–44.
4. Huang B, Yang WQ, Liu XT, Liu HJ, Li PJ, Lu HK. Basilar artery atherosclerotic plaques distribution in symptomatic patients: a 3.0T high-resolution MRI study. Eur J Radiol. 2013;82:e199–203.
5. Vidal A, Bureau Y, Wade T, Spence JD, Rutt BK, Fenster A, et al. Scan-rescan and intra-observer variability of magnetic resonance imaging of carotid atherosclerosis at 1.5 T and 3.0 T. Phys Med Biol. 2008;53:6821–35.
6. Mossa-Basha M, Shibata DK, Hallam DK, de Havenon A, Hippe DS, Becker KJ, et al. Added value of Vessel Wall magnetic resonance imaging for differentiation of nonocclusive intracranial Vasculopathies. Stroke. 2017;48: 3026–33.
7. Harteveld AA, van der Kolk AG, van der Worp HB, Dieleman N, Zwanenburg JJM, Luijten PR, et al. Detecting intracranial Vessel Wall lesions with 7T-magnetic resonance imaging: patients with posterior circulation ischemia versus healthy controls. Stroke. 2017;48:2601–4.
8. Yang WJ, Wong KS, Chen XY. Intracranial atherosclerosis: from microscopy to high-resolution magnetic resonance imaging. J Stroke. 2017;19:249–60.
9. Kim JM, Jung KH, Sohn CH, Moon J, Shin JH, Park J, et al. Intracranial plaque enhancement from high resolution vessel wall magnetic resonance imaging predicts stroke recurrence. Int J Stroke. 2016;11:171–9.
10. Wu F, Song H, Ma Q, Xiao J, Jiang T, Huang X, et al. Hyperintense plaque on intracranial Vessel Wall magnetic resonance imaging as a predictor of artery-to-artery embolic infarction. Stroke. 2018;49:905–11.
11. Alkhalil M, Edmond E, Edgar L, Digby JE, Omar O, Robson MD, et al. The relationship of perivascular adipose tissue and atherosclerosis in the aorta and carotid arteries, determined by magnetic resonance imaging. Diab Vasc Dis Res. 2018. http://sci-hub.tw/10.1177/1479164118757923.
12. Watase H, Sun J, Hippe DS, Balu N, Li F, Zhao X, et al. Carotid artery remodeling is segment specific: an in vivo study by Vessel Wall magnetic resonance imaging. Arterioscler Thromb Vasc Biol. 2018;38:927–34.
13. Lu M, Peng P, Cui Y, Qiao H, Li D, Cai J, et al. Association of Progression of carotid Artery Wall volume and recurrent transient ischemic attack or stroke: a magnetic resonance imaging study. Stroke. 2018;49:614–20.
14. Zhao X, Hippe DS, Li R, Canton GM, Sui B, Song Y, et al. Prevalence and characteristics of carotid artery high-risk atherosclerotic plaques in Chinese patients with cerebrovascular symptoms: a Chinese atherosclerosis risk evaluation II study. J Am Heart Assoc. 2017;6.
15. Lin R, Chen S, Liu G, Xue Y, Zhao X. Association between carotid atherosclerotic plaque calcification and Intraplaque hemorrhage: a magnetic resonance imaging study. Arterioscler Thromb Vasc Biol. 2017;37:1228–33.

16. Abd-Elmoniem KZ, Ramos N, Yazdani SK, Ghanem AM, Holland SM, Freeman AF, et al. Coronary atherosclerosis and dilation in hyper IgE syndrome patients: depiction by magnetic resonance vessel wall imaging and pathological correlation. Atherosclerosis. 2017;258:20–5.
17. Dweck MR, Puntman V, Vesey AT, Fayad ZA, Nagel E. MR imaging of coronary arteries and plaques. JACC Cardiovasc Imaging. 2016;9:306–16.
18. Makowski MR, Henningsson M, Spuentrup E, Kim WY, Maintz D, Manning WJ, et al. Characterization of coronary atherosclerosis by magnetic resonance imaging. Circulation. 2013;128:1244–55.
19. Xie G, Zhang N, Xie Y, Nguyen C, Deng Z, Bi X, et al. DANTE-prepared three-dimensional FLASH: a fast isotropic-resolution MR approach to morphological evaluation of the peripheral arterial wall at 3 tesla. J Magn Reson Imaging. 2016;43:343–51.
20. Langham MC, Desjardins B, Englund EK, Mohler ER, 3rd, Floyd TF, Wehrli FW. Rapid high-resolution, self-registered, dual lumen-contrast MRI method for vessel-wall assessment in peripheral artery disease:: A Preliminary Investigation Acad Radiol 2016;23:457–467.
21. Isbell DC, Meyer CH, Rogers WJ, Epstein FH, DiMaria JM, Harthun NL, et al. Reproducibility and reliability of atherosclerotic plaque volume measurements in peripheral arterial disease with cardiovascular magnetic resonance. J Cardiovasc Magn Reson. 2007;9:71–6.
22. Zhou C, Qiao H, He L, Yuan C, Chen H, Zhang Q, et al. Characterization of atherosclerotic disease in thoracic aorta: a 3D, multicontrast vessel wall imaging study. Eur J Radiol. 2016;85:2030–5.
23. Kim YS, Lim SH, Oh KW, Kim JY, Koh SH, Kim J, et al. The advantage of high-resolution MRI in evaluating basilar plaques: a comparison study with MRA. Atherosclerosis. 2012;224:411–6.
24. Zhu XJ, Du B, Lou X, Hui FK, Ma L, Zheng BW, et al. Morphologic characteristics of atherosclerotic middle cerebral arteries on 3T high-resolution MRI. AJNR Am J Neuroradiol. 2013;34:1717–22.
25. Feng C, Hua T, Xu Y, Liu XY, Huang J. Arterial remodeling of basilar atherosclerosis in isolated pontine infarction. Neurol Sci. 2015;36:547–51.
26. Ma N, Jiang WJ, Lou X, Ma L, Du B, Cai JF, et al. Arterial remodeling of advanced basilar atherosclerosis: a 3-tesla MRI study. Neurology. 2010;75: 253–8.
27. Chen L, Liu Q, Zhan Q, Zhang X, Lu J. Comparison of two different measurement methods in evaluating basilar atherosclerotic plaque using high resolution MRI at 3T. Honolulu: International Society for Magnetic Resonance in Medicine; 2017.
28. Underhill HR, Yarnykh VL, Hatsukami TS, Wang J, Balu N, Hayes CE, et al. Carotid plaque morphology and composition: initial comparison between 1. 5- and 3.0-T magnetic field strengths. Radiology. 2008;248:550–60.
29. Shrout PE, Fleiss JL. Intraclass correlations: uses in assessing rater reliability. Psychol Bull. 1979;86:420–8.
30. Bland JM, Altman DG. Statistical methods for assessing agreement between two methods of clinical measurement. Lancet. 1986;1:307–10.
31. Lim SH, Choi H, Kim HT, Kim J, Heo SH, Chang DI, et al. Basilar plaque on high-resolution MRI predicts progressive motor deficits after pontine infarction. Atherosclerosis. 2015;240:278–83.
32. Ryu CW, Kwak HS, Jahng GH, Lee HN. High-resolution MRI of intracranial atherosclerotic disease. Neurointervention. 2014;9:9–20.
33. Cai JM, Hatsukami TS, Ferguson MS, Small R, Polissar NL, Yuan C. Classification of human carotid atherosclerotic lesions with in vivo multicontrast magnetic resonance imaging. Circulation. 2002;106:1368–73.
34. Felmlee JP, Ehman RL. Spatial presaturation: a method for suppressing flow artifacts and improving depiction of vascular anatomy in MR imaging. Radiology. 1987;164:559–64.
35. Li L, Miller KL, Jezzard P. DANTE-prepared pulse trains: a novel approach to motion-sensitized and motion-suppressed quantitative magnetic resonance imaging. Magn Reson Med. 2012;68:1423–38.
36. Wang J, Yarnykh VL, Hatsukami T, Chu B, Balu N, Yuan C. Improved suppression of plaque-mimicking artifacts in black-blood carotid atherosclerosis imaging using a multislice motion-sensitized driven-equilibrium (MSDE) turbo spin-echo (TSE) sequence. Magn Reson Med. 2007;58:973–81.
37. Yarnykh VL, Yuan C. Multislice double inversion-recovery black-blood imaging with simultaneous slice reinversion. J Magn Reson Imaging. 2003; 17:478–83.
38. Yang WQ, Huang B, Liu XT, Liu HJ, Li PJ, Zhu WZ. Reproducibility of high-resolution MRI for the middle cerebral artery plaque at 3T. Eur J Radiol. 2014;83:e49–55.

24

Repeatability and variation of region-of-interest methods using quantitative diffusion tensor MR imaging of the brain

Ullamari Hakulinen[1,2*], Antti Brander[1†], Pertti Ryymin[1†], Juha Öhman[3†], Seppo Soimakallio[1,4†], Mika Helminen[5†], Prasun Dastidar[1,4†] and Hannu Eskola[1,2†]

Abstract

Background: Diffusion tensor imaging (DTI) is increasingly used in various diseases as a clinical tool for assessing the integrity of the brain's white matter. Reduced fractional anisotropy (FA) and an increased apparent diffusion coefficient (ADC) are nonspecific findings in most pathological processes affecting the brain's parenchyma. At present, there is no gold standard for validating diffusion measures, which are dependent on the scanning protocols, methods of the softwares and observers. Therefore, the normal variation and repeatability effects on commonly-derived measures should be carefully examined.

Methods: Thirty healthy volunteers (mean age 37.8 years, SD 11.4) underwent DTI of the brain with 3T MRI. Region-of-interest (ROI) -based measurements were calculated at eleven anatomical locations in the pyramidal tracts, corpus callosum and frontobasal area. Two ROI-based methods, the circular method (CM) and the freehand method (FM), were compared. Both methods were also compared by performing measurements on a DTI phantom. The intra- and inter-observer variability (coefficient of variation, or CV%) and repeatability (intra-class correlation coefficient, or ICC) were assessed for FA and ADC values obtained using both ROI methods.

Results: The mean FA values for all of the regions were 0.663 with the CM and 0.621 with the FM. For both methods, the FA was highest in the splenium of the corpus callosum. The mean ADC value was 0.727 $\times 10^{-3}$ mm^2/s with the CM and 0.747 $\times 10^{-3}$ mm^2/s with the FM, and both methods found the ADC to be lowest in the corona radiata. The CV percentages of the derived measures were < 13% with the CM and < 10% with the FM. In most of the regions, the ICCs were excellent or moderate for both methods. With the CM, the highest ICC for FA was in the posterior limb of the internal capsule (0.90), and with the FM, it was in the corona radiata (0.86). For ADC, the highest ICC was found in the genu of the corpus callosum (0.93) with the CM and in the uncinate fasciculus (0.92) with FM.

Conclusions: With both ROI-based methods variability was low and repeatability was moderate. The circular method gave higher repeatability, but variation was slightly lower using the freehand method. The circular method can be recommended for the posterior limb of the internal capsule and splenium of the corpus callosum, and the freehand method for the corona radiata.

* Correspondence: ullamari.hakulinen@pshp.fi
[†]Equal contributors
[1]Department of Radiology, Medical Imaging Center of Pirkanmaa Hospital District, Teiskontie 35 PL 2000, 33521, Tampere, Finland
[2]Department of Biomedical Engineering, Tampere University of Technology, Tampere, Finland
Full list of author information is available at the end of the article

Background

Diffusion tensor imaging (DTI) is an MRI technique that has been increasingly used as both a scientific and a clinical tool in the past decade [1]. DTI is based on the diffusion characteristics of water molecules and it enables investigation of the architecture of the biological environment [2] that cannot be seen by conventional magnetic resonance MRI techniques. In the brain area, DTI is used for visualizing and characterizing white matter tracts in which water diffusion follows the direction of fibers. The diffusion metrics such as fractional anisotropy (FA) and apparent diffusion coefficient (ADC) are often used in the diffusion analysis. FA is a measure of the degree of diffusion anisotropy, and ADC describes the average diffusion [3]. Decreased FA values and increased ADC values are related to the disruption of the tissue microstructure, including the axons in white matter tracts [4].

The diffusion measures have been used to evaluate the integrity of white matter tracts in pathological conditions [5-7] and in healthy brains [8-11]. FA and ADC changes have been found in several white matter diseases [12-16], but it is known that age affects both FA and ADC values, and small changes occur across the lifespan and even in different ways with men and women [17].

The quantitative DTI is still a relatively new method, and therefore it is essential to be aware of the variables and limitations relating to technique. For example, low signal-to-noise ratio (SNR), many artifacts [18-20] as well as partial volume effects impact on derived measures. The diffusion measures are also dependent on angular resolution and spatial resolutions [21] which affect the particular values of FA. In order to interpret the findings correctly observers need to realize these factors.

Region-of-interest (ROI) -based [1,11,22] and voxel-based methods [23,24] are the most commonly used quantitative approaches. The ROI-based method has been available for a longer time, and therefore, most clinical softwares include only this approach. In this method, the measurements are performed on the original slices, thus avoiding post-processing calculation errors, but the method suffers from the lack of normal values, and relatively low repeatability [22] and high variability [25]. Voxel-based methods are increasingly used in the research and they are more automated and are not dependent on the observer, but these methods require inter-subject registration and image smoothing [26]. One of the recent methods "tract-based spatial statistics" (TBSS) is fully automated, simple to use and investigates the whole brain. It aims to solve voxel-based statistics across subjects on the skeleton-space FA data.

An alternative technique to ROI measurements is fiber tracking (tractography). With this method, the FA and ADC values are averaged for the fiber bundles. Most commonly, tractography is based on convential DTI, but it suffers from difficulties with complex fiber architecture like crossing fiber tracts [27,28]. New techniques, such as high angular resolution diffusion imaging (HARDI), are able to solve these difficulties by measuring the diffusion attenuation in more angular directions. HARDI reconstruction techniques, such as Q-ball imaging [29], are particularly useful for reproducing complex fiber geometries and can lead to an SNR even lower than that of DTI [28].

Although various other methods have been suggested for neuroradiological quantifications, we have applied the ROI-based methods in this study. This is because these methods have wide availability and easiness to use in individual patients. The aim of our study was to evaluate these quantitative methods and to give preferences for the two ROI approaches. The analysis was based on intra- and inter-observer variation and repeatability. According to the medical literature no other studies with comparison of two specific DTI-based ROI methods have been measured in normal adults.

Methods

Subjects

Thirty healthy adults were scanned with a 3T Siemens Trio (Siemens Healthcare, Erlangen, Germany). The volunteer group consisted of 21 women and 9 men with an age range of 18 – 60 years and a mean age of 37.8 years [11]. MRI scans were performed during the autumn of 2008. The criteria for selecting the control group were age, sex and intelligence matching with patients enrolled in a mild traumatic brain injury study [30]. The volunteers included hospital staff and their relatives with no history of neurological or psychiatric diseases. The ethics committee of the hospital approved the study, and an informed consent was received from each volunteer.

DTI phantom

The DTI phantom consisted of winding polyamide fibers (polyfil, 15-μm fibers, 50 dtex, Filamentgarn TYPE 611, Trevira GmbH, Bobingen, Germany) around an acrylic glass spindle [31]. The fluid portion consisted of an aqueous sodium chloride solution and distilled water (83 g NaCl per kilogram of water). The concentration of sodium chloride was matched to the susceptibility of the fluid and fibers [32]. According to the information provided by the manufacturer, the reference values were FA = 0.820 and ADC = 0.832 $\times 10^{-3}$ mm^2/s.

MRI acquisition

The MRI protocol included sagittal T1-weighted 3D IR-prepared gradient echo, axial T2-weighted turbo spin echo, conventional axial and high-resolution sagittal

FLAIR (Fluid Attenuation Inversion Recovery), axial T2*-weighted, and axial SWI (Susceptibility Weighted Imaging) series. The DTI data were collected by a single-shot, spin echo-based, and diffusion-weighted echo planar imaging sequence. The parameters for the DTI sequence were TR 5144 ms, TE 92 ms, FOV 230 mm, matrix 128 × 128, 3 averages, slice/gap 3.0/0.9 mm, voxel dimension 1.8×1.8×3.0 mm, b-factor 0 and 1000 s/mm^2, and 20 diffusion gradient orientations. A 12-channel head matrix coil was used. The DTI phantom was imaged using the same protocol and equipment as with the volunteers. Two 7 cm loop coils were used with the 12-channel head matrix coil to increase the SNR of the measurement.

Data analysis

Multi directional diffusion data was first analysed visually for distortions and artifacts. Eddy current distortion was qualitatively estimated by drawing the brain contours to b_0 images, and copying them to diffusion weighted images. We did not find significant eddy current distortions due to diffusion gradients.

Two observers, a physicist (UH) and a neuroradiologist (AB), separately performed the volunteer ROI measurements on a workstation using the commercially available software Neuro3D (Siemens Healthcare, Malvern, USA). With the circular (CM) and the freehand method (FM), ROIs were manually placed on axial images of the color-coded FA maps [33] and automatically transferred on the non-diffusion-weighted b_0 images and ADC maps. The ROIs of the corpus callosum were drawn onto the median-line sagittal images. The ROIs were centered in the region using color-coded directions while taking care to avoid border areas, such as areas overlapping with cerebrospinal fluid spaces and neighboring tracts. The size of the ROI was chosen by using the subject´s own anatomical knowledge of regions. The measurements were similar to those performed in ordinary clinical conditions; for example, the levels of the slices were chosen each time the measurement was performed. The time between the first and repeat measurements was at least four weeks.

The FA and ADC values were measured in eleven separate regions. The ROIs for the pyramidal tracts included the basal pons, cerebral peduncle, posterior limb of the internal capsule, corona radiata and centrum semiovale (Figure 1). In the frontobasal area, the regions of interest were the uncinate fasciculus, forceps minor and anterior corona radiata (Figure 2). In the corpus callosum, the ROIs included the genu, body and splenium (Figure 3).

With the phantom measurements, the ROIs were placed in four different regions (Figure 4).

Signal-to-Noise Ratio (SNR) was determined according the NEMA Standards 1–2008, including the following expression for SNR:

$$SNR = \frac{S}{\text{image\_noise}}$$

where S = signal, and image noise is estimated with Rayleigh distribution:

$$\text{image\_noise} = \frac{SD}{0.66}$$

The SNR measurements were used from the images of three subjects. The ROI was placed on the left side of the each region of the b = 0 s/mm^2 image. The standardized ROI of the background noise (9.7 cm^2) was placed outside the anatomical structures. SNR measurements were also performed in the DTI phantom. These four measurements were placed at similar locations as the actual measurements.

Statistical analyses

The statistical analyses were performed using the SPSS software package (SPSS, Chicago, IL). The normality of the distributions was tested using the Kolmogorov-Smirnov test. The regional mean values were calculated from the mean values of the right and left hemispheres (N = 30). The FA and ADC values of the left and right hemispheres were compared using paired t-tests with the two-tailed significance set at $p < 0.05/11$. It was used Bonferroni correction for 11 regions instead of 22, because FA and ADC are relative independent. The right and left hemisphere asymmetries were evaluated according to the formula (A) = (left-right)/ ((left+right)/2) [25]. The differences between repeat measurements and measurements made by two different ROI-methods were compared using the standard deviation of the differences. These d ± 2s limits for the difference are known as the 95% limits of agreement, and these limits can be displayed as horizontal lines. This graphical representation is called a Bland-Altman plot [34]. The coefficient of variation (CV%) was calculated according the following equation (with SD = standard deviation and d = mean):

$$CV\% = \frac{SD}{d} \cdot 100\%.$$

The intra– and inter-observer repeatability values were assessed using the averages of intra-class correlation coefficients (ICCs) with absolute agreement. The ICC values were considered to indicate excellent agreement if they were greater than 0.8 and substantial agreement if they were from 0.60 to 0.79 [35]. The absolute p values were also defined, the statistical significance of which was set to $p < 0.05/11$ with Bonferroni correction for 11

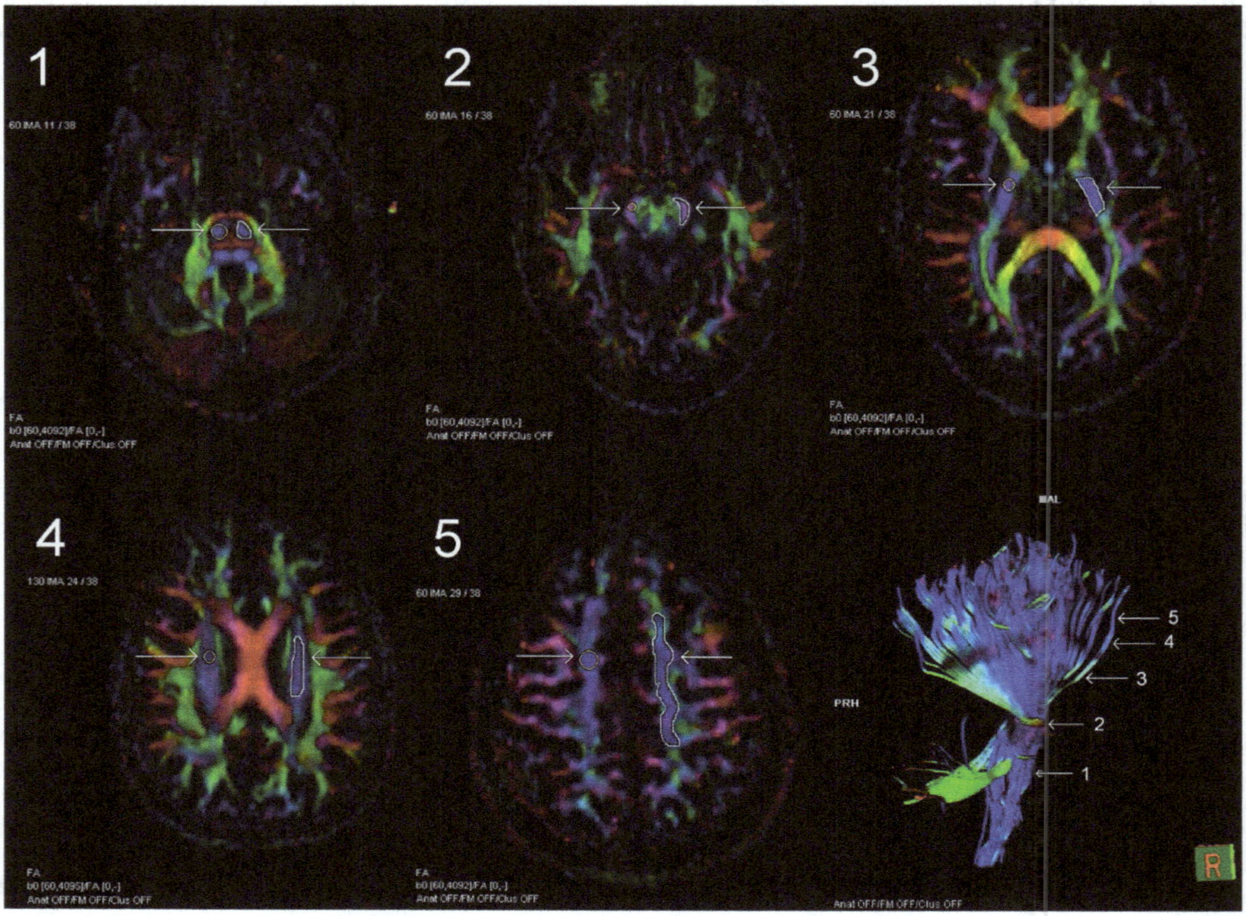

Figure 1 ROIs in the pyramidal tracts. Axial FA color maps with the circular and freehand ROIs (region-of-interest), and tractography of the pyramidal tract with five locations of the measurements: basal pons [**1**], cerebral peduncle [**2**], posterior limb of the internal capsule [**3**], corona radiata [**4**] and centrum semiovale [**5**].

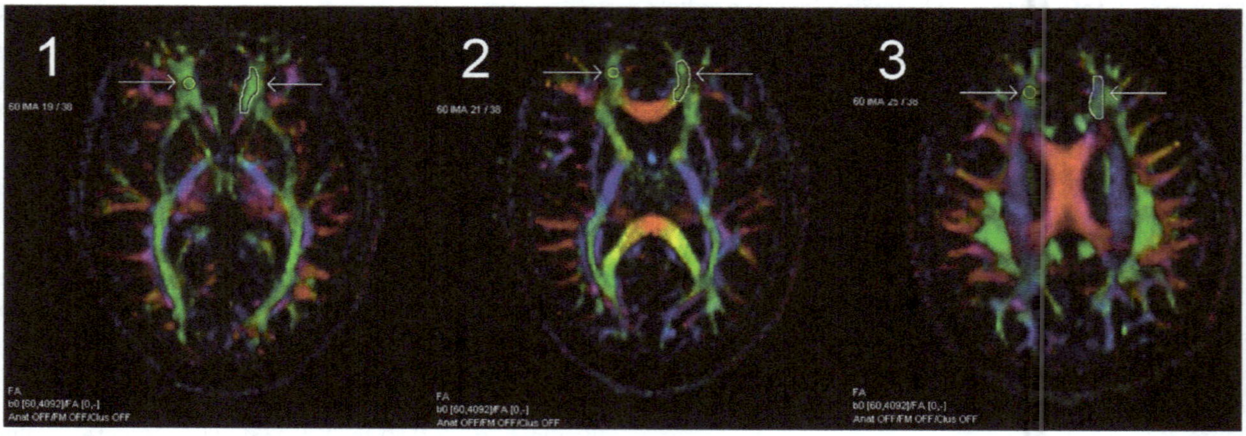

Figure 2 ROIs in the frontobasal area. ROI placements on axial FA color maps with circular and freehand methods in the frontobasal area: uncinate fasciculus [**1**], forceps minor [**2**] and anterior corona radiata [**3**].

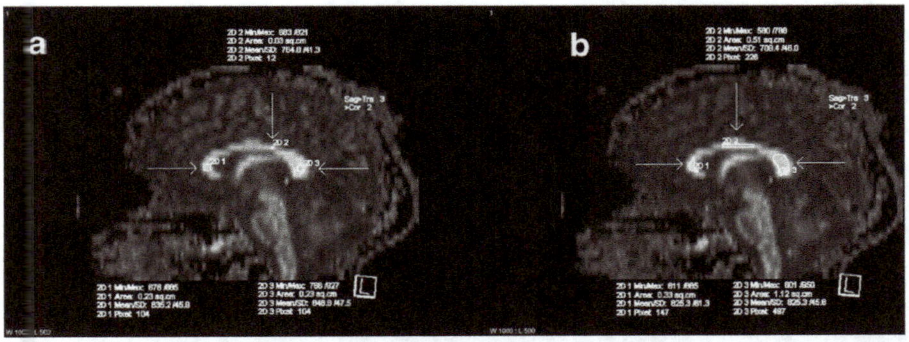

Figure 3 ROIs in the corpus callosum. ROI placements on sagittal FA maps in the corpus callosum with the circular (**a**) and freehand (**b**) methods: genu, body and splenium.

regions. The results of the DTI phantom were compared with the values supplied by the manufacturer using the equation (with MV = measured value and RV = reference value):

$$Change\% = \frac{MV - RV}{RV} \cdot 100\%$$

Results

The preliminary results on the part of the pyramidal tract have been presented in our previous study [33], but in this study, the results are a part of a wider context. Using visual inspection the data quality was excellent in most cases, except in certain regions of the basal pons (Figure 5a), cerebral peduncle (Figure 5b) and the body of the corpus callosum, which had artifacts caused by air-filled cavities, pulsation or water containing tissues.

Mean values for FA and ADC

The Kolmogorov–Smirnov test found that all mean values (N = 30) were normally distributed ($p > 0.10$). The intra-observer mean values, with the CM and the FM for FA and ADC, are shown in Table 1. The mean FA values were highest in the splenium of the corpus callosum with both methods; they were lowest in the corona radiata with CM and in the forceps minor with FM. The mean ADC values were highest in the body of the corpus callosum and lowest in the corona radiata with both methods. The values were 2.8% lower for FA and 0.4% higher for ADC with the FM compared to the CM.

Statistically significant differences were found between right and left hemisphere in the four regions. These regions were the posterior of the internal capsule with the CM, uncinate fasciculus and forceps minor with the FM, and the corona radiata with both methods.

Table 2 shows the observer 2 results for the mean FA and ADC values. Using CM, observer 2 had 1.0% higher average FA and 0.6% higher average ADC mean values than did observer 1. Using FM, observer 2 had 2.9% lower FA values and 2.4% higher ADC values than observer 1.

SNR analysis

The mean SNR value (± standard deviation) of $b = 0\ s/mm^2$ images for all regions in vivo measurements was 25.4 ± 3.9, for the pyramidal tract 25.3 ± 3.7, for the corpus callosum 25.4 ± 5.1 and for the frontobasal area 25.4 ± 2.6. The mean SNR of the four regions of the DTI phantom was 27.9 ± 6.0.

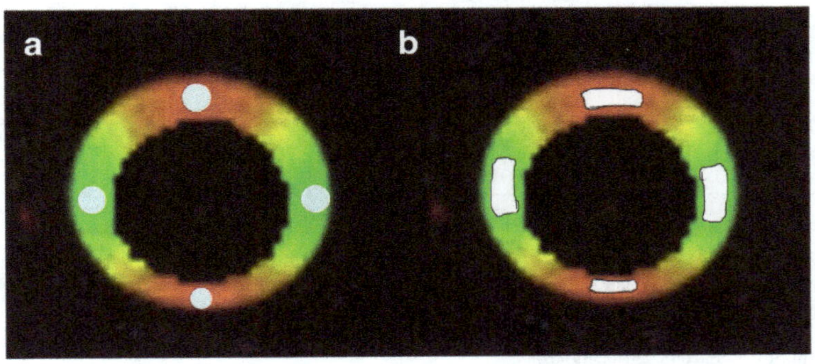

Figure 4 ROIs in the phantom images. ROI placements on axial FA color maps in the phantom with the circular (**a**) and freehand (**b**) methods.

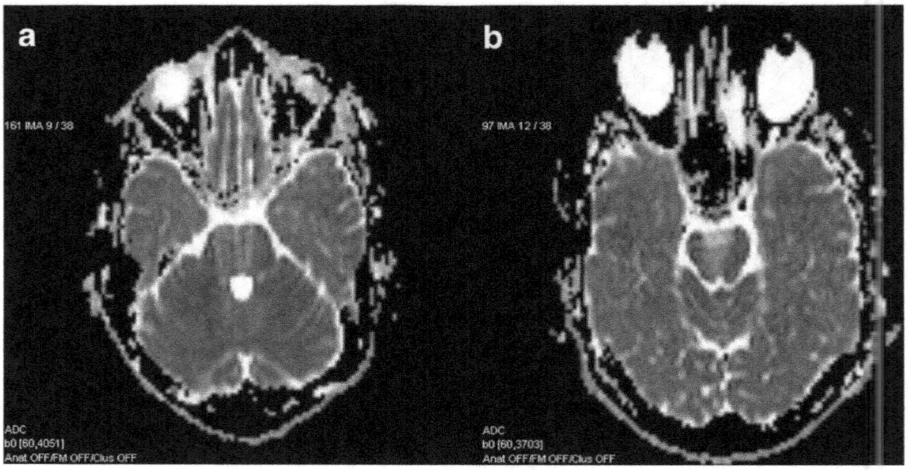

Figure 5 Artifacts. Axial ADC maps with the artifacts in the basal pons (**a**) and cerebral peduncle (**b**).

Table 1 The intra-observer regional mean FA and ADC ($10^{-3}mm^2/s$) values (mean ± sd) for the circular and freehand ROI methods (N = 30)

		Circular ROI		Freehand ROI	
Region	Parameter	1st meas.	2nd meas.	1st meas.	2nd meas.
Basal pons	FA	0.653 ± 0.065	0.637 ± 0.070	0.573 ± 0.060	0.634 ± 0.054
	ADC	0.708 ± 0.052	0.709 ± 0.060	0.709 ± 0.044	0.705 ± 0.041
Cerebral peduncle	FA	0.853 ± 0.052	0.847 ± 0.049	0.779 ± 0.049	0.817 ± 0.041
	ADC	0.711 ± 0.057	0.710 ± 0.051	0.758 ± 0.058	0.728 ± 0.033
Internal capsule, post	FA	0.734 ± 0.043	0.737 ± 0.038	0.671 ± 0.042	0.714 ± 0.037
	ADC	0.685 ± 0.024 [a]	0.679 ± 0.024	0.685 ± 0.015	0.688 ± 0.017
Corona radiata	FA	0.508 ± 0.053 [b]	0.504 ± 0.050 [c]	0.511 ± 0.049	0.524 ± 0.046 [d]
	ADC	0.644 ± 0.027	0.648 ± 0.027	0.671 ± 0.025	0.663 ± 0.022
Centrum semiovale	FA	0.505 ± 0.053	0.516 ± 0.081	0.507 ± 0.047	0.558 ± 0.055
	ADC	0.688 ± 0.034	0.693 ± 0.042	0.698 ± 0.021	0.692 ± 0.022
Uncinate fasciculus	FA	0.542 ± 0.051	0.535 ± 0.064	0.501 ± 0.039 [e]	0.552 ± 0.041
	ADC	0.773 ± 0.032	0.773 ± 0.032	0.774 ± 0.025	0.777 ± 0.032
Forceps minor	FA	0.539 ± 0.059	0.548 ± 0.074	0.466 ± 0.044 [f]	0.511 ± 0.045
	ADC	0.764 ± 0.039	0.765 ± 0.031	0.761 ± 0.029	0.760 ± 0.027
Ant corona radiata	FA	0.551 ± 0.066	0.542 ± 0.073	0.472 ± 0.038	0.508 ± 0.043
	ADC	0.742 ± 0.027	0.759 ± 0.028	0.747 ± 0.027	0.750 ± 0.027
CC genu	FA	0.834 ± 0.041	0.826 ± 0.036	0.673 ± 0.049	0.810 ± 0.033
	ADC	0.758 ± 0.067	0.766 ± 0.051	0.858 ± 0.056	0.770 ± 0.049
CC body	FA	0.750 ± 0.048	0.723 ± 0.038	0.616 ± 0.054	0.683 ± 0.063
	ADC	0.755 ± 0.073	0.839 ± 0.084	0.896 ± 0.076	0.810 ± 0.090
CC splenium	FA	0.856 ± 0.055	0.855 ± 0.050	0.742 ± 0.051	0.836 ± 0.044
	ADC	0.713 ± 0.055	0.714 ± 0.040	0.792 ± 0.047	0.732 ± 0.042

Regions with significant differences between right and left cerebral hemispheres (p< 0.05/11):

[a] Posterior limb of the internal capsule ADC (circular): a) right 0.699±0.028, left 0.671±0.037.

[b,c] Corona radiata FA (circular): b) right 0.484±0.055, left 0.533±0.063, c) right 0.490±0.055, left 0.518±0.058.

[d] Corona radiata FA (freehand): d) right 0.508±0.048, left 0.539±0.054.

[e] Uncinate fasciculus FA (freehand): e) right 0.512±0.045, left 0.490±0.039.

[f] Forceps minor FA (freehand): f) right 0.481±0.046, left 0.452 ±0.048.

Table 2 Measurements by observer 2 (mean ± sd), inter-observer repeatability (Obs. 1: 2. meas.) and variation (N = 30) for FA and ADC ($10^{-3}mm^2/s$)

		Circular ROI				Freehand ROI			
Region	Parameter	Mean ± SD	ICC	p	CV(%)	Mean ± SD	ICC	p	CV(%)
Basal pons	FA	0.705 ± 0.044	0.44	0.004*	8.6	0.621 ± 0.061	0.73	< 0.001*	9.2
	ADC	0.726 ± 0.069	0.24	0.226	8.9	0.730 ± 0.080	0.01	0.487	8.4
Cerebral peduncle	FA	0.850 ± 0.035	0.62	0.006	4.9	0.788 ± 0.062	0.14	0.319	6.4
	ADC	0.706 ± 0.048	0.56	0.018	7.0	0.772 ± 0.070	0.49	0.008	6.8
Internal capsule, post	FA	0.767 ± 0.046	0.67	< 0.001*	5.6	0.728 ± 0.036	0.80	< 0.001*	5.0
	ADC	0.696 ± 0.034	0.63	0.001*	4.2	0.693 ± 0.021	0.84	< 0.001*	2.8
Corona radiata	FA	0.508 ± 0.038	0.54	0.023	8.6	0.515 ± 0.047	0.78	< 0.001*	9.0
	ADC	0.648 ± 0.030	0.64	0.005	4.5	0.665 ± 0.025	0.93	< 0.001*	3.6
Centrum semiovale	FA	0.501 ± 0.067	0.64	0.004*	14.5	0.509 ± 0.051	0.47	0.007	9.9
	ADC	0.700 ± 0.042	0.75	< 0.001*	6.0	0.693 ± 0.024	0.86	< 0.001*	3.3
Uncinate fasciculus	FA	0.529 ± 0.060	0.62	0.007	11.7	0.517 ± 0.050	0.74	< 0.001*	8.5
	ADC	0.779 ± 0.036	0.55	0.018	4.4	0.768 ± 0.025	0.84	< 0.001*	3.7
Forceps minor	FA	0.545 ± 0.057	0.64	0.004*	12.0	0.499 ± 0.051	0.83	< 0.001*	9.5
	ADC	0.762 ± 0.046	0.17	0.319	5.1	0.757 ± 0.029	0.88	< 0.001*	3.7
Ant corona radiata	FA	0.551 ± 0.073	0.84	< 0.001*	13.7	0.497 ± 0.040	0.86	< 0.001*	8.3
	ADC	0.754 ± 0.029	0.45	0.060	3.8	0.748 ± 0.024	0.82	< 0.001*	3.5
CC genu	FA	0.836 ± 0.034	0.80	< 0.001*	4.2	0.785 ± 0.051	0.51	0.013	5.3
	ADC	0.765 ± 0.044	0.80	< 0.001*	6.2	0.846 ± 0.069	0.37	0.012	7.3
CC body	FA	0.696 ± 0.057	0.39	0.066	6.7	0.654 ± 0.069	0.62	0.003*	9.8
	ADC	0.821 ± 0.164	0.61	0.008	15	0.862 ± 0.114	0.65	0.001*	12.2
CC splenium	FA	0.864 ± 0.047	0.90	< 0.001*	5.6	0.838 ± 0.043	0.88	< 0.001*	5.2
	ADC	0.717 ± 0.038	0.81	< 0.001*	5.4	0.739 ± 0.039	0.80	< 0.001*	5.5

* = the statistical significance $p < 0.05/11$ with Bonferroni correction for 11 regions.
ICC = intra-class correlation coefficient; CV = coefficient of variation.

Intra- and inter-observer variation

The intra-observer variation (CV%) results are shown in Table 3. Using CM, the CV percentage for FA was below 10% in 5 of 11 regions. Using FM, this percentage was below 10% in all of the regions. For ADC, the CV percentage was below 10% in all of the regions with both methods. The mean variation of the FA results was 9% with the CM and 8% with the FM. For ADC, the variation was 6% with the CM and 5% with the FM. For FA, the highest variation was in the centrum semiovale with the CM and the basal pons with the FM. The lowest variation was found in the genu of the corpus callosum with the CM and in the cerebral peduncle with the FM. For ADC, both methods had the highest variation in the body of the corpus callosum and the lowest in the posterior limb of the internal capsule.

The inter-observer CV% was below 10% in most of the regions; for FA measured with the CM, 7 of 11 regions had a CV% below 10%, and the FA in all of the regions measured with the FM had a CV percentage below 10%. For ADC, 9 of 11 regions had a CV percentage below 10% with both methods. The mean variation of the FA results was 9% with the CM and 7% with the FM, and for ADC, the variation was 8% with the CM and 6% with the FM.

The differences versus the sum (as measured by the FM and CM) for the FA and ADC values are shown in Figure 6. The Bland–Altman plots show minimum differences in the genu of the corpus callosum for FA and in the posterior limb of internal capsule for ADC and maximum differences in the centrum semiovale for FA and in the basal pons for ADC.

Intra- and inter-observer repeatability

The intra-observer repeatability (ICC) results are shown in Table 3. For FA, the average ICC was higher with the CM (0.70) than with the FM (0.52); for ADC, however, the FM had a higher ICC (0.67) than the CM (0.61). The ICC results for FA were above 0.8 in 3 of 11 regions with the CM and in 1 of 11 regions with the FM. For ADC, the corresponding results were 3 of 11 with the CM and 5 of 11 with the FM. The best ICC for FA values was in the posterior limb of the internal capsule (0.90) with the CM and in the corona radiata (0.86) with the FM. For

Table 3 The intra-observer repeatability and variability (N = 30) for FA and ADC (10^{-3}mm2/s) (N = 30)

		Circular ROI				Freehand ROI			
					Mean diff. ± 2sd				Mean diff. ± 2sd
Region	Parameter	ICC	p	CV (%)		ICC	p	CV (%)	
Basal pons	FA	0.74	< 0.001*	10.4	0.020 ± 0.093	0.63	< 0.001*	9.5	−0.061 ± 0.085
	ADC	0.83	< 0.001*	7.9	−0.010 ± 0.038	0.70	0.001*	6.0	0.004 ± 0.082
Cerebral peduncle	FA	0.74	< 0.001*	5.9	0.006 ± 0.092	0.42	0.025	5.6	−0.038 ± 0.101
	ADC	0.19	0.297	7.6	0.001 ± 0.145	0.29	0.141	6.[illegible]	0.030 ± 0.120
Internal capsule, post	FA	0.90	< 0.001*	5.5	−0.002 ± 0.049	0.66	< 0.001*	5.7	−0.043 ± 0.051
	ADC	0.76	< 0.001*	3.5	0.006 ± 0.042	0.78	< 0.001*	2.3	−0.002 ± 0.027
Corona radiata	FA	0.84	< 0.001*	10.2	0.005 ± 0.077	0.86	< 0.001*	9.2	−0.013 ± 0.063
	ADC	0.76	< 0.001*	4.2	−0.004 ± 0.048	0.86	< 0.001*	3.5	0.008 ± 0.030
Centrum semiovale	FA	0.48	0.041	13.1	−0.001 ± 0.160	0.26	0.121	9.5	−0.051 ± 0.128
	ADC	0.63	0.005	5.5	−0.005 ± 0.079	0.87	< 0.001*	3.1	0.005 ± 0.028
Uncinate fasciculus	FA	0.67	0.002*	10.7	0.007 ± 0.116	0.61	< 0.001*	7.5	−0.051 ± 0.051
	ADC	0.69	0.001*	4.1	0.000 ± 0.063	0.92	< 0.001*	3.7	−0.003 ± 0.031
Forceps minor	FA	0.76	< 0.001*	12.2	−0.009 ± 0.118	0.65	< 0.001*	9.1	−0.044 ± 0.067
	ADC	0.64	0.005	4.6	−0.001 ± 0.073	0.89	< 0.001*	3.7	0.001 ± 0.035
Ant corona radiata	FA	0.71	0.001*	12.8	0.009 ± 0.133	0.61	< 0.001*	8.3	−0.036 ± 0.073
	ADC	0.27	0.169	3.7	−0.017 ± 0.071	0.85	< 0.001*	3.7	−0.002 ± 0.040
CC genu	FA	0.67	0.002*	4.7	0.008 ± 0.078	0.15	0.002*	5.7	−0.137 ± 0.082
	ADC	0.93	< 0.001*	7.7	−0.008 ± 0.062	0.37	0.001*	6.5	0.089 ± 0.102
CC body	FA	0.23	0.203	5.8	0.027 ± 0.112	0.59	< 0.001*	9.0	−0.067 ± 0.091
	ADC	0.26	0.107	9.8	−0.085 ± 0.195	0.50	0.002*	9.3	0.087 ± 0.166
CC splenium	FA	0.89	< 0.001*	6.1	0.002 ± 0.066	0.27	0.006	6.0	−0.094 ± 0.100
	ADC	0.82	< 0.001*	6.6	−0.001 ± 0.075	0.34	0.015	5.9	0.060 ± 0.099

ICC = intra-class correlation coefficient; CV = coefficient of variation; Mean diff. ± 2sd = 95% limits of agreement, * = the statistical significance $p < 0.05/11$ with Bonferroni correction for 11 regions.

ADC, the best ICC was in the genu of the corpus callosum (0.93) with the CM and in the uncinate fasciculus (0.92) with the FM.

The best 95% limit for FA intra-observer agreement was found in the posterior limb of the internal capsule for the CM and in the uncinate fasciculus for the FM. The lowest level of agreement was in the centrum semiovale with both ROI methods. For ADC, both methods had the highest observed agreement in the posterior limb of internal capsule and the lowest in the body of the corpus callosum. With the FA and ADC measurements, statistically significant of the ($p < 0.05/11$) repeatability was found in 68% of the regions with the CM and 78% in the regions with the FM.

Table 2 shows the inter-observer repeatability (ICC) results. The ICC of the FA measurement was 0.65 with the CM and 0.67 with the FM, and for the ADC measurements it was 0.56 with the CM and 0.68 with the FM. For FA, the ICC results were 0.8 or above in 3 of 11 regions with the CM and in 4 of 11 regions with the FM. For ADC, the results were found in 2 of 11 regions with the CM and 7 of 11 regions with the FM. The best ICC results of the FA was found in the splenium of the corpus callosum with both methods (ICC for CM = 0.90 and ICC for FM = 0.88). For the ADC, the highest ICC was in the splenium of the corpus callosum (0.81) with the CM and in the corona radiata (0.93) with the FM.

Phantom measurements

Using the CM method in phantom studies resulted in a mean FA value of 0.836 ± 0.017 (range 0.823 – 0.861) and a mean ADC value of 0.837 ± 0.016 $\times 10^{-3}$ mm^2/s (range 0.823 – 0.857 $\times 10^{-3}$ mm^2/s). Similarly, the FM results gave a mean FA value of 0.818 ± 0.010 (range 0.806 – 0.830) and a mean ADC value of 852 ± 0.009 $\times 10^{-3}$ mm^2/s (range 0.841 – 0.862 $\times 10^{-3}$ mm^2/s). For FA, the CM result differed from reference value CV% = 2.1, and for ADC it was CV% = 1.9. The corresponding FM results were CV% = 1.3 for FA and CV% = 1.0 for ADC. The SNR result of the phantom was presented above.

Discussion

In this study, we investigated the mean values, variation and repeatability in an intra- and inter-observer study on MRI´s of 30 healthy volunteers using two methods based on circular and freehand regions of interests. The

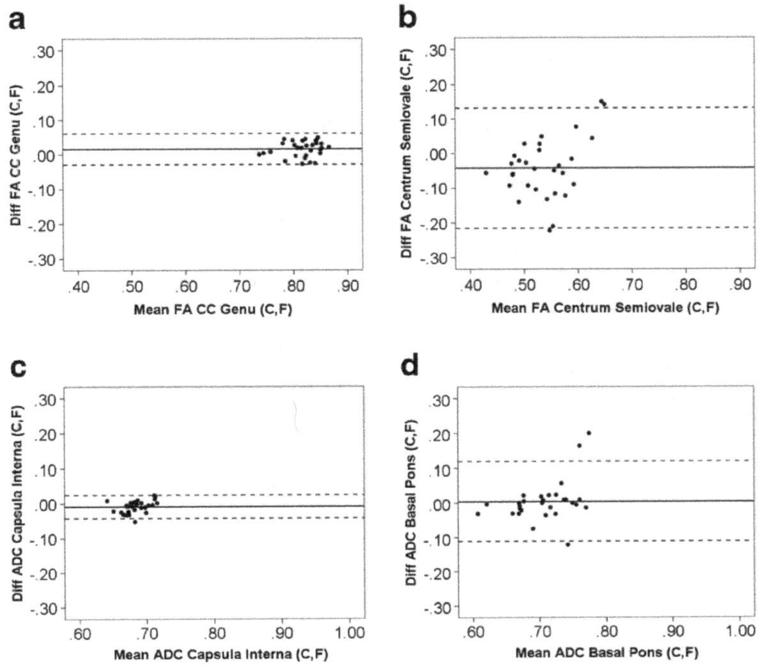

Figure 6 The Bland–Altman plots. Difference versus sum for FA (scaled 0–1) and ADC ($10^{-3}mm^2/s$) measured by circular (C) and freehand (F) methods. The Bland–Altman plots show maximum and minimum differences of regions with 95% limits of agreement (dotted lines): genu of the corpus callosum (FA) (**a**), centrum semiovale (FA) (**b**), posterior limb of the internal capsule (ADC) (**c**) and basal pons (ADC) (**d**).

SNR and phantom measurements showed that the image quality was good and adequate for analysis purposes.

Regional variation of the FA and ADC absolute values was large, which has also been found in previous studies [11,33,36]. In our study the highest values were obtained in the corpus callosum, in concordance with Lee et al. 2009 and Brander et al. 2010. The high FA reflects the microstructure of corpus callosum in which the fibers are tightly packed and parallel to each other. The highest FA value within the pyramidal tract was found in the cerebral peduncle, which we have reported also in our previous study [33]. The results of the frontobasal regions were very close to each other in each region.

Brain asymmetries were noticed in some regions. They were found in the corona radiata for FA, and in the posterior limb of the internal capsule for ADC, which agree with previous findings [11]. In addition, asymmetries were found in the frontobasal area such as the uncinate fasciculus and forceps minor. Recently, Bonekamp et al. 2007 and Snook et al. 2005 have reported the existence of asymmetry in the centrum semiovale. Generally, the brain asymmetries have also been observed with other imaging modalities such as computed tomography (CT) [37].

The variation of the FA and ADC mean values were lower for the FM than for the CM. The results agree with the study by Bonecamp et al. 2009 and our earlier study, which included regions of the pyramidal tracts [33]. The repeatability was better with the CM than with the FM because the freehand ROIs included the border-zones of the tracts, which have lower FA than the central tracts. However, the results were highly dependent on the region.

The interregional variation was due to the location. It depended on the density of the tracts and also the artifacts, which were represented above. In addition, relative low spatial resolution effects especially in the small regions. Variation may also be caused by several factors such as noise level, gradient stability, motion and slice position between subjects [25]. The SNR of the b = 0 s/mm^2 should be at least 20 in order to derive relatively reliable FA values [20]. In our study, the SNR was well above 20 in all regions expect basal pons (SNR = 19.2), and measured SNR are comparable to earlier study [38]. The variability of the intra-observer and inter-observer was relatively low at all regions. It was higher in the FA values than in the ADC values, as has been found in previous studies [1,11,19,25,39,40]. It is known that ADC values are homogeneous throughout the healthy brain, whereas FA values change depending on the location [41]. However, increased ADC variability was found in such regions as the cerebral peduncle and the corpus callosum, which is consistent with the study by Bonekamp [25]. In this study, the high variability in the body of the corpus callosum resulted from the effect of cerebrospinal fluid and the small ROI diameter. On average, the intra- and inter-observer variabilities were lower with the FM than with the CM.

According to 95% limits of agreement the differences between two methods was the smallest in the genu and splenium of the corpus callosum and in the posterior limb of the pyramidal tract for FA. The result can be explained by these regions being small, compact and usually without artifacts, so that the locations and size of the ROIs were almost the same. The differences were larger in the other regions because the ROI size between circle and freehand methods varied considerably. The CM represented a small sample area, whereas the freehand ROI covers the entire area of the measured tract. In the case of the basal pons and cerebral peduncle, the sources of variation were artifacts such as air-filled cavities, which affect the FM more than the CM.

The level of repeatability was moderate in most of the regions, as has been found in previous studies [11,22]. We found an excellent FA agreement in the posterior limb of the internal capsule and corona radiata, such as in the splenium of the corpus callosum, when using the CM [22]. The repeatability of the FA results was lower than that of the ADC results [19,25] because the partial volume effects and border areas had more effect on the FA values. Our results were consistent with the FM findings with the exception of the region of the body of the corpus callosum that was close to the cerebrospinal fluid. In general, the results were region-dependent. In most regions, repeatability was acceptable at the group level, but only few regions at the single-subject level.

The FA results of the DTI phantom showed more variation from the reference values when the CM was used than when the FM was used. In addition, the FA and ADC values were more variable for the FM than for the CM. Generally, the variability of both methods resembled that of the similar phantoms in previous studies [31]. The results of SNR were a bit higher for the phantom in comparison with in vivo measures. This difference is due to the fact that it we used two loop coils with the acquisition.

The repeatability of the results was decreased by the level being chosen separately each time, but this practice is a reality in the clinical environment. In addition, the examiner displayed learning effects, for example learning to avoid the artifacts and the border areas.

More investigations are needed to characterize different methods with a larger group of volunteers. These investigations should not concentrate only on ROI-based methods, but also studies comparing them to voxel-based methods would be important. These kinds of studies could also give rise to optimal combinations of different methods producing valuable new tools for the neuroradiologists.

Conclusions

Both methods, the circular and freehand method, had low variability and moderate repeatability in most regions. Slightly less variation was found with the freehand method, but the repeatability was higher with the circular method. Based on our study, the circular method can be recommended for the posterior limb of the internal capsule and splenium of the corpus callosum, and the freehand method for the corona radiata.

Competing interests

The authors assure that they have no competing interest.

Authors' contributions

Guarantors of integrity of entire study, UH; study concepts/study design, all authors; data acquisition, PR, JÖ, SS, PD; data analysis/interpretation, UH, AB; manuscript drafting, UH; manuscript revision, all authors; approval of final version of submitted manuscript, all authors; literature research, UH; statistical analysis, UH, MH; and manuscript editing, UH, AB, PR, HE. All authors read and approved the final manuscript.

Acknowledgements

We are grateful to the hospital staff of the Department of Radiology of the Tampere University Hospital for enabling this research.

Author details

[1]Department of Radiology, Medical Imaging Center of Pirkanmaa Hospital District, Teiskontie 35 PL 2000, 33521, Tampere, Finland. [2]Department of Biomedical Engineering, Tampere University of Technology, Tampere, Finland. [3]Department of Neurosurgery, Tampere University Hospital, Tampere, Finland. [4]Tampere Medical School, University of Tampere, Tampere, Finland. [5]Science Center of Pirkanmaa Hospital District, Tampere, Finland.

References

1. Lee CE, Danielian LE, Thomasson D, Baker EH: **Normal regional fractional anisotropy and apparent diffusion coefficient of the brain measured on a 3 T MR scanner.** *Neuroradiology* 2009, **51**:3–9.
2. Farrell JA, Landman BA, Jones CK, Smith SA, Prince JL, van Zijl PC, Mori S: **Effects of signal-to-noise ratio on the accuracy and reproducibility of diffusion tensor imaging-derived fractional anisotropy, mean diffusivity, and principal eigenvector measurements at 1.5 T.** *J Magn Reson Imaging* 2007, **26**:756–767.
3. Basser PJ: **Inferring microstructural features and the physiological state of tissues from diffusion-weighted images.** *NMR Biomed* 1995, **8**:333–344.
4. Pierpaoli C, Barnett A, Pajevic S, Chen R, Penix LR, Virta A, Basser P: **Water diffusion changes in Wallerian degeneration and their dependence on white matter architecture.** *Neuroimage* 2001, **13**:1174–1185.
5. Basser PJ, Mattiello J, LeBihan D: **Estimation of the effective self-diffusion tensor from the NMR spin echo.** *J Magn Reson B* 1994, **103**:247–254.
6. Zhang Y, Schuff N, Jahng GH, Bayne W, Mori S, Schad L, Mueller S, Du AT, Kramer JH, Yaffe K, Chui H, Jagust WJ, Miller BL, Weiner MW: **Diffusion tensor imaging of cingulum fibers in mild cognitive impairment and Alzheimer disease.** *Neurology* 2007, **68**:13–19.
7. Newcombe VF, Williams GB, Scoffings D, Cross J, Carpenter TA, Pickard JD, Menon DK: **Aetiological differences in neuroanatomy of the vegetative state: insights from diffusion tensor imaging and functional implications.** *J Neurol Neurosurg Psychiatry* 2010, **81**:552–561.
8. Hunsche S, Moseley ME, Stoeter P, Hedehus M: **Diffusion-tensor MR imaging at 1.5 and 3.0 T: initial observations.** *Radiology* 2001, **221**:550–556.
9. Wakana S, Jiang H, Nagae-Poetscher LM, van Zijl PC, Mori S: **Fiber tract-based atlas of human white matter anatomy.** *Radiology* 2004, **230**:77–87.

10. Huisman TA, Loenneker T, Barta G, Bellemann ME, Hennig J, Fischer JE, Il'yasov KA: **Quantitative diffusion tensor MR imaging of the brain: field strength related variance of apparent diffusion coefficient (ADC) and fractional anisotropy (FA) scalars.** *Eur Radiol* 2006, **16**:1651–1658.
11. Brander A, Kataja A, Saastamoinen A, Ryymin P, Huhtala H, Ohman J, Soimakallio S, Dastidar P: **Diffusion tensor imaging of the brain in a healthy adult population: normative values and measurement reproducibility at 3 T and 1.5 T.** *Acta Radiol* 2010, **51**:800–807.
12. Cassol E, Ranjeva JP, Ibarrola D, Mékies C, Manelfe C, Clanet M, Berry I: **Diffusion tensor imaging in multiple sclerosis: a tool for monitoring changes in normal-appearing white matter.** *Mult Scler* 2004, **10**:188–196.
13. Kubicki M, Park H, Westin CF, Nestor PG, Mulkern RV, Maier SE, Niznikiewicz M, Connor EE, Levitt JJ, Frumin M, Kikinis R, Jolesz FA, McCarley RW, Shenton ME: **DTI and MTR abnormalities in schizophrenia: analysis of white matter integrity.** *Neuroimage* 2005, **26**:1109–1118.
14. Niogi SN, Mukherjee P, Ghajar J, Johnson C, Kolster RA, Sarkar R, Lee H, Meeker M, Zimmerman RD, Manley GT, McCandliss BD: **Extent of microstructural white matter injury in postconcussive syndrome correlates with impaired cognitive reaction time: a 3T diffusion tensor imaging study of mild traumatic brain injury.** *AJNR Am J Neuroradiol* 2008, **29**:967–973.
15. Li W, Liu J, Skidmore F, Liu Y, Tian J, Li K: **White matter microstructure changes in the thalamus in Parkinson disease with depression: a diffusion tensor MR imaging study.** *AJNR Am J Neuroradiol* 2010, **31**:1861–1866.
16. Rossi ME, Jason E, Marchesotti S, Dastidar P, Ollikainen J, Soimakallio S: **Diffusion tensor imaging correlates with lesion volume in cerebral hemisphere infarctions.** *BMC Med Imaging* 2010, **10**:21.
17. Sullivan EV, Adalsteinsson E, Hedehus M, Ju C, Moseley M, Lim KO, Pfefferbaum A: **Equivalent disruption of regional white matter microstructure in ageing healthy men and women.** *Neuroreport* 2001, **12**:99–104.
18. Basser PJ, Jones DK: **Diffusion-tensor MRI: theory, experimental design and data analysis—a technical review.** *NMR Biomed* 2002, **15**:456–467.
19. Heim S, Hahn K, Sammann PG, Fahrmeir L, Auer DP: **Assessing DTI data quality using bootstrap analysis.** *Magn Reson Med* 2004, **52**:582–589.
20. Mukherjee P, Chung SW, Berman JI, Hess CP, Henry RG: **Diffusion tensor MR imaging and fiber tractography: technical considerations.** *AJNR Am J Neuroradiol* 2008, **29**:843–852.
21. Zhan L, Jahanshad N, Ennis DB, Jin Y, Bernstein MA, Borowski BJ, Jack CR Jr, Toga AW, Leow AD, Thompson PM: **Angular versus spatial resolution trade-offs for diffusion imaging under time constraints.** *Hum Brain Mapp* 2012.
22. Bisdas S, Bohning DE, Besenski N, Nicholas JS, Rumboldt Z: **Reproducibility, interrater agreement and age-related changes of fractional anisotropy measures at 3 T in healthy subjects: effect of the applied b-value.** *Am J Neuroradiol* 2008, **29**:1128–1133.
23. Barnea-Goraly N, Menon V, Eckert M, Tamm L, Bammer R, Karchemskiy A, Dant CC, Reiss AL: **White matter development during childhood and adolescence: a cross-sectional diffusion tensor imaging study.** *Cereb Cortex* 2005, **5**:1848–1854.
24. Tang J, Liao Y, Zhou B, Tan C, Liu T, Hao W, Hu D, Chen X: **Abnormal anterior cingulum integrity in first episode, early-onset schizophrenia: a diffusion tensor imaging study.** *Brain Res* 2010, **1343**:199–205.
25. Bonekamp D, Nagae LM, Degaonkar M, Matson M, Abdalla WM, Barker PB, Mori S, Horská A: **Diffusion tensor imaging in children and adolescents: repeatability, hemispheric, and age-related differences.** *Neuroimage* 2007, **34**:733–742.
26. Smith SM, Jenkinson M, Johansen-Berg H, Rueckert D, Nichols TE, Mackay CE, Watkins KE, Ciccarelli O, Cader MZ, Matthews PM, Behrens TE: **Tract-based spatial statistics: voxelwise analysis of multi-subject diffusion data.** *Neuroimage* 2006, **31**:1487–1505.
27. Wahl M, Strominger Z, Jeremy RJ, Barkovich AJ, Wakahiro M, Sherr EH, Mukherjee P: **Variability of homotopic and heterotopic callosal connectivity in partial agenesis of the corpus callosum: a 3T diffusion tensor imaging and Q-ball tractography study.** *AJNR Am J Neuroradiol* 2009, **30**:282–289.
28. Raj A, Hess C, Mukherjee P: **Spatial HARDI: improved visualization of complex white matter architecture with Bayesian spatial regularization.** *Neuroimage* 2011, **54**:396–409.
29. Tuch DS: **Q-ball imaging.** *Magn Reson Med* 2004, **52**:1358–1372.
30. Iverson GL, Hakulinen U, Wäljas M, Dastidar P, Lange RT, Soimakallio S, Öhman J: **To exclude or not to exclude: White matter hyperintensities in diffusion tensor imaging research.** *Brain Inj* 2011, **25**:1325–1332.
31. Laun FB, Huff S, Stieltjes B: **On the effects of dephasing due to local gradients in diffusion tensor imaging experiments: relevance for diffusion tensor imaging fiber phantoms.** *Magn Reson Imaging* 2009, **27**:541–548.
32. Laun FB, Stieltjes B, Huff S, Schad LR: **Investigations of a DTI—phantom with properties similar to in vivo neuronal tissue.** *ISMRM Proceedings* 2007, **15**:1526.
33. Hakulinen U, Brander A, Ryymin P, Öhman J, Soimakallio S, Dastidar P, Eskola H: **Intra- and inter-observer variation of region-of-interest methods in quantitative clinical diffusion tensor imaging.** *IFMBE Proceedings* 2011, **37**:551–554.
34. Bland JM, Altman DG: **Statistical methods for assessing agreement between two methods of clinical measurements.** *Lancet* 1986, **8**:307–310.
35. Shrout PE, Fleiss JL: **Intra-class correlations: uses in assessing rater reliability.** *Psychol Bull* 1979, **86**:420–428.
36. Marenco S, Rawlings R, Rohde GK, Barnett AS, Honea RA, Pierpaoli C, Weinberger DR: **Regional distribution of measurement error in diffusion tensor imaging.** *Psychiatry Res* 2006, **147**:69–78.
37. Zipursky RB, Lim KO, Pfefferbaum A: **Volumetric assessment of cerebral asymmetry from CT scans.** *Psychiatry Res* 1990, **35**:71–89.
38. Polders DL, Leemans A, Hendrikse J, Donahue MJ, Luijten PR, Hoogduin JM: **Signal to noise ratio and uncertainty in diffusion tensor imaging at 1.5, 3.0, and 7.0 Tesla.** *J Magn Reson Imaging* 2011, **33**:1456–1463.
39. Snook L, Paulson LA, Roy D, Phillips L, Beaulieu C: **Diffusion tensor imaging of neurodevelopment in children and young adults.** *Neuroimage* 2005, **26**:1164–1173.
40. Ozturk A, Sasson AD, Farrell JA, Landman BA, da Motta AC, Aralasmak A, Yousem DM: **Regional differences in diffusion tensor imaging measurements: assessment of intrarater and interrater variability.** *AJNR Am J Neuroradiol* 2008, **29**:1124–1127.
41. Basser PJ, Pajevic S: **Statistical artifacts in diffusion tensor MRI (DT-MRI) caused by background noise.** *Magn Reson Med* 2000, **44**:41–50.

Proton nuclear magnetic resonance and pattern recognition analysis of liver extracts from rats under different anesthetics

Tomoyuki Tajima[1*], Keiko Hirakawa[2], Hiroshi Kawaguchi[1] and Atsuhiro Sakamoto[1]

Abstract

Background: Although general anesthesia is widely used in the surgical arena, the mechanisms by which general anesthetics act remain unclear. We previously described alterations in gene expression ratios in hepatic tissue taken from rats treated with anesthetics. Consequently, it is considered that anesthetics influence liver metabolism. Thus, the goal of this study was to use pattern recognition analysis of proton nuclear magnetic resonance spectra to visualize changes in liver metabolic phenotypes in response to widely used intravenous anesthetics (propofol and dexmedetomidine) and inhalational anesthetics (sevoflurane and isoflurane).

Methods: Rats were randomized into 13 groups (n = 6 in each group), and each group received one of following agents: propofol, dexmedetomidine, sevoflurane, isoflurane, or no anesthetic (control group). The liver was directly removed from rats immediately after or 24 h or 48 h after a 6-h period of anesthesia. Hydrophilic compounds were extracted from the liver and were analyzed with proton nuclear magnetic resonance spectroscopy. All spectral data were processed and analyzed by principal component analysis for comparison of metabolite profiles.

Results: Data were visualized by plotting principal component (PC) scores. In the plots, each point represents an individual sample. Each group was clustered separately on the plots, and the PC scores of the propofol group were clearly distinct from those of the control group and other anesthetic groups. The difference in PC scores was more pronounced immediately after completion of anesthesia when compared with 24 or 48 h after completion of anesthesia. Although the effect of intravenous anesthetics on the liver dissipated over time, the effect of inhalational anesthetics persisted.

Conclusions: Propofol, dexmedetomidine, sevoflurane and isoflurane exert different effects on liver metabolism. In particular, liver metabolism was markedly altered after exposure to propofol. The effect of anesthesia on the liver under propofol or dexmedetomidine resolved rapidly when compared with the effect under sevoflurane or isoflurane.

Background

General anesthesia is widely used in the surgical arena, with good efficacy and safety demonstrated for a variety of agents, including sevoflurane [1], isoflurane [2], propofol [3], and dexmedetomidine [4]. However, the mechanisms by which these agents act remain unclear. We previously reported that anesthetic agents altered the gene expression ratios in rat livers [5], which suggest that these agents can influence hepatic metabolism.

* Correspondence: ta-ji-tom@nms.ac.jp
[1]Department of Anesthesiology, Nippon Medical School, Bunkyo-ku, Tokyo, Japan
Full list of author information is available at the end of the article

Sevoflurane and isoflurane are inhalational anesthetics. They have low solubilities in blood and tissues (resulting in rapid recovery from anesthesia), and are frequently used. Propofol is the most commonly used intravenous anesthetic and is administered as an alkylphenol formulated in a lipid emulsion [6]. Propofol provides rapid and smooth induction of anesthesia and exhibits rapid clearance from the body. Dexmedetomidine is an ideal intravenous anesthetic. It is a highly selective α_2-adrenergic agonist, produces sedation, hypnosis, and analgesia, and has a minimal effect on respiration. Dexmedetomidine is rapidly metabolized in the liver and is excreted in both the urine and feces.

We previously used microarray analyses to show that anesthesia under sevoflurane affected expression ratios of 177 of 10,000 genes in various organs from rats [7]. The highest number of altered genes was detected in the liver and included several genes encoding drug-metabolizing enzymes (DMEs). Furthermore, we investigated the expression ratios of eight genes encoding DMEs that showed the greatest alterations among the affected genes in the liver [5]. We also investigated changes in brain metabolic phenotypes in response to anesthetics by means of a metabolomics study and demonstrated that intravenous and inhalational anesthetics exert differential effects on brain metabolism under anesthesia [8].

Metabolomics is defined as "the exhaustive analysis of endogenous metabolites". Metabolomics can reveal profiles of endogenous low molecular weight metabolites and can measure dynamic multiparametric responses of living systems to internal and external influences [9]. The main analytical techniques employed for metabolomic studies are based on proton nuclear magnetic resonance (^{1}H-NMR) spectroscopic analysis. To interpret ^{1}H-NMR digitized spectra data, pattern recognition analysis was used in the present study. One of the most useful and easily applied pattern recognition analyses is principal component analysis (PCA). Moreover, ^{1}H-NMR spectroscopy is the only method that can measure many types of metabolites in a tissue or in an organism noninvasively and nondestructively.

The liver plays an important role in drug metabolism, and anesthetics change liver metabolism. Clarification of the different effects of different anesthetics on liver metabolism is important and could provide useful information with regards to the rational selection of anesthetics for clinical use. The purpose of this study was to compare metabolic responses of the liver to anesthesia with representative inhalational (sevoflurane, isoflurane) and intravenous (propofol, dexmedetomidine) anesthetics using pattern recognition ^{1}H-NMR spectroscopy with multivariate analyses.

Methods

The flow chart of the experimental protocol is shown in Figure 1. A previous study model [8] on acquisition of data, data processing and statistical analysis of ^{1}H-NMR data was used.

Animals and preparation

The animal protocol was approved by the Animal Experimental Ethics Review Committee of Nippon Medical School and involved 9-week-old male Wistar rats weighing 300 ± 20 g (Saitama Experimental Animals Supply, Saitama, Japan). A venous catheter was inserted into the tail vein of all rats, and rats was housed in individual plastic cages (45 × 32 × 23 cm). Rats were anesthetized for 6 h with sevoflurane, isoflurane, propofol or dexmedetomidine, and animals were sacrificed immediately after completion of anesthesia (0-h time-point) or 24 or 48 h later (24 or 48-h time-points). Rats undergoing inhalational anesthesia were placed in plastic boxes supplied with sevoflurane (Maruishi Pharmaceutical, Osaka, Japan; 2.4% gas-air mixture) [10] or isoflurane (Abbot Japan, Tokyo, Japan; 1.5% gas-air mixture) [11] at a rate of 6 L/min (33% oxygen), and normal saline was administered via a venous catheter at a rate of 1 mL/h. Rats undergoing intravenous anesthesia were housed in plastic boxes supplied with 33% oxygen at a rate of 6 L/min and were administered propofol (AstraZeneca, Osaka, Japan; 600 μg/kg/min) [12] or dexmedetomidine (Hospira Japan, Osaka, Japan; 1 μg/kg/min) [13] via a venous catheter at a rate of 1 mL/h. All rats were allowed to breathe spontaneously.

Rats were randomly assigned to 1 of 13 groups (n = 6 per group; one control group and 12 anesthesia groups). Four anesthesia groups (sevoflurane, isoflurane, propofol or dexmedetomidine group) were divided into three subgroups, according to the time of animal sacrifice (immediately after completion of anesthesia or 24 or 48 h later). In the control group, rats were housed in individual plastic cages (45 × 32 × 23 cm) and were not given any anesthetics. These animals were not given access to feed, and they were sacrificed 6 h later. The left lateral lobe of the liver was extracted from each sacrificed rat within 1 min after death, and livers were immediately frozen in liquid nitrogen and stored at −80°C.

Physiological parameters

Physiological variables were measured in the five separate groups not taken for liver metabolic evaluation (n = 6 each), including those treated with isoflurane, sevoflurane, propofol, dexmedetomidine, or no anesthetic (control group) (Figure 1B). For all rats, a catheter was inserted into the tail vein, and lactated Ringer's solution was infused continuously at 10 mL/kg/h. During the experiment, each rat was placed into a plastic cage (45 × 32 × 23 cm). All rats were supplied with 33% oxygen and were allowed to breathe spontaneously. Body temperature was maintained at 37°C with a heat lamp. Anesthetics were administered as described above. An arterial catheter was placed in the left femoral artery in all rats to draw blood samples for measurement of arterial PO_2, arterial PCO_2, arterial blood pH, plasma glucose concentrations and to monitor heart rate and arterial blood pressure. Anesthesia groups were anesthetized for 6 h. In the control group, rats were placed in a rat tunnel and allowed to recover from anesthesia. Blood samples were taken 2 h later. In the anesthesia groups,

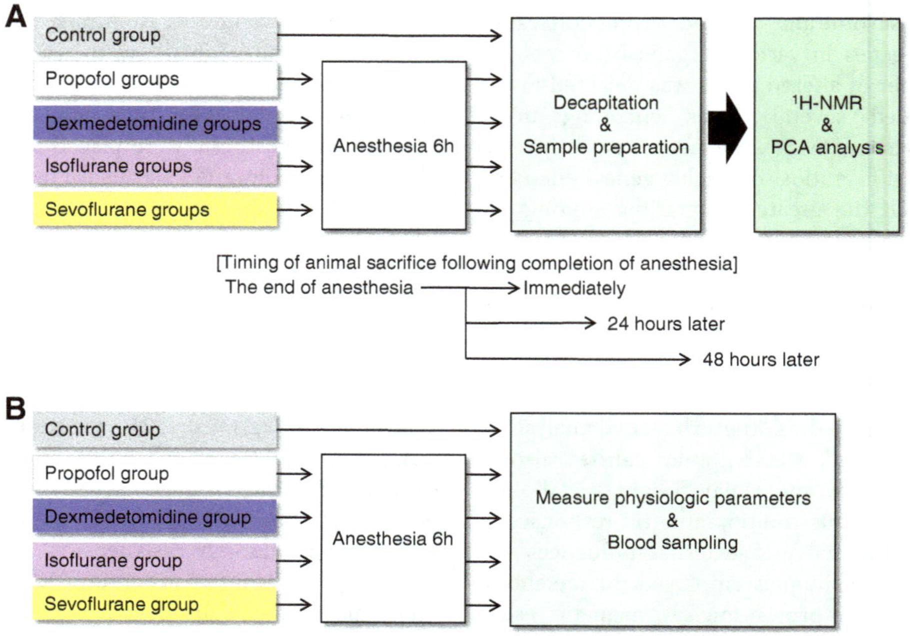

Figure 1 Flow chart of the experimental protocol. (A) Experimental protocol of ^{1}H-NMR and PC analysis. **(B)** Experimental protocol for measurement of physiologic parameters.

blood samples were taken 6 h after the induction of anesthesia.

Sample preparation

Neutral extraction was performed according to the method described by Yoshioka et al. [14]. The method described by Folch [15] was originally designed for extraction of hydrophobic substances, but this method is also useful for extracting low molecular weight hydrophilic organic compounds, essentially without any in vitro modifications, oxidation hydrolysis or decomposition. Frozen tissue samples were ground and pulverized into a fine powder in liquid nitrogen using a frozen cell crusher (Cryo-Press^{TM}, Microtec, Chiba, Japan) and some of the fine powder (approximately 1.0 g) was then homogenized in 10 mL of a chloroform/methanol (2:1) mixture. After removing the residues by filtration, 1 mL of distilled water was then added to the filtrates. After thoroughly mixing, they were left to stand for 24 h at 4° C to separate the hydrophilic phase layer from the hydrophobic phase. The hydrophilic phase was evaporated in an evacuated centrifuge overnight. Dried extracts were reconstituted in 0.6 mL of deuterium oxide (D_2O) (ISOTEC Inc., Laurenceville, NJ, USA) containing 0.25 mM sodium (3-trimethylsilyl) tetradeuteriopropionate-2,2,3,3-d4 (TMSP) (MSD Isotopes, Montreal, Canada) and then were pipette into 5-mm NMR tubes (Wilmad-LabGlass, Buena, NJ, USA) for subsequent NMR measurements. D_2O provided a deuterium field frequency lock for the NMR spectrometer, while TMSP provided an internal chemical shift reference ($\delta = 0.00$). The pH of the sample solutions was 7.2 to 7.4.

Acquisition of proton nuclear magnetic resonance data

Solution state ^{1}H NMR spectroscopy was performed at a proton resonance frequency of 300 MHz using an ECX NMR spectrometer interfaced with a TH5 probe (normal geometry, auto tunable type) equipped with an automatic 16-position sample changer and Delta^{TM} NMR processing and control software (version 4.3.2, JEOL Ltd., Tokyo, Japan). Two different ^{1}H NMR spectra were acquired for each sample. In all cases, the water resonance was suppressed using a conventional presaturation pulse sequence for the water (HDO) proton signal suppression based on homo-gated irradiation and dante pulse sequence (presaturation time = 2 s, dante pulse = 8 μs, dante interval = 0.1 ms, dante loop = 185, dante attenuator = 24dB). Standard one-dimensional (1D) spectra were acquired using a 45° pulse, 5,580-Hz spectral width, a relaxation delay of 2.0 s between pulses (repetition time = 3.47 s), and 400 transients. Two-dimensional J RES spectra were collected using a double spin echo sequence with 48 transients. This method yields good information on the multiplicity and coupling patterns of resonances, which facilitates molecule identification. The appropriate projection of this spectrum onto the chemical shift axis yields a fingerprint of peaks from only the most highly mobile small molecules, with the added benefit that all of the spin coupling peak multiplicities have been removed.

Data processing and reduction

The resultant spectra were processed using Alice2™, version 5.5 (JEOL DATUM Ltd., Tokyo, Japan). Free induction decays (FIDs) were subjected to an exponential weighting function of 0.5 Hz, Fourier transformed from the time to frequency domain, and then phased manually, followed by linear baseline correction and referencing to the TMSP singlet at 0.00 ppm.

To simplify the ^{1}H NMR spectra of the tissues by means of data compression, all spectra were integrated between 0.5 and 9.5 ppm using an integration macro written within the Alice2 for Metabolome™, version 1.0 (JEOL DATUM Ltd., Tokyo, Japan) software package, which integrated the spectrum into 215 segments (buckets) with 0.04 ppm integral regions. Regions containing resonances of residual water (4.6 ppm to 5.0 ppm) were excluded before integration. Close inspection of the important integral regions for pattern recognition identified some cases where one resonance straddled two or more integral buckets, and therefore, these integral regions were corrected manually combining or extending the regions to include one resonance in a single integral region. Other regions that largely consisted of noise were excluded to produce more significant multivariate mapping. Finally, all the spectral data were reduced into 186 buckets. To account for the bulk mass differences between samples, each spectral region was normalized to the sum of all of the integrals of the buckets.

Assignments of metabolites in the ^{1}H NMR spectra were made by comparing the proton chemical shifts with literature values [16,17] and by comparison with spectra of authentic compounds via an in-house spectral database.

Multivariate analysis and statistical analysis

Calculated results obtained from all measured spectra were exported to a spreadsheet as a text file, which was then used as the input into the pattern recognition/multivariate statistics software package for non-biased metabolic profiling. Datasets were imported into the ADMEWORKS/ModelBuilder™ software, version 4.5 (Fujitsu Kyushu Systems Ltd., Fukuoka, Japan) software package. All data were mean-centered, and a multicollinearity test and genetic-algorithm were used to identify the buckets that included the resonances from key metabolites that differed among the groups. Using the selected bucket data, PCA was performed to discern the presence of inherent similarities between spectral profiles. Data were visualized using the PC score and loading plots. PCA was used to examine trends and clustering in an unsupervised manner. In this analysis, the algorithm calculates the maximum amount of correlated variation in a data set and scores each spectrum according to this variation along PC1. This procedure is repeated for other components until the majority of the variations in the data set are described. Being an unsupervised method, spectra are grouped according to the highest amount of variance in the data set, regardless of the group of each sample. For each type of analysis, data were visualized by plotting PC scores. In the plots, each point represents an individual sample. The plots allow the recognition of clusters of samples with similar scores. Each score plot has an associated loading profile, which helps in identifying the spectral regions (metabolites responsible for the sample clustering observed).

An analysis of variance (ANOVA) test was used to compare physiological variables between the experimental and control groups. $P < 0.01$ was considered to be statistically significant. Data are given as the mean ± standard deviation (SD).

Results

Physiological parameters in control and anesthetized rats

Physiologic parameters were observed in control and anesthetized rats (Table 1). There were no significant differences in pH, PaO2, PaCO2, heart rate, mean arterial pressure or plasma glucose concentration between groups.

Table 1 Physiological Parameters in Control and Anesthetized Rats

	Control	Propofol	Dexmedetomidine	Isoflurane	Sevoflurane
pH	7.45 ± 0.01	7.42 ± 0.02	7.42 ± 0.02	7.41 ± 0.03	7.41 ± 0.02
PaO_2 (mm Hg)	107.1 ± 7.5	102 ± 10.0	109 ± 8.2	103 ± 10.1	106 ± 6.5
$PaCO_2$ (mm Hg)	37.5 ± 1.4	43.5 ± 3.6	39.5 ± 3.7	43.5 ± 2.0	41.5 ± 2.9
HR (beats/min)	301 ± 25	285 ± 25	294 ± 18	292 ± 25	295 ± 24
MAP (mm Hg)	111 ± 6.0	95 ± 10	100 ± 9.0	95 ± 9	97 ± 8.5
GLU (mg/dL)	143 ± 18.0	157 ± 23.0	144 ± 20.7	148 ± 15.6	142 ± 10.8

Data represent mean ± SD for six animals in each group. Low mean blood pressure and high PCO_2 were observed following the administration of anesthetic drugs. However, there were no significant differences between the anesthetized groups and the control group. HR: heart rate; MAP: mean arterial pressure; and GLU: plasma glucose concentration.

Proton NMR of hydrophilic liver extracts in control rats

A typical proton NMR spectrum of hydrophilic extracts from rat livers in the control group is shown in Figure 2. Assignments of metabolites in the ^1H NMR spectra were made by comparing the proton chemical shifts with literature values [16,17] and by comparison with spectra of authentic compounds via an in-house spectral database.

PCA score plots

A PCA score plot (PC1 vs. PC2) of hydrophilic liver extracts from rats sacrificed immediately after anesthesia is shown in Figure 3A. PCA is a multivariate technique that reduces highly dimensional data into only a few PCs, which are variables created from the linear combinations of the starting variables with appropriate weighting coefficients. The first PC (PC1) contains the largest part of the variance of the data set. In this manner, the data can be reduced into two dimensions, which allows graphic representation of data trends. The plots for the intravenous anesthetic groups (propofol and dexmedetomidine) and inhalational anesthetic groups (isoflurane and sevoflurane) were divided into separate clusters. In particular, the propofol group was separated from the other groups in the direction to PC1 dominantly. The dexmedetomidine group was separated from the other groups in the direction to PC2. By contrast, the separation of data clusters was subtler when comparing the inhalational anesthetic groups and the control group.

PC loading plots of individual data sets

Loading plots for PC1 vs. PC2 corresponding to Figure 3A are shown in Figure 3B and Figure 3C, respectively. Loading plots show the relative contribution to the PCs of the original variable. The numbers in the loading plots indicate the center value of each of the integral area as follows: 1.19 and 1.22 ppm (3-D-hydroxybutyrate (3-D-HB)), 1.32 and 1.35 ppm (lactate), 2.40 ppm (succinate), 2.46 ppm (glutamine), 3.20 ppm (choline), 3.22 ppm (choline, phosphocholine), 3.24 ppm (glycerophosphorylcholine (GPC)), 3.28 ppm (trimethylamine-N-oxide (TMAO)), 3.43 ppm (taurine), 3.75 (mannitol), 3.91 (betaine) and 3.30-4.00 ppm (glucose). TMAO was most effective metabolite that separated the PC scores in the PC1 direction. GPC was also effective in separation in the PC2 direction.

PCA score plots over time

Changes in liver metabolism were observed over time. The PCA score plot revealed that the differences between anesthetized groups get into trifle with time (Figure 4A-4C). Consequently, liver metabolism was compared among different groups at the 0-h time-point. On the other hand, the PC scores at the 24-h time-point

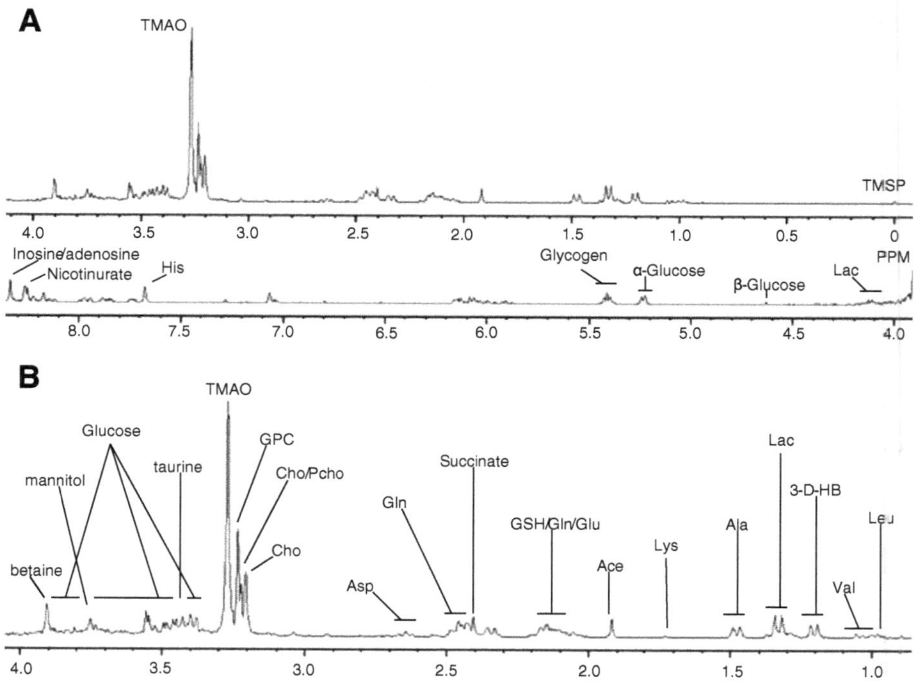

Figure 2 Proton NMR spectrum of a hydrophilic liver extract in a control rat. (A) 0.00 ppm to 9.00 ppm and **(B)** 1.00 ppm to 4.00 ppm (Ace: acetate; Ala: alanine; Asp: aspartate; Cho: choline; Gln: glutamine; Glu: glutamate; GPC: glycerophosphorylcholine; GSH: glutathione; His: histidine; Lac: lactate; Lys: lysine; PCho: phosphocholine; TMAO: trimethylamine-N-oxide; Val: valine; and 3-D-HB: 3-D-hydroxybutyrate.).

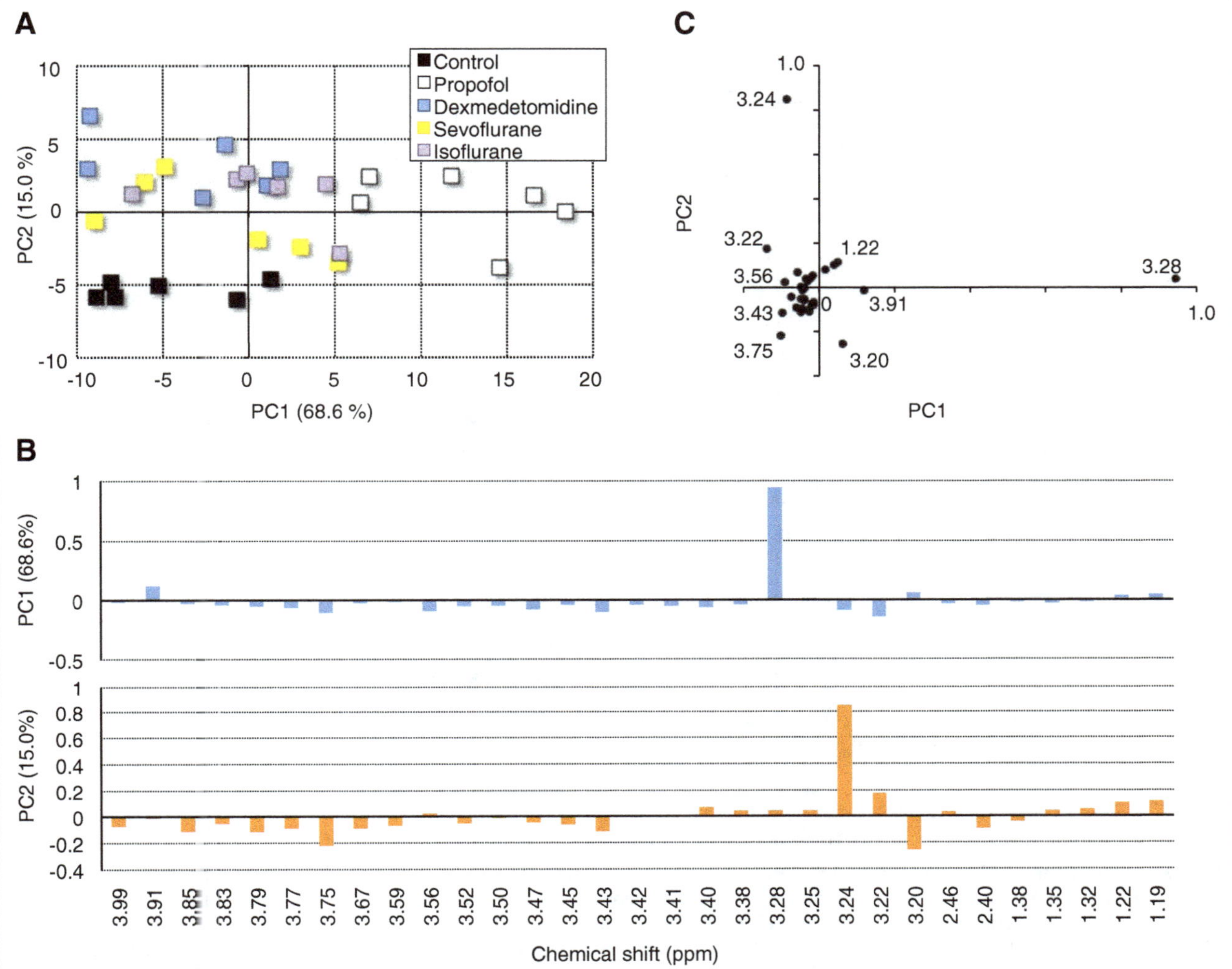

Figure 3 PCA score plot of hydrophilic liver extracts from the rats sacrificed immediately after anesthesia. (A) Each plot represents the metabolic data set from an individual rat. Groups are delineated as follows: control (black), propofol (white), dexmedetomidine (blue), sevoflurane (yellow), isoflurane (purple). The plot for each group was clearly divided into separate clusters. In particular, the propofol group was separated from the other groups in the direction of PC1 dominantly. The dexmedetomidine group was separated from the other groups in the direction of PC2. The separation in data clusters was subtler when comparing the inhalational anesthetic groups and the control group. Variables (n = 31 reduced from 186). **(B)** PC loading plot versus chemical shift are graphically illustrated. The numbers indicate the center value of the integral area of each of the conditions as follows: 1.19 and 1.22 ppm (3-D-hydroxybutyrate (3-D-HB)), 1.32 and 1.35 ppm (lactate), 2.40 ppm (succinate), 2.46 ppm (glutamine), 3.20 ppm (choline), 3.22 ppm (choline, phosphocholine), 3.24 ppm (glycerophosphorylcholine (GPC)), 3.28 ppm (trimethylamine-N-oxide (TMAO)), 3.43 ppm (taurine), 3.75 (mannitol), 3.91 (betaine) and 3.30-4.00 ppm (glucose). **(C)** Each plot represents the PC loading plot of individual data sets to distinguish single putative NMR peaks responsible for the clustering pattern observed in the PCA score plot. The 3.28 ppm (TMAO) peak was an effective metabolite used to separate the PC scores in the PC1 direction. The 3.24 ppm (GPC) peak was also effective for separation in the PC2 direction.

showed that the effect of intravenous anesthetics on the liver resolved quickly when compared to the effect of inhalational anesthetics (Figure 4B).

Discussion

The present study demonstrated that different liver metabolic phenotypes result from exposure to different types of anesthetic agents. In particular, the liver metabolic phenotype after exposure to propofol was markedly different from that after exposure to other anesthetic agents. However, the differences in liver metabolic phenotype between anesthetics decreased over time.

In this study, experiments were conducted using intravenous anesthetics (propofol and dexmedetomidine) and inhaled anesthetics (isoflurane and sevoflurane). These anesthetics are extensively used in everyday clinical practice. Metabolomic changes in the livers of rats anesthetized with one minimum alveolar concentration of inhaled

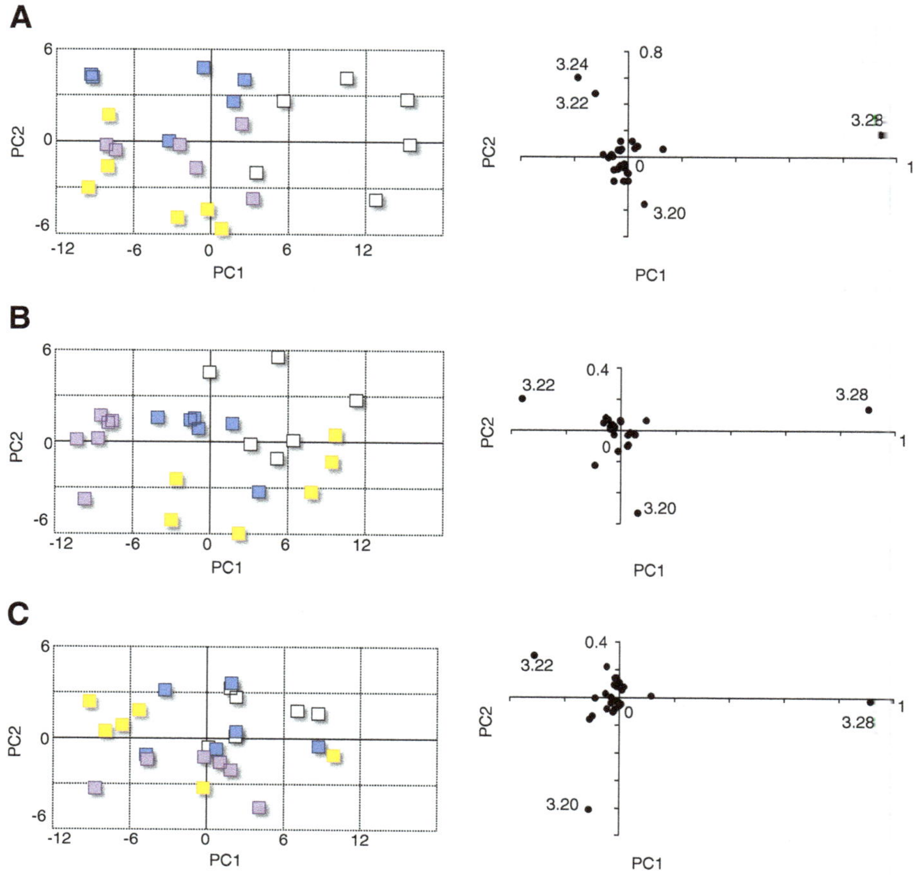

Figure 4 Time course of PCA score plot. Graphs located on the left side represent PCA score plots of each group, and graphs on the right side represent PC loading plots corresponding to each graph on the left. Graphs indicate the data from rats sacrificed immediately after anesthesia **(A)**, 24 h after completion of anesthesia **(B)**, and 48 h after completion of anesthesia **(C)**. Variables of each graph are **(A)** n = 31 reduced from 186, **(B)** n = 31 reduced from 186, **(C)** n = 31 reduced from 186. The different marks represent each group: propofol (white), dexmedetomidine (blue), sevoflurane (yellow), and isoflurane (purple). The PCA scores plot revealed that the differences between anesthetized groups decreased with time. The effect of propofol and dexmedetomidine resolved by the 24-h time-point; however, the effect of sevoflurane and isoflurane persisted **(B)**.

anesthetics (sevoflurane at 2.4%, isoflurane at 1.5%) [10,11] or with continuous infusion of intravenous anesthetics (propofol at 600 μg/kg/min, dexmedetomidine at 1 μg/kg/min) [12,13] were investigated. Infusion of propofol at 600 μg/kg/min is a median effective dose (ED50) for rats. These doses were chosen because lower doses may not induce adequate anesthesia and because higher doses can produce hemodynamic changes that can independently alter liver metabolism. In a previous study of changes in brain metabolism over time in response to anesthetics, rats were anesthetized for 2 h and at 6 h [8]; the 6-h anesthesia groups exhibited clear metabolic changes. Therefore, in the present study, it was thought that 6 h was a sufficient time period to produce metabolic changes, but sufficiently short to prevent any toxicity.

Separation of PCA scores between the different groups was related to differences in 3-D-HB, choline, phosphocholine, GPC, TMAO, taurine, mannitol, betaine and glucose levels (Figure 3C). 3-D-HB is a ketone body derived from fatty acids metabolism in liver mitochondria (lipid β-oxidation). In the context of hepatic insufficiency, lipid β-oxidation and gluconeogenesis accelerates, and acetyl-coenzyme A (acetyl-CoA) derived from glycolysis and lipid β-oxidation exceeds the capacity of the Krebs cycle [18,19]. Normally, ketone bodies are transported from the liver to other tissues, where they can be reconverted to acetyl-CoA to produce energy; impairment of the Krebs cycle leads to increased release of ketone bodies from the liver as fuel for other tissues [20].

A change in the level of hepatic glucose in anesthetized rats suggests an alteration in the rate of glycogenolysis and glycolysis that is consistent with mitochondrial impairment, and can lead to an inability to use pyruvate in the Krebs cycle and to enhancement of anaerobic metabolism [21]. Thus, the changes of 3-D-

HB and glucose likely reflect a general decrease in energy metabolism.

In addition, rats were not fed during this study. Thus, it is possible that changes in the level of glucose, mannitol and taurine may have resulted from the fasting state. Among the four anesthetics administered in this study, only propofol can provide calories due to its fat content. Indeed, propofol is a 1% fat preparation, which corresponds with 1.1 kcal/mL and a total of 7.3 kcal administered to rats during this study. Mannitol is a sugar alcohol, while taurine is related to bile acids and digestion. Thus, the fasting state may also affect levels of those substances.

Choline and phosphocholine are metabolic products of phosphatidylcholine, which is a major membrane constituent. GPC is also a membrane constituent, while TMAO is a product of choline degradation. Betaine helps to maintain cellular osmotic pressure when the cell membrane damaged. Increased levels of choline, phosphocholine, GPC, TMAO and betaine are associated with cell membrane disruption [22].

Changes of endogenous metabolites in hepatic tissue suggest that propofol was the most influential anesthetic on hepatic energy metabolism among the four anesthetics administered in the present study. PC scores showed that TMAO was the most effective metabolite that separated the propofol group from the other groups in the PC1 direction (Figure 3A, 3B, 3C). The dexmedetomidine group was separately clustered from the other groups, but the extent of the difference on the PCA plot was smaller than the difference between the propofol group and the other groups. PC scores showed that GPC was effective in separation of the dexmedetomidine group from the other groups in the PC2 direction (Figure 3A, 3B, 3C). It is possible that the intravenous anesthetics affected the metabolism in the liver by different mechanisms. There was little difference in hepatic metabolites when comparing the inhalational anesthetic groups to the control group. However, the effect of inhalational anesthetics persisted at the 24-h time point while the effect of intravenous anesthetics on the liver resolved over time (Figure 4B), suggesting that propofol and dexmedetomidine were metabolized rapidly when compared with sevoflurane and isoflurane. The loading plot included in Figure 4A-4C remained static over time, and at the 48-h time-point, PCA plots were mixed, and the difference between groups became unclear (Figure 4C).

Sevoflurane and isoflurane are metabolized by hepatic cytochrome P450 CYP2E1 [23], and hepatotoxicity is rarely seen with these two agents [24-27]. In a previous study, there were no significant differences in liver function or total hepatic blood flow when comparing sevoflurane and isoflurane anesthesia [28]. This finding is consistent with observations from the present study, in which PCA scores were relatively similar when comparing the inhalational anesthetic groups and the control group. Indeed, investigators have suggested that liver function is relatively preserved with inhalational anesthetics when compared with intravenous anesthetics [29,30].

Propofol is rapidly metabolized in the liver by conjugation to glucuronide and sulfate to produce water-soluble compounds, and 68.3% of these compounds are excreted in the urine within 24 h [31]. Dexmedetomidine is rapidly distributed and extensively metabolized in the liver. It undergoes conjugation (41%), N-methylation (21%) or hydroxylation followed by conjugation, and 85% of the resulting compounds are excreted in the urine within 24 h [32,33]. Some reports suggest that dexmedetomidine preserves blood flow to the most vital organs (e.g., brain, heart, liver, kidneys) [34] and that there is no difference in clearance of indocyanine green or hepatic blood flow when comparing propofol and dexmedetomidine [32,35]. By contrast, the PCA scores in the present study suggest that propofol has a larger effect on hepatic metabolism when compared with dexmedetomidine.

In previous studies, propofol administration did not affect hepatic arterial blood flow [36], but increase total liver blood flow, portal tributary blood flow, and hepatic oxygen consumption [37]. The increase in oxygen consumption may reflect an increase in hepatic metabolic activity during the clearance of propofol and reflect propofol-induced changes in hepatic metabolism. Previous studies reported that the expression ratios of genes encoding DMEs were elevated under anesthesia and that the expression ratio of Ugt1a7 (a gene encoding DME) was elevated under propofol anesthesia. Ugt1a7 is biotransformation enzyme of the glucuronidation pathway that transforms small lipophilic molecules into water-soluble excretable metabolites [38], and propofol is mainly metabolized by glucuronidation in the liver. In addition, propofol is administered as an emulsion consisting of soybean oil, glycerol, and purified egg phosphatide, which may also affect hepatic metabolism. Further, propofol delivers calories in the form of fat, which may result in differences from other anesthetics and control groups on PCA in this study.

To investigate the utility of ^{1}H-NMR for clinical applications, the hydrophilic fraction of the rat liver extracts were analyzed in this study. When the metabolic state is investigated for clinical purposes, the major target is the hydrophilic fraction. The extracted endogenous metabolites in the present study may have utility as a marker of liver metabolism, thereby enhancing the clinical utility of ^{1}H-NMR.

Metabolomics is an exhaustive analysis, and we did not attempt to accurately quantitate individual NMR peaks in this study. Our main purpose was to compare the patterns of spectra using chemometric methods to visualize the metabolic phenotypes of the samples. Further investigations that target individual metabolites with refined analysis may be of benefit.

In the present study, metabolite profiling of the liver showed that anesthesia with propofol, dexmedetomidine, sevoflurane and isoflurane exerted different effects on rat liver metabolism. Although analysis of metabolic substances from the liver after exposure to various drugs has been conducted [39], an exhaustive analysis of liver metabolites after exposure to anesthetics has not previously been reported. Thus, the results from this study may enhance the clinical use of anesthetics.

Conclusions

In conclusion, pattern recognition analysis of ^{1}H-NMR of liver tissue under anesthesia revealed that propofol, dexmedetomidine, sevoflurane and isoflurane exert different effects on rat liver metabolism. In particular, liver metabolism was markedly altered after exposure to propofol. The inclusion of fat within the propofol preparation may contribute to this finding. Further, the effects of intravenous anesthetics (propofol, dexmedetomidine) resolved rapidly when compared with the effects of inhalational anesthetics (sevoflurane, isoflurane).

Abbreviations

DMEs: Drug-metabolizing enzymes; GPC: Glyserophosphorylcholine; H-NMR: Proton nuclear magnetic resonance; PCA: Principal component analysis; 3-D-HB: 3-D-hydroxybutyrate; TMAO: Trimethylamine-N-oxide; TMSP: Tetradeuteriopropionate-2,2,3,3-d4.

Competing interests

The authors declare that they have no competing interests.

Authors' contributions

TT and AS conceived and designed the experiments. TT, KH and HK performed the experiments. TT and KH analyzed the data. TT contributed reagents, materials, and analysis tools. TT wrote the paper. All authors read and approved the final manuscript.

Acknowledgements

We are grateful to Prof. K. Koike (Kyoto University), Prof. Y. Ohno (Nippon Medical School) and the technical staff of the NMR laboratory at Nippon Medical School for their advice.

This study was supported by a Grant-in-Aid for Scientific Researches (20591820) from the Ministry of Education, Culture, Sports, Science and Technology (MEXT), Japan.

Author details

[1]Department of Anesthesiology, Nippon Medical School, Bunkyo-ku, Tokyo, Japan. [2]NMR Laboratory and Department of Legal Medicine, Nippon Medical School, Bunkyo-ku, Tokyo, Japan.

References

1. Mazze RI: **The safety of sevoflurane in humans.** *Anesthesiology* 1992, **77:**1062–1063.
2. Levy WJ: **Clinical anaesthesia with isoflurane. A review of the multicentre study.** *Br J Anaesth* 1984, **56**(Suppl 1):101S–112S.
3. Marik PE: **Propofol: therapeutic indications and side-effects.** *Curr Pharm Des* 2004, **10:**3639–3649.
4. Gerlach AT, Dasta JF: **Dexmedetomidine: an updated review.** *Ann Pharmacother* 2007, **41:**245–252.
5. Nakazato K, Yoshida Y, Takemori K, Kobayashi K, Sakamoto A: **Expressions of genes encoding drug-metabolizing enzymes are altered after sevoflurane, isoflurane, propofol or dexmedetomidine anesthesia.** *Biomed Res* 2009, **30:**17–24.
6. Simons PJ, Cockshott ID, Douglas EJ, Gordon EA, Hopkins K, Rowland M: **Disposition in male volunteers of a subanaesthetic intravenous dose of an oil in water emulsion of 14C-propofol.** *Xenobiotica* 1988, **18:**429–440.
7. Sakamoto A, Imai J, Nishikawa A, Honma R, Ito E, Yanagisawa Y, Kawamura M, Ogawa R, Watanabe S: **Influence of inhalation anesthesia assessed by comprehensive gene expression profiling.** *Gene* 2005, **356:**39–48.
8. Kawaguchi H, Hirakawa K, Miyauchi K, Ohno Y, Sakamoto A: **Pattern recognition analysis of proton nuclear magnetic resonance spectra of brain tissue extracts from rats anesthetized with propofol or isoflurane.** *PLoS One* 2010, **5:**e11172.
9. Nicholson JK, Lindon JC, Holmes E: **'Metabonomics': understanding the metabolic responses of living systems to pathophysiological stimuli via multivariate statistical analysis of biological NMR spectroscopic data.** *Xenobiotica* 1999, **29:**1181–1189.
10. Obal D, Preckel B, Scharbatke H, Mullenheim J, Hoterkes F, Thamer V, Schlack W: **One MAC of sevoflurane provides protection against reperfusion injury in the rat heart in vivo.** *Br J Anaesth* 2001, **87:**905–911.
11. Shichino T, Murakawa M, Adachi T, Adrai T, Miyazaki Y, Mori K: **Effects of inhalation anaesthetics on the release of acetylcholine in the rat cerebral cortex in vivo.** *Br J Anaesth* 1998, **80:**365–370.
12. Orth M, Barter L, Dominguez C, Atherley R, Carstens E, Antognini JF: **Halothane and propofol differentially affect electroencephalographic responses to noxious stimulation.** *Br J Anaesth* 2005, **95:**477–484.
13. Bol CJJG, Danhof M, Stanski DR, Mandema JW: **Pharmacokinetic-pharmacodynamic characterization of the cardiovascular, hypnotic, EEG and ventilatory responses to dexmedetomidine in the rat.** *J Pharmacol Exp Ther* 1997, **283:**1051–1058.
14. Yoshioka Y, Masuda T, Nakano H, Miura H, Nakaya S, Itazawa S, Kubokawa M: **In vitro 1H-NMR spectroscopic analysis of metabolites in fast- and slow-twitch muscles of young rats.** *Magn Reson Med Sci* 2002, **1:**7–13.
15. Folch J, Rebaron FN: **The chemistry of the phosphoinositides.** *Can J Biochem Physiol* 1956, **34:**305–319.
16. Bollard ME, Garrod S, Holmes E, Lindon JC, Humpfer E, Spraul M, Nicholson JK: **High-resolution (1)H and (1)H-(13)C magic angle spinning NMR spectroscopy of rat liver.** *Magn Reson Med* 2000, **44:**201–207.
17. Martinez-Granados B, Monleon D, Martinez-Bisbal MC, Rodrigo JM, del Olmo J, Lluch P, Ferrandez A, Marti-Bonmati L, Celda B: **Metabolite identification in human liver needle biopsies by high-resolution magic angle spinning 1H NMR spectroscopy.** *NMR Biomed* 2006, **19:**90–100.
18. McGarry JD, Boyd ME, Foster DW: **Regulation of hepatic fatty acid oxidation and ketone body production.** *Annu Rev Biochem* 1980, **49:**395–420.
19. Wu H, Zhang X, Li Z, Wu Y, Pei F: **Comparison of metabolic profiles from serum from hepatotoxin-treated rats by nuclear-magnetic-resonance-spectroscopy-based metabonomic analysis.** *Anal Biochem* 2005, **340:**99–105.
20. Knowles SE, Jarrett IG, Filsell OH, Ballard FJ: **Production and utilization of acetate in mammals.** *Biochem J* 1974, **142:**01–411.
21. Solanky KS, Bailey NJ, Beckwith-Hall BM, Davis A, Bingham S, Holmes E, Nicholson JK, Cassidy A: **Application of biofluid 1H nuclear magnetic resonance-based metabonomic techniques for the analysis of the biochemical effects of dietary isoflavones on human plasma profile.** *Anal Biochem* 2003, **323:**197–204.
22. Griffin JL, Mann CJ, Scott J, Shoulders CC, Nicholson JK: **Choline containing metabolites during cell transfection: an insight into magnetic resonance spectroscopy detectable changes.** *FEBS Lett* 2001, **509:**263–266.
23. Kharasch ED, Thummel KE: **Identification of cytochrome P450 2E1 as the predominant enzyme catalyzing human liver microsomal defluorination of sevoflurane, isoflurane, and methoxyflurane.** *Anesthesiology* 1993, **79:**795–807.
24. Shichinohe Y, Masuda Y, Takahashi H, Kotaki M, Omote T, Shichinohe M, Namiki A: **A case of postoperative hepatic injury after sevoflurane anesthesia.** *Masui* 1992, **41:**1802–1805.

25. Watanabe K, Hatakenaka S, Ikemune K, Chigyo Y, Kubozono T, Arai T: **A case of suspected liver dysfunction induced by sevoflurane anesthesia.** *Masui* 1993, **42**:902–905.
26. Carrigan TW, Straughen WJ: **A report of hepatic necrosis and death following isoflurane anesthesia.** *Anesthesiology* 1987, **67**:581–583.
27. Sinha A, Clatch RJ, Stuck G, Blumenthal SA, Patel SA: **Isoflurane hepatotoxicity: a case report and review of the literature.** *Am J Gastroenterol* 1996, **91**:2406–2409.
28. Nishiyama T, Tokoyama T, Hanaoka K: **Effects of sevoflurane and isoflurane anesthesia on arterial ketone body ratio and liver function.** *Acta Anaesthesiol Scand* 1999, **43**:347–351.
29. Tao KM, Yang LQ, Liu YT, Tao Y, Song JC, Wu FX, Yu WF: **Volatile anesthetics might be more beneficial than propofol for postoperative liver function in cirrhotic patients receiving hepatectomy.** *Med Hypotheses* 2010, **75**:555–557.
30. Fukuda I, Uchihashi Y, Ira M, Ogura T, Shizukuishi M, Kazama T, Sugiura Y: **Effects of propofol on hepatic venous oxygen saturation–a comparison with isoflurane or sevoflurane anesthesia.** *Masui* 2005, **54**:736–741.
31. Guitton J, Buronfosse T, Desage M, Flinois JP, Perdrix JP, Brazier JL, Beaune P: **Possible involvement of multiple human cytochrome P450 isoforms in the liver metabolism of propofol.** *Br J Anaesth* 1998, **80**:788–795.
32. Gertler R, Brown HC, Mitchell DH, Silvius EN: **Dexmedetomidine: a novel sedative-analgesic agent.** *Proc (Bayl Univ Med Cent)* 2001, **14**:13–21.
33. Kaivosaari S, Toivonen P, Aitio O, Sipila J, Koskinen M, Salonen JS, Finel M: **Regio- and stereospecific N-glucuronidation of medetomidine: the differences between UDP glucuronosyltransferase (UGT) 1A4 and UGT2B10 account for the complex kinetics of human liver microsomes.** *Drug Metab Dispos* 2008, **36**:1529–1537.
34. Lawrence CJ, Prinzen FW, de Lange S: **The effect of dexmedetomidine on nutrient organ blood flow.** *Anesth Analg* 1996, **83**:1160–1165.
35. Memis D, Kargi M, Sut N: **Effects of propofol and dexmedetomidine on indocyanine green elimination assessed with LIMON to patients with early septic shock: a pilot study.** *J Crit Care* 2009, **24**:603–608.
36. Haberer JP, Audibert G, Saunier CG, Muller C, Laxenaire MC, Hartemann D: **Effect of propofol and thiopentone on regional blood flow in brain and peripheral tissues during normoxia and hypoxia in the dog.** *Clin Physiol* 1993, **13**:197–207.
37. Carmichael FJ, Crawford MW, Khawam N, Saldivia V: **Effect of propofol infusion on splanchnic hemodynamics and liver oxygen consumption in the rat. A dose–response study.** *Anesthesiology* 1993, **79**:1051–1060.
38. Shelby MK, Cherrington NJ, Vansell NR, Klaassen CD: **Tissue mRNA expression of the rat UDP-glucuronosyltransferase gene family.** *Drug Metab Dispos* 2003, **31**:326–333.
39. Bedirli N, Ofluoglu E, Kerem M, Utebey G, Alper M, Yilmazer D, Bedirli A, Ozlu O, Pasaoglu H: **Hepatic energy metabolism and the differential protective effects of sevoflurane and isoflurane anesthesia in a rat hepatic ischemia-reperfusion injury model.** *Anesth Analg* 2008, **106**:830–837.

Artifact quantification and tractography from 3T MRI after placement of aneurysm clips in subarachnoid hemorrhage patients

Faraz Khursheed[1], Fiona Rohlffs[1], Shuichi Suzuki[2,3], Dong H Kim[1] and Timothy M Ellmore[1*]

Abstract

Background: The application of advanced 3T MRI imaging techniques to study recovery after subarachnoid hemorrhage (SAH) is complicated by the presence of image artifacts produced by implanted aneurysm clips. To characterize the effect of these artifacts on image quality, we sought to: 1) quantify extent of image artifact in SAH patients with implanted aneurysm clips across a range of MR sequences typically used in studies of volumetry, blood oxygen level dependent signal change (BOLD-fMRI), and diffusion-weighted imaging (DW-MRI) and 2) to explore the ability to reconstruct white matter pathways in these patients.

Methods: T1- and T2-weighted structural, BOLD-fMRI, and DW-MRI scans were acquired at 3T in two patients with titanium alloy clips in ACOM and left ACA respectively. Intensity-based planimetric contouring was performed on aligned image volumes to define each artifact. Artifact volumes were quantified by artifact/clip length and artifact/brain volume ratios and analyzed by two-way (scan-by-rater) ANOVAs. Tractography pathways were reconstructed from DW-MRI at varying distances from the artifacts using deterministic methods.

Results: Artifact volume varied by MR sequence for length ($p = 0.007$) and volume ($p < 0.001$) ratios: it was smallest for structural images, larger for DW-MRI acquisitions, and largest on fMRI images. Inter-rater reliability was high ($r = 0.9626$, $p < 0.0001$), and reconstruction of white matter connectivity characteristics increased with distance from the artifact border. In both patients, reconstructed white matter pathways of the uncinate fasciculus and inferior fronto-occipital fasciculus were clearly visible within 2 mm of the artifact border.

Conclusions: Advanced 3T MR can successfully image brain tissue around implanted titanium aneurysm clips at different spatial ranges depending on sequence type. White matter pathways near clip artifacts can be reconstructed and visualized. These findings provide a reference for designing functional and structural neuroimaging studies of recovery in aSAH patients after clip placement.

Keywords: artifact, BOLD-fMRI, diffusion-weighted imaging, inferior fronto-occipital fasciculus, intracranial aneurysm clip, magnetic resonance imaging, subarachnoid hemorrhage, titanium alloy, uncinate fasciculus

Background

Recent advances in aneurysmal subarachnoid hemorrhage (aSAH) management have led to consistent improvement in survival, with case fatality rates decreasing 0.9% every year without a rebound increase in the proportion of survivors with severe disabilities [1]. Most published data on aSAH use the Glasgow Outcome Scale (GOS) and modified Rankin Scale (mRS) that place patients with mild disabilities in a 'Good Recovery' category. However, even patients who make a good recovery based on these outcome scales suffer from varying degrees of cognitive deficits, including most prominently problems with memory [2,3]. These deficits impair day-to-day functioning, impact workplace productivity, and affect social interactions often during the most productive years of patients' lives. While a growing body of literature documents these cognitive deficits in aSAH

* Correspondence: Timothy.Ellmore@uth.tmc.edu
[1]The Vivian L. Smith Department of Neurosurgery and Mischer Neuroscience Institute, The University of Texas Medical School at Houston, 6431 Fannin St., Houston TX 77030, USA
Full list of author information is available at the end of the article

survivors using objective batteries of neuropsychological tests [2-6], far fewer studies have attempted to relate cognitive deficits to specific neurobiological changes.

The acquisition of advanced neuroimaging sequences and application of recently developed analysis techniques promises to shed more light on the relationship between brain changes following aSAH and specific cognitive deficits. Such techniques include 1) high spatial resolution (1 mm^3) structural MRI volumes to measure cortical thickness and gray/white matter density using voxel based morphometric techniques [7,8], 2) high temporal resolution (1-2 sec) blood oxygen level dependent functional MRI [9] to measure rest-state [10,11] and task-evoked hemodynamic changes [12], and 3) diffusion-weighted MRI (DW-MRI) to measure white matter integrity and connectivity [13-16]. A recent set of voxel-based morphometric studies employed structural MRI acquired at 1.5 tesla and demonstrated gray matter atrophy in multiple brain areas following aSAH that, in some cases, correlate with neuropsychological deficits [17-20]. However, many more systematic imaging studies will be required to unravel the complex set of brain changes caused by accumulation of subarachnoid blood, lesions induced by intraparenchymal hemotomas frequently seen with aneurysm rupture (Fisher Grade 4 [21]), vasospasm-induced ischemic damage, and surgical retraction/manipulation of local tissue. The widespread availability of high-field (3 tesla and greater) in clinical and research MRI centers will reduce the time to acquire advanced sequences and provide increased signal-to-noise ratios compared to lower field scanners [22-24].

Treatment of many aSAH patients involves the surgical placement of non-ferromagnetic (e.g., titanium alloy) intracranial aneurysm clips [25,26]. These patients are routinely scanned clinically at 1.5 tesla field strength [27,28] if the implanted clips are confirmed by written record to be made from titanium or other non-metallic materials that have been tested [29-37]. Clips made with ferromagnetic materials are unsafe even at low field strengths [38,39] and if operative records indicate these are implanted then patients cannot be scanned. Recent studies have assessed various characteristic (e.g., torque and translational attraction, MRI-related heating, and artifacts) in high-field strength MR environments of clips made from a range of non-ferromagnetic materials, including titanium alloy, at high field strengths from 3 up to 8 tesla [40-44]. While it may be routine clinical practice to obtain MRI scans in patients with these clips, the implants produce a noticeable artifact in the images. These artifacts have never been quantitatively described *in vivo* at high field (> 1.5 tesla) in aSAH patients, although basic characteristics of artifacts have been reported for imaging obtained with clips in phantoms at 1.5 tesla and higher [29,34,45,46].

Given previous studies of MRI artifacts from aneurysm clip implants in humans conducted at low field strength and studies at both low and high field strengths conducted with phantoms, we expected at the outset of this study to find that artifact size depends on the type of pulse sequence. The novelty of our study is that it is conducted at 3T *in vivo* with patients who have a history of SAH, and that artifact size is quantified across a range of acquisitions using parameters that are typically found in advanced research MRI studies of cognitive function. The major motivation to characterizing the MR artifact *in vivo* rather than in phantoms is that the results can be interpreted from a clinically-relevant perspective in order to give neurosurgeons, neuroradiologists and researchers alike an idea of how much signal loss varies across these acquisitions before they embark on large-sample imaging studies of neurocognitive recovery after SAH. A description of artifact characteristics obtained *in vivo* across a range of advanced image acquisition sequences is necessary in order to understand the extent of signal integrity around the aneurysm clip. Only after the boundary of signal loss around the clip is quantified can the signal changes arising from damage due to the hemorrhage, normal signal change from healthy brain tissue, and connectional neuroanatomy near implanted clips, like that made possible by DW-MRI tractography, be adequately summarized.

Objectives

Image artifact due to the presence of titanium alloy aneurysm clips is generally acknowledged to be minimal. Yet no *in vivo* data is available from aSAH patients to guide clinicians and researchers in estimating the extent of aneurysm clip artifact in images reconstructed from advanced high-field (> 1.5 tesla) MR sequences. In this paper, we test the null hypothesis that the resulting artifact from implanted titanium alloy clips is spatially similar across high-resolution T1- and T2-weighted structural, T2* echo-planar BOLD-fMRI, and DW-MRI images when clinical characteristics related to the extent of aSAH and clip characteristics are similar. We also explore the ability to reconstruct temporal and frontal lobe white matter fiber pathways reconstructed using deterministic tractography methods from the DW-MRI acquisitions, and quantify pathway density at different distances from the artifact border.

Methods

Patients

Two patients with a history of SAH who were treated by placement of titanium alloy aneurysm clips were imaged after giving informed verbal and written consent for enrollment in the study. Patients gave informed consent for their brain images to be published. This research study was approved by The Committee for the Protection of Human Subjects of The University of Texas Health Science Center at Houston (HSC-MS-09-0497). The two patients were similar in terms of the degree and distribution of SAH, its intraparenchymal component, the degree and severity of vasospasm [47], the surgical approach taken, and characteristics of implanted clips, including composition, *in-vivo* clip orientation, and dimensions (for details of each, see Table 1). We did not study patients with clips made from Phynox, MP35N, and Elgiloy, as these clips are not routinely implanted at our institution, nor did we study patients with curved, right-angle or other more complicated clip configurations.

Image Acquisition

The following brain scans were obtained using a 3T Philips Intera scanner (Philips Medical Systems, Bothell WA; 8-channel SENSE acquisition): (1) T2-weighted turbo-spin echo 3D volume acquisition (repetition [TR]/echo time [TE] = 2500/367 ms; ETL 120, pixel bandwidth 380, FA = 90 degrees, matrix size = 256 × 256; field of view [FOV] = 240 mm, 186 0.94 mm thick contiguous, sagittal slices), (2) high-resolution 3D T1-weighted magnetization-prepared rapid acquisition turbo field echo sequence (TR/TE = 8.4/3.9ms; FA = 8 deg; matrix size = 256 × 256; FOV = 240 mm; slice thickness = 1.0 mm thick sagittal slices), (3) a set of diffusion-weighted image volumes (32-directions high angular resolution) using the gradient overplus option with one B0 (non-diffusion weighted) image volume acquired before the acquisition of one repetition of the diffusion-weighted scans (TR/TE = 8500/67 ms; FA = 90 deg; matrix size 128 × 128; FOV = 224 mm; 2 mm thick axial slices, b-value of 800 s/mm^2), (4) a set of functional images obtained with a gradient-recalled echo-planar imaging (EPI) sequence sensitive to the blood-oxygen level dependent (BOLD) signal (TR/TE = 2000/30 ms; FA = 90 deg; matrix size = 80 × 80; FOV = 220 mm; 3 mm thick axial slices, 150 dynamics). These

Table 1 Patient Demographics and Aneurysm Clip Characteristics

	Patient A	*Patient B*
Patient Demographics		
Age	62	36
Sex	F	F
Hunt and Hess Grade	3	4
Fisher's Grade	4	4
SAH Distribution	Bilateral, L > R	Bilateral, L > R
Aneurysm location	ACOM	Left ACA
Intraparenchymal Component	Left Frontal	Left Frontal
Focal Neurological Deficits	Yes	Yes
Vasospasm	Clinically significant requiring endovascular intervention	Clinically significant requiring endovascular intervention
Surgery		
Approach	Left Pterional	Left Pterional
Operative findings	Hemosiderin deposition on brain surface	Significant subarachnoid blood
Time between SAH and Surgery	11 months	9 days
Time between Surgery and 3T MR Scan	5 months	15 months
Clip Specifications		
Manufacturer	Aesculap Yasargil FT720T (Aesculap, Germany)	Aesculap Yasargil FT760T (Aesculap, Germany)
Composition	Titanium Alloy Ti6A14V ISO 5823-3	Titanium Alloy Ti6A14V ISO 5823-3
Size	7 mm (mini)	11 mm (Standard)
Weight	0.08 g	0.19 g
Width	0.95 mm	1.35 mm
Shape	Straight	Straight

particular sequence parameters were selected for use here because they are commonly applied in structural and functional studies of cognition in both healthy controls [48] and different patient groups [49,50]. Identical MR parameters were used to scan both patients; no attempt was made to adjust these parameters on an individual patient basis to minimize artifact extent.

Image Analysis

Image visualization and artifact quantification was performed using the AFNI package [51]. Two raters with fellowship training in neuroimage analysis and who were blind to each other's results performed intensity-based planimetric contouring to define each artifact. The T2, EPI and DW image volumes were aligned to the T1 volume using the 3dAlineate alignment algorithm with a mutual information cost function in AFNI. Each rater created 3D binary masks on the aligned volumes that encompassed the entire spatial extent of the artifact on each patient's T1, T2, mean EPI, and the B0 diffusion-weighted scans. The artifact was clearly visible in each of the four different acquisitions, and verified numerically to consist of a low intensity (i.e., black) region wherein the highest intensity image value at the center of the artifact was verified across all patients and all scans to never exceeded 10% of the global image maximum. The consistent behavior of the artifact intensity allowed for the choice of an intensity-based threshold to be automatically chosen during 3D contouring of the artifact border. After the artifact was delineated, the long-axis and total volume for each of these binary masks was then measured by summing mask voxel volumes. Most importantly, for comparison across patients and MR sequences, artifact volume was expressed as a percentage of whole brain volume, defined as the total gray and white matter of the brain as computed in Freesurfer v4.5 [52,53].

To determine whether the clip artifact differed significantly as a function of scan sequence and rater, two 2-way analyses of variance were conducted using SPSS (v.13). In the first ANVOA, the dependent variable was the artifact length/clip length ratio, and the two fixed factors were rater (2-levels: rater 1 & 2) and scan sequence (4-levels: T1, T2, EPI, and DW). In the second ANOVA, the dependent variable was the artifact volume/brain volume ratio, and the two fixed factors were rater (2-levels: rater 1 & 2) and scan sequence (4-levels: T1, T2, EPI, and DW). These ANOVAs had 3 and 15 numerator and denominator degrees of freedom, allowing for *a priori* $p < 0.05$ statistical threshold for the fixed effects of rater and scan sequence. Due to the few patients studied, no statistical interpretation about the random effect of patient was possible.

To quantify how the number of white matter tractography pathways varied as a function of distance from the artifact, diffusion tractography pathways were computed from the set of aligned diffusion-weighted images according to previously described methods [54,55]. Then, the artifact mask delineated on the diffusion-weighted scan was morphologically dilated in three dimensions by increments of the native-space DW voxel resolution (2 mm), and all pathways intersecting with the dilated mask were saved and visualized in DTI Query [56].

Results

The means and standard deviations of the two raters' measurements of each patient's artifact are listed by imaging sequence in Table 2.

For both patients, the artifact appeared smallest on T2-weighted structural volume (0.21% to 0.45% of whole brain volume, artifact/clip length ratio of 2.82 to 2.89) and the largest on the EPI functional image (3.21% to 3.94% of whole brain volume, artifact/clip length ratio of 4.75 to 6.55).

Significant main effects of scan type were found by the ANOVA of artifact length/clip length ratio ($F_{(3,15)} = 8.51$, $p = 0.007$), and the ANOVA of artifact volume/brain volume ratio ($F_{(3,15)} = 22.25$, $p < 0.001$) supporting the hypothesis the artifact size varies among the different MR acquisition sequences. Further evidence was found by computing post-hoc tests for significant ($p < 0.05$) differences among the means (Bonferroni corrected for multiple comparisons). These showed differences between the structural (T1 and T2) and EPI sequences for the artifact length/clip length ratios, and between the structural (T1 and T2) and EPI and DW sequences for the artifact volume/brain volume ratios. Differences between the EPI and DW artifact volume/brain volume ratios trended toward but failed to reach significance ($p = 0.11$).

Inter-rater reliability for all measurements (artifact volume, artifact as percentage of brain volume, and artifact length) was very high ($r = 0.9626$, $p < 0.0001$) demonstrating objective differentiation between raters of the artifact size as a function of MR sequence. In general, inter-rater variability in estimation of artifact length was low (Range: 0.21-1.80 mm for T2, 4.41-4.72 mm for EPI) and artifact volume was relatively high (Range: 101-185 mm^3 for T2, 2728-4767 mm^3 for EPI). There were no significant main effects of rater found in either the ANOVA of artifact length/clip length ratio or the ANOVA of artifact volume/brain volume ratio, showing that estimates of artifact size were consistent and did not differ systematically by individual rater.

Artifact size differences are easily visualized by comparing an image plane across different MR sequences taken through the center of the artifact (Figure 1). On all sequences in both patients, the maximum length

Table 2 Artifact Measurements as a Function of MR Sequence

	Sequence	Artifact Volume mm^3	% Of Brain Volume	Artifact Length mm	Artifact/Clip Length Ratio
Patient A	*T1*	1038 (366)	0.45 (0.16)	25.31 (0.09)	3.61
(7 mm clip)	*T2*	484 (185)	0.21 (0.08)	20.28 (1.80)	2.89
	EPI	7366 (4767)	3.21 (2.08)	45.91 (4.72)	6.55
	DW	3792 (168)	1.65 (0.07)	36.62 (2.39)	5.23
Patient B	*T1*	2223 (428)	0.92 (0.18)	34.52 (1.19)	3.18
(11 mm clip)	*T2*	1093 (101)	0.45 (0.04)	31.05 (0.21)	2.82
	EPI	9557 (2728)	3.94 (1.13)	52.33 (4.41)	4.75
	DW	6897 (2644)	2.85 (1.09)	42.97 (0.36)	3.90

The mean of the two raters' estimates is listed with standard deviation in parentheses.

measured along the long axis of the artifact was larger than the actual clip length, ranging from 2.82 times the length of the clip for the T2 structural sequence to 6.5 times the length of the clip for the EPI sequence.

Computed whole-brain volumes were 229,705 and 242,419 mm^3 for patient's A and B respectively. These values are in line with an average of whole brain volumes, 235,821 (SD 22,571), computed from a group of similar aged controls (N = 7, 3F, 1LH, 54.0 years, SD 7.8) published recently [49]. To help aide visualization of clip artifact volume in relation to brain size, example artifact volume reconstructions from the range of MR sequences are shown in relation to patient cortical surface models in Figure 2.

The ability to reconstruct nearby white matter fiber pathways as a function of distance from the artifact border was examined in both patients. The artifact mask delineated on the diffusion-weighted sequence was expanded by 3D morphological dilation incrementally in 2 mm steps (Figure 3) and the volume of the white matter tracts intersecting the dilated mask was found to increase markedly from the border, from 592 micro liters within 2 mm of the artifact border to 2752 micro liters within 6 mm of the border for Patient A with the 7 mm clip, and from 1348 to 4556 in Patient B with the larger 11 mm clip. After just one increment of dilation, pathways of the uncinate fasciculus (connecting anterior temporal and ventral frontal lobe) and pathways of the inferior fronto-occipital fasciculus, connecting parieto-occipital and ventral frontal lobe [57-59], were visible in the data of both patients (Figure 3).

Discussion

Widespread application of advanced imaging techniques to investigate changes in brain structure, function, and connectivity following SAH is presently slowed by the fact that interpretation of the images obtained from patients with implanted aneurysm clips is complicated by the presence of an artifact in and around the clip. The spatial extent of the artifact with respect to clip size and type of MR sequence has not been previously described from images collected from aSAH patients *in vivo*. The main objective in conducting this study was to describe the extent of image artifact produced by implanted titanium aneurysm clips in aSAH patients across a set of advanced MR sequences necessary to quantify structural, functional, and connectivity patterns. A secondary objective was to describe using DW-MRI tractography methods how well white matter connectional patterns could be reconstructed around the clip artifact. This second objective is critical, we believe, for beginning to understanding how well modern neuroimaging approaches to studying white matter can be applied in SAH patients who have implanted aneurysm clips.

We focused on just two subarachnoid hemorrhage patients with similar clinical characteristics, including surgical approach, aneurysm location, Fisher's SAH grade [21], global distribution of subarachnoid blood, and implanted clip size and orientation. We acknowledge several limitations of this approach. First, the clinical characteristic of these patients were not matched exactly. Second, the small number of patients studied does not allow generalization of the findings to the entire population of aSAH patients who are treated neurosurgically with clips. We cannot predict for certain based on the findings presented here how artifact will manifest in patients with clips placed on, for example, the middle cerebral or basilar arteries. However, the two patients imaged in this study had clips placed after rupture of ACOM and ACA. Estimates based on large sample studies of western [60] and eastern [61,62] patient populations indicate that these locations account for between 29 to 38 percent of total intracranial aneurysm ruptures. This suggests that, despite the limited scope of our study, our findings may be generalizable to a sizeable subset of the population with titanium clips placed at these locations. Finally, we studied patients implanted only with straight titanium alloy clips. Patients with

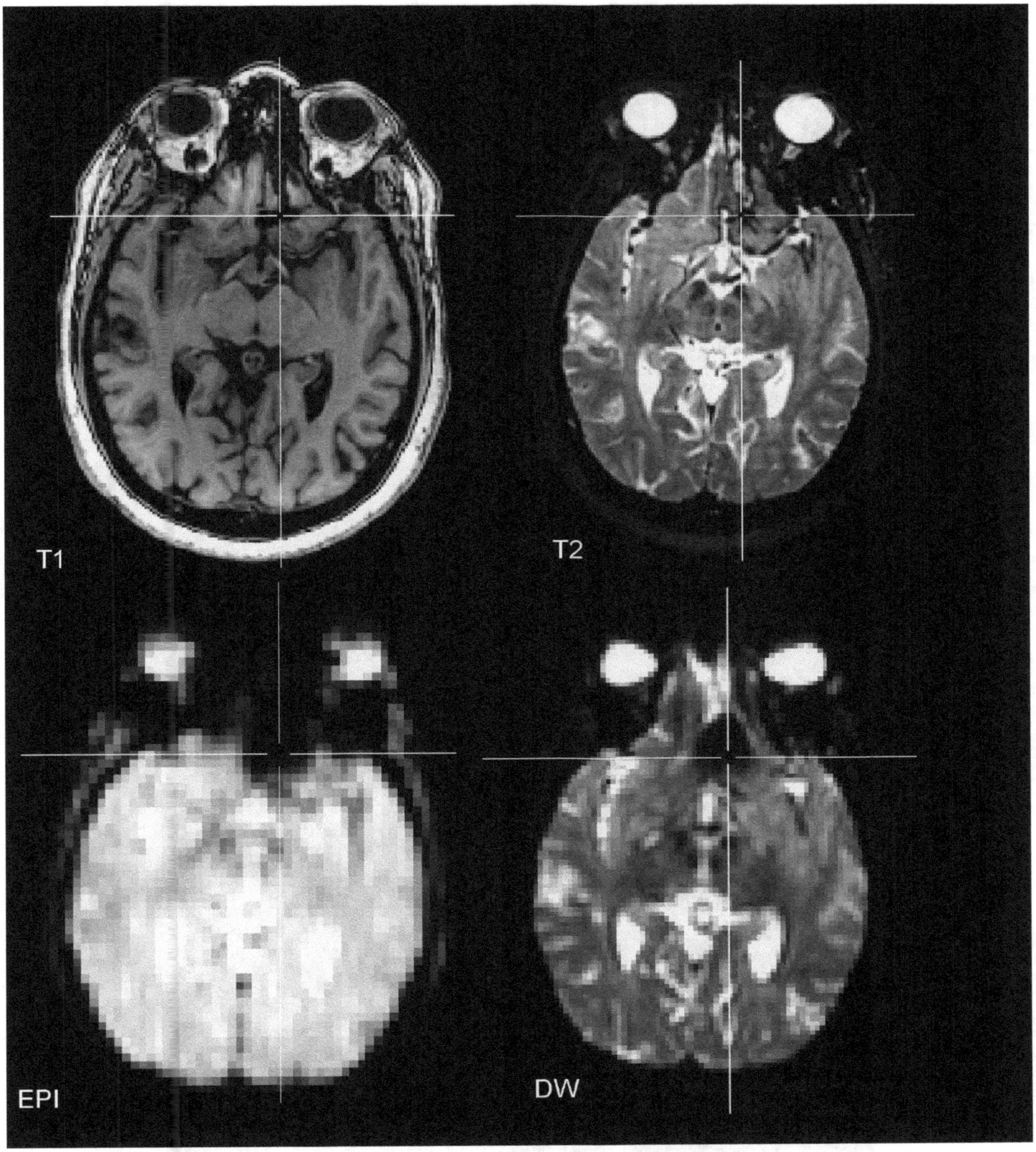

Figure 1 Appearance of Aneurysm Clip Artifact on Different Aligned MRI Sequences. Axial slices taken in the same imaging plane for Patient A are displayed in the axial plane (radiological convention) with the crosshair placed in the center of the clip artifact.

more complex clip configurations might demonstrate a larger artifact relative to a straight clip of same size and weight. Furthermore, more SAH blood distribution around the clip, more aggressive surgical manipulation of surrounding tissue and more complex clip configuration would likely increase artifact size relative to the estimates presented here. In our limited study, two patients studied were scanned at 3 tesla, and high

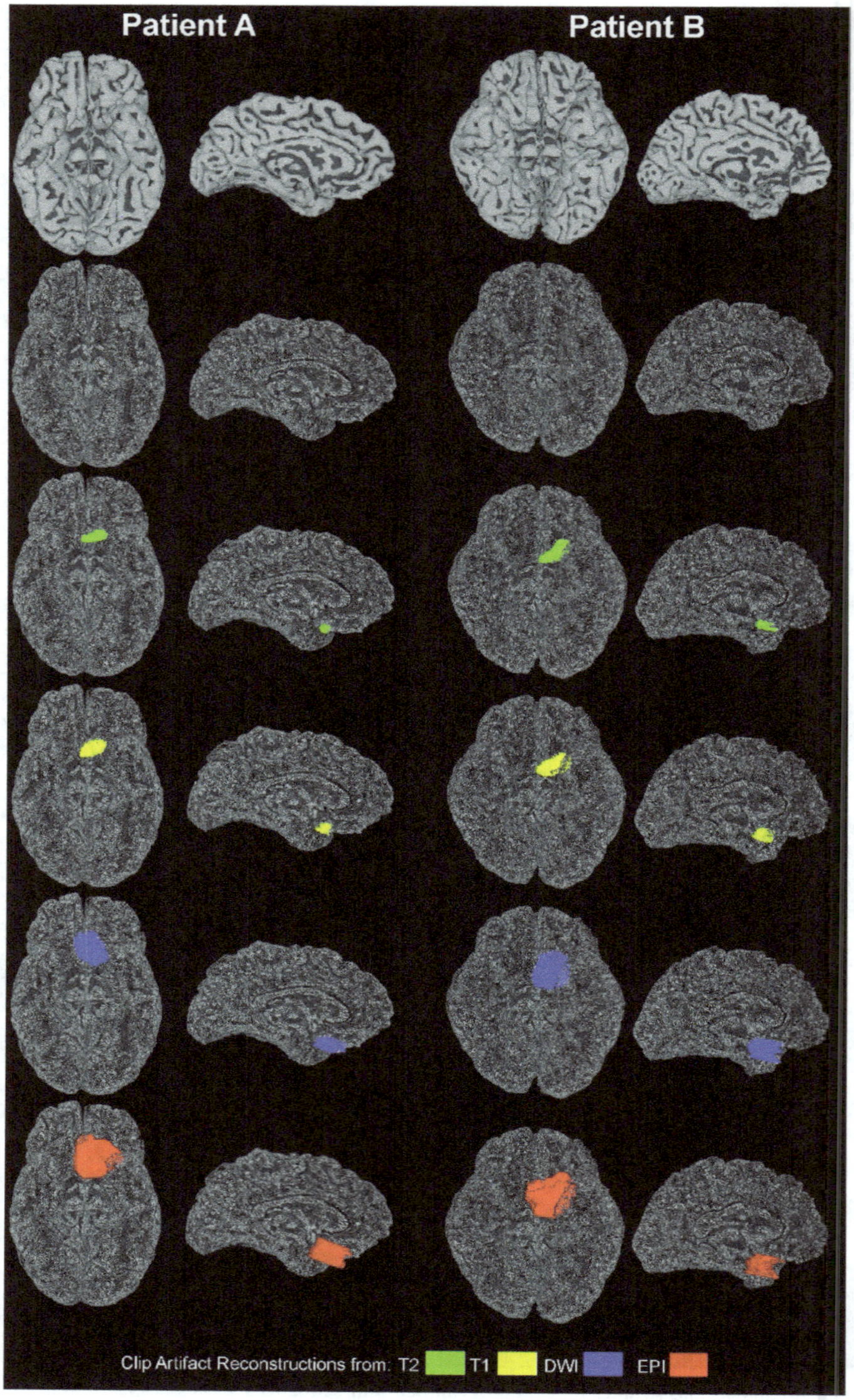

Figure 2 Example Clip Artifact Volume Reconstructions in Relation to Cortical Surface Models. Basal and mid-sagittal views of each patient's cortical surface model are shown shaded by curvature (top row) and as a point cloud (second row). Superimposed on the point could displays to aide artifact visualization are the reconstructed clip artifact volumes colored according to MR sequence in descending order by clip volume as percentage of brain volume (T2 = green, T1 = yellow, DWI = blue, EPI = red). These artifact volumes are 0.27%, 0.56%, 1.70%, and 4.67% respectively for Patient A (two columns on left), and 0.48%, 1.04%, 3.62%, and 4.74% respectively for Patient B (two columns on right).

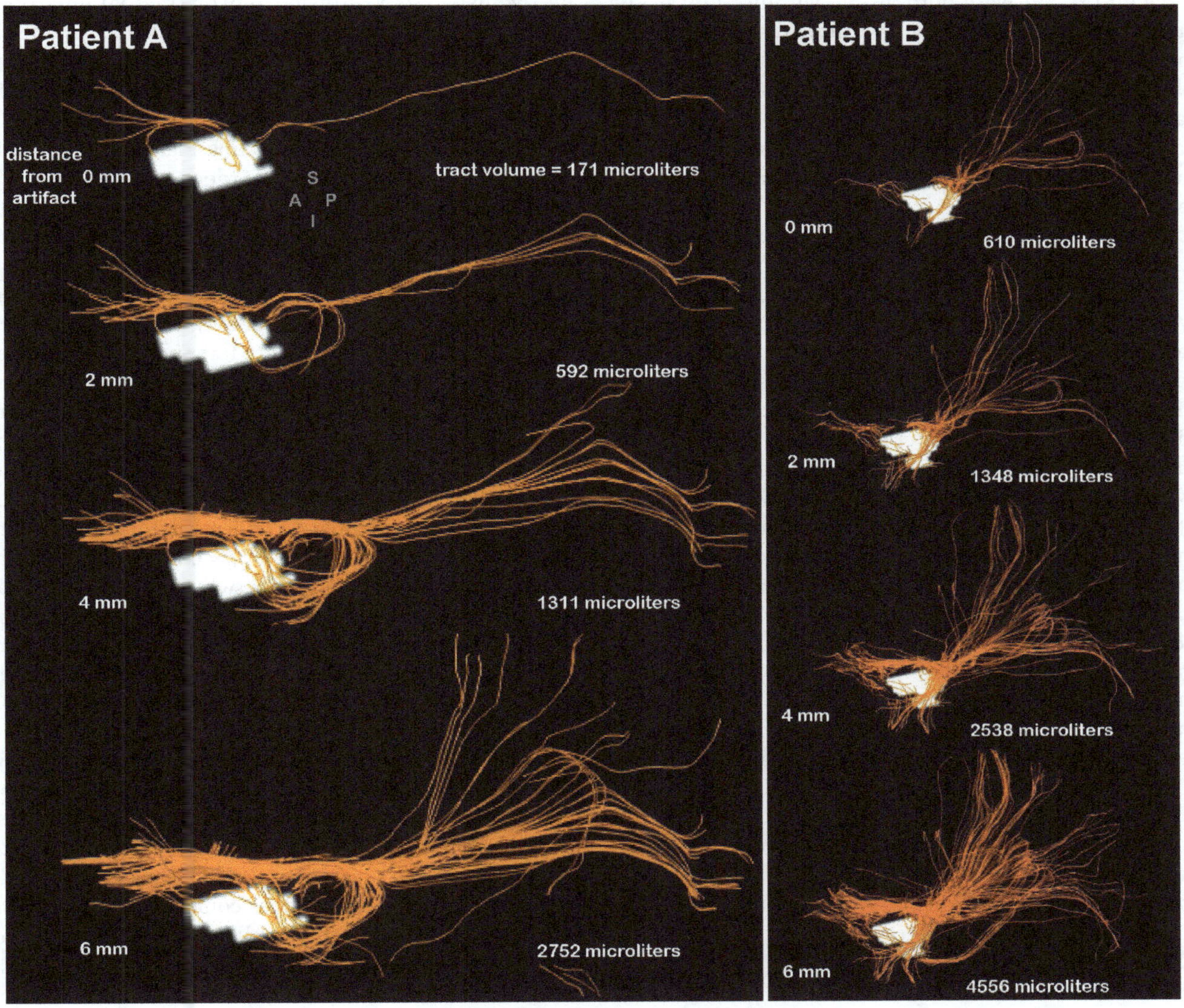

Figure 3 White Matter Tractography Reconstruction Ability Increases as a Function of Distance from Artifact Border. The artifact masks derived from the diffusion-weighted image volume were dilated in 2 mm increments, and the volume of white matter tracts that intersected any component of the dilated mask was computed. Components of the uncinate fasciculus (loop from temporal to ventral frontal) and inferior fronto-occipital fasciculus (occipital to temporal) in both patients' left hemisphere can be resolved within 2 mm of the artifact border by visual inspection of the orange tractography pathways. Both views are sagittal left hemisphere where A, P, S, and I indicate anterior, posterior, superior and inferior directions

resolution T1- and T2-weighted structural, BOLD-fMRI, and DW-MRI sequences were acquired. The image volumes were aligned to the native image space of the high resolution T1 anatomical scan, and experienced raters used semi-automated tracing methods to delineate the image artifact around the aneurysm clip on each set of image volumes. For each sequence, a 3D mask of the artifact was produced. Mask volumes were compared across sequences and between raters. Inter-rater reliability was highly significant, indicating that the extent of the image artifact was reproducible across sequences. Most importantly, we found evidence to reject our initial null hypothesis that the spatial extent of the image artifact is the same across 3T MR acquisition sequences. Our main result is that the size of the clip artifact varies considerably; it is smallest in volume on the structural scans and largest on the echo-planar BOLD-fMRI scans, with the artifact on the DW-MRI sequence falling in between.

The result from our second objective is that we were surprised to learn that it is possible to reconstruct white matter pathways very close to the artifact border using DW-MRI data. For the two patients studied here, pathways comprising uncinate and inferior fronto-occipital fasciculi [57-59] were both visible within 2 mm of the artifact border. After applying a three dimensional artifact mask generation method, we also provide multiple objective measures, including an artifact/clip-length ratio and artifact volume/brain tissue volume ratio that can be used to guide neuroimaging researchers in estimating the size of the artifact if clip characteristics like length are known.

In hindsight, it is not too surprising that the clip artifact differs considerably in size given that the sequences required to measure structural, functional, and diffusion-weighted connectivity information differ according to radiofrequency pulse design, gradient readout times, and spatial resolution. It is necessary that these parameters differ in order for scanners to be capable of measuring different MR signal characteristics, and it is important to know how clip artifact size will differ as a function of type of imaging sequence. In this study, we made no attempt to adjust parameters in individual patients to minimize artifact. This was a deliberate choice made to minimize signal variance as a function of acquisition parameters so that within-group (SAH) analyses and between-group (SAH vs. matched control) can be conducted in future larger-sample studies. For functional imaging, there is a necessary tradeoff between high spatial and temporal resolution when acquiring fMRI-BOLD sequences. In our echo-planar fMRI sequence, we used a 2 second repetition time, meaning that hemodynamic activity throughout 34 slices representing the entire volume of the brain is captured every two seconds. This acquisition speed is common for task-evoked and rest state designs. Fast fMRI acquisitions require larger voxel sizes of ~ 3 mm in order to image most of the brain. Advances in head coil design, including the number of channels to record the signal, will in the future allow acquisition of higher spatial resolution scans in a shorter time, but the spatial-temporal tradeoff will remain.

Artifact size in the fMRI-BOLD sequence acquired here is also significantly magnified by a susceptibility artifact at the base of the brain, near where many aneurysm clips are likely to be placed. This well-known dropout of signal due to a large static magnetic field inhomogeneity that occurs near air/brain interfaces is also present in echo-planar acquisitions in healthy controls. The interaction between clip location and signal dropout due to the brain tissue/air cavity susceptibility complicated delineation of the clip artifact because both artifacts appeared as low intensity regions and overlapped to some extent. However, the tissue-air artifact extends outside the border of the brain, so by constraining our artifact delineation to within-brain borders as defined by the high-resolution anatomical images we were able to minimize this error to some extent.

Outside the boundary of our artifact masks, imaging signal integrity recovers quickly. This was demonstrated by reconstructing diffusion tensor tractography fiber pathways as the artifact mask volumes were parametrically dilated in three dimensions. As we used standard diffusion tensor imaging methods here with relatively few gradient orientations, future investigations should evaluate the feasibility of collecting higher direction diffusion-weighted sequences in order to more accurately reconstruct white matter pathways in SAH patients using methods like Q-ball [63] and diffusion spectrum techniques [64]. Nevertheless, during dilation, the mask volume was expanded to include tissue outside the artifact and the number of tractography pathways increased rapidly as the mask was dilated at successively higher iterations, indicating an increase in our ability to examine connectivity characteristics just a few millimeters away from the artifact mask. This is critically important as aSAH may involve subtle damage to brain tissue near the rupture site. The damage may cause atrophy of nearby gray matter, altered connectivity of nearby white matter to other brain areas, or a combination of both. Altered network connectivity between brain regions near the rupture site (i.e., hippocampal complex) and regions distal to the rupture site (i.e., ventrolateral prefrontal cortex) is one hypothesis that could account for complex deficits [4], like those of memory, mood, and decision making, that have been reported in aSAH patients. To adequately test this hypothesis, white matter connectivity, for tracts thought to be important for memory like the uncinate fasciculus (shown in Figure 3 for both patients) must be reconstructed, and the extent of artifact due to the aneurysm clip must be quantifiable and reproducible in order to know in which areas connectivity information is reliable. The results presented here show how this may be achieved through construction of a spatial confidence boundary of signal integrity, represented numerically by an artifact mask volume. These volumes should be constructed from the MR imaging data obtained from each aSAH patient. Across patients, the spatial extent of these artifact masks may be considered in a group analysis of the imaging data. Using this approach, it would be possible to quantify the degree of uncertainty across patients about whether signal in a particular region of the brain is completely or partially affected by clip artifact. Importantly, this method is also generalizable to other methods of assessing connectivity, like functional connectivity computed from rest-state fMRI [65].

Conclusions

In summary, we show that artifact due to the presence of titanium clips differs across a range of advanced high-field (3 tesla) MR imaging sequences in aneurysmal subarachnoid hemorrhage patients. This artifact is easily quantifiable and 3D volumes of confidence can be produced outside of which the MR signal for measuring structure, function, and diffusion-weighted connectivity information may be obtained. We also show that DW-MRI tractography can reveal white matter pathways in close proximity to the artifact borders. These results have important methodological implications for studying brain changes with advanced neuroimaging tools in patients who recover from subarachnoid hemorrhage after neurosurgical treatment.

Funding

This project was supported by the Brain Aneurysm Foundation and the Vivian L. Smith Foundation for Neurological Research. Partial funding for the purchase of the Philips 3T scanner used to collect the imaging data was provided by NIH S10 RR19186. No funding was provided by manufacturers of clips studied.

Abbreviations

3T: three tesla; AFNI: Analysis of Functional Neuroimages; ANOVA: analysis of variance; ACA: anterior cerebral artery; ACOM: anterior communicating artery; aSAH: aneurysmal subarachnoid hemorrhage; BOLD: blood oxygen level dependent; DTI: diffusion tensor imaging; DW-MRI: diffusion-weighted magnetic resonance imaging; EPI: echo-planar imaging; ETL: echo train length; FA: flip angle; fMRI: functional magnetic resonance imaging; FOV: field of view; GOS: Glasgow Outcome Scale; mRS: modified Rankin Scale; MRI: magnetic resonance imaging; TE: echo time; TR: repetition time

Acknowledgements

We thank Vipulkumar S. Patel for help collecting the MRI data, Vicki Massie and Jamie Yost from Aesculap, USA, for providing detailed technical specifications about the aneurysm clips, Yuxiang Zhou, Ph.D. for help interpreting imaging data, and Florencia Leyton for help with patient scheduling.

Author details

[1]The Vivian L. Smith Department of Neurosurgery and Mischer Neuroscience Institute, The University of Texas Medical School at Houston, 6431 Fannin St., Houston TX 77030, USA. [2]Department of Diagnostic and Interventional Imaging, The University of Texas Medical School at Houston, 6431 Fannin St., Houston TX 77030, USA. [3]Neurointerventional/Neuro Endovascular, Radiological Sciences, University of California, Irvine, 101 The City Drive South, Rt. 140, South Bldg. 56, Mail Code: 5005, Orange, CA 92868, USA.

Authors' contributions

FK, FR, and TME collected the MRI data. DK did the surgeries and referred patients for research. FK and TME analyzed the data. SS helped interpret the imaging data. FK and TME wrote the paper. All authors read and approved the final manuscript.

Competing interests

The authors declare that they have no competing interests.

References

1. Lovelock CE, Rinkel GJ, Rothwell PM: **Time trends in outcome of subarachnoid hemorrhage: Population-based study and systematic review.** *Neurology* 2010, **74(19)**:1494-1501.
2. Hackett ML, Anderson CS: **Health outcomes 1 year after subarachnoid hemorrhage: An international population-based study. The Australian Cooperative Research on Subarachnoid Hemorrhage Study Group.** *Neurology* 2000, **55(5)**:658-662.
3. Orbo M, Waterloo K, Egge A, Isaksen J, Ingebrigtsen T, Romner B: **Predictors for cognitive impairment one year after surgery for aneurysmal subarachnoid hemorrhage.** *J Neurol* 2008, **255(11)**:1770-1776.
4. Al-Khindi T, Macdonald RL, Schweizer TA: **Cognitive and functional outcome after aneurysmal subarachnoid hemorrhage.** *Stroke* 2010, **41(8)**: e519-536.
5. Schweizer TA, Macdonald RL: **Brain hemorrhage: assessing outcome after subarachnoid hemorrhage.** *Nat Rev Neurol* 2010, **6(8)**:427-428.
6. Haug T, Sorteberg A, Finset A, Lindegaard KF, Lundar T, Sorteberg W: **Cognitive functioning and health-related quality of life 1 year after aneurysmal subarachnoid hemorrhage in preoperative comatose patients (Hunt and Hess Grade V patients).** *Neurosurgery* 2010, **66(3)**:475-484, discussion 484-475.
7. Ashburner J, Friston KJ: **Voxel-based morphometry–the methods.** *Neuroimage* 2000, **11(6 Pt 1)**:805-821.
8. Good CD, Johnsrude IS, Ashburner J, Henson RN, Friston KJ, Frackowiak RS: **A voxel-based morphometric study of ageing in 465 normal adult human brains.** *Neuroimage* 2001, **14(1 Pt 1)**:21-36.
9. Ogawa S, Tank DW, Menon R, Ellermann JM, Kim SG, Merkle H, Ugurbil K: **Intrinsic signal changes accompanying sensory stimulation: functional brain mapping with magnetic resonance imaging.** *Proc Natl Acad Sci USA* 1992, **89(13)**:5951-5955.
10. Shehzad Z, Kelly AM, Reiss PT, Gee DG, Gotimer K, Uddin LQ, Lee SH, Margulies DS, Roy AK, Biswal BB, *et al*: **The resting brain: unconstrained yet reliable.** *Cereb Cortex* 2009, **19(10)**:2209-2229.
11. Zhang D, Johnston JM, Fox MD, Leuthardt EC, Grubb RL, Chicoine MR, Smyth MD, Snyder AZ, Raichle ME, Shimony JS: **Preoperative sensorimotor mapping in brain tumor patients using spontaneous fluctuations in neuronal activity imaged with functional magnetic resonance imaging: initial experience.** *Neurosurgery* 2009, **65(6 Suppl)**:226-236.
12. Amiez C, Kostopoulos P, Champod AS, Collins DL, Doyon J, Del Maestro R, Petrides M: **Preoperative functional magnetic resonance imaging assessment of higher-order cognitive function in patients undergoing surgery for brain tumors.** *J Neurosurg* 2008, **108(2)**:258-268.
13. Basser PJ: **Inferring microstructural features and the physiological state of tissues from diffusion-weighted images.** *NMR in biomedicine* 1995, **8(7-8)**:333-344.
14. Basser PJ, Pajevic S, Pierpaoli C, Duda J, Aldroubi A: **In vivo fiber tractography using DT-MRI data.** *Magn Reson Med* 2000, **44(4)**:625-632.
15. Beaulieu C: **The basis of anisotropic water diffusion in the nervous system - a technical review.** *NMR in biomedicine* 2002, **15(7-8)**:435-455.
16. Behrens TE, Woolrich MW, Jenkinson M, Johansen-Berg H, Nunes RG, Clare S, Matthews PM, Brady JM, Smith SM: **Characterization and propagation of uncertainty in diffusion-weighted MR imaging.** *Magn Reson Med* 2003, **50(5)**:1077-1088.
17. Bendel P, Koivisto T, Hanninen T, Kolehmainen A, Kononen M, Hurskainen H, Pennanen C, Vanninen R: **Subarachnoid hemorrhage is followed by temporomesial volume loss: MRI volumetric study.** *Neurology* 2006, **67(4)**:575-582.
18. Bendel P, Koivisto T, Kononen M, Hanninen T, Hurskainen H, Saari T, Vapalahti M, Hernesniemi J, Vanninen R: **MR imaging of the brain 1 year after aneurysmal subarachnoid hemorrhage: randomized study comparing surgical with endovascular treatment.** *Radiology* 2008, **246(2)**:543-552.
19. Bendel P, Koivisto T, Niskanen E, Kononen M, Aikia M, Hanninen T, Koskenkorva P, Vanninen R: **Brain atrophy and neuropsychological outcome after treatment of ruptured anterior cerebral artery aneurysms: a voxel-based morphometric study.** *Neuroradiology* 2009, **51(11)**:711-722.
20. Martinaud O, Perin B, Gerardin E, Proust F, Bioux S, Gars DL, Hannequin D, Godefroy O: **Anatomy of executive deficit following ruptured anterior communicating artery aneurysm.** *Eur J Neurol* 2009, **16(5)**:595-601.
21. Claassen J, Bernardini GL, Kreiter K, Bates J, Du YE, Copeland D, Connolly ES, Mayer SA: **Effect of cisternal and ventricular blood on risk of delayed cerebral ischemia after subarachnoid hemorrhage: the Fisher scale revisited.** *Stroke* 2001, **32(9)**:2012-2020.
22. Alvarez-Linera J: **3T MRI: advances in brain imaging.** *Eur J Radiol* 2008, **67(3)**:415-426.
23. Blamire AM: **The technology of MRI–the next 10 years?** *Br J Radiol* 2008, **81(968)**:601-617.
24. Okada T, Yamada H, Ito H, Yonekura Y, Sadato N: **Magnetic field strength increase yields significantly greater contrast-to-noise ratio increase: Measured using BOLD contrast in the primary visual area.** *Acad Radiol* 2005, **12(2)**:142-147.

25. Colby GP, Coon AL, Tamargo RJ: **Surgical management of aneurysmal subarachnoid hemorrhage.** *Neurosurgery clinics of North America* 2010, **21(2)**:247-261.
26. Dujovny M, Agner C, Ibe O, Perlin A: **Self-closing aneurysm clip: a historical review.** *Neurol Res* 2010, **32(10)**:1011-1020.
27. Ferris NJ, Kavnoudias H, Thiel C, Stuckey S: **The 2005 Australian MRI safety survey.** *AJR Am J Roentgenol* 2007, **188(5)**:1388-1394.
28. Evans JC, Smith ET, Nixon TE: **A national survey of attitudes towards the use of MRI in patients known to have intracranial aneurysm clips.** *Br J Radiol* 2001, **74(888)**:1118-1120.
29. Olsrud J, Latt J, Brockstedt S, Romner B, Bjorkman-Burtscher IM: **Magnetic resonance imaging artifacts caused by aneurysm clips and shunt valves: dependence on field strength (1.5 and 3 T) and imaging parameters.** *J Magn Reson Imaging* 2005, **22(3)**:433-437.
30. Ooka K, Shibuya M, Suzuki Y: **Motion and image artifacts of various intracranial aneurysm clips in a magnetic field.** *Acta Neurochir (Wien)* 1996, **138(10)**:1241-1245.
31. Pride GL Jr, Kowal J, Mendelsohn DB, Chason DP, Fleckenstein JL: **Safety of MR scanning in patients with nonferromagnetic aneurysm clips.** *J Magn Reson Imaging* 2000, **12(1)**:198-200.
32. Shellock FG, Kanal E: **Yasargil aneurysm clips: evaluation of interactions with a 1.5-T MR system.** *Radiology* 1998, **207(3)**:587-591.
33. Shellock FG, Tkach JA, Ruggieri PM, Masaryk TJ, Rasmussen PA: **Aneurysm clips: evaluation of magnetic field interactions and translational attraction by use of "long-bore" and "short-bore" 3.0-T MR imaging systems.** *AJNR Am J Neuroradiol* 2003, **24(3)**:463-471.
34. Shellock FG, Valencerina S: **In Vitro Evaluation of MR Imaging Issues at 3T for Aneurysm Clips Made from MP35N: Findings and Information Applied to 155 Additional Aneurysm Clips.** *AJNR Am J Neuroradiol* 2009.
35. Kanal E, Shellock FG: **MR imaging of patients with intracranial aneurysm clips.** *Radiology* 1993, **187(3)**:612-614.
36. Kanal E, Shellock FG: **Aneurysm clips: effects of long-term and multiple exposures to a 1.5-T MR system.** *Radiology* 1999, **210(2)**:563-565.
37. Sutherland GR, Kelly JJ, Boehm DW, Klassen JB: **Ceramic aneurysm clips.** *Neurosurgery* 2008, **62(5 Suppl 2)**:ONS400-405, discussion ONS405-406.
38. Becker RL, Norfray JF, Teitelbaum GP, Bradley WG Jr, Jacobs JB, Wacaser L, Rieman RL: **MR imaging in patients with intracranial aneurysm clips.** *Ajnr* 1988, **9(5)**:885-889.
39. Klucznik RP, Carrier DA, Pyka R, Haid RW: **Placement of a ferromagnetic intracerebral aneurysm clip in a magnetic field with a fatal outcome.** *Radiology* 1993, **187(3)**:855-856.
40. Kangarlu A, Shellock FG: **Aneurysm clips: evaluation of magnetic field interactions with an 8.0 T MR system.** *J Magn Reson Imaging* 2000, **12(1)**:107-111.
41. Kakizawa Y, Seguchi T, Horiuchi T, Hongo K: **Cerebral aneurysm clips in the 3-tesla magnetic field. Laboratory investigation.** *J Neurosurg* 2010, **113(4)**:859-869.
42. Watanabe A, Seguchi T, Koyama J, Aoyama T, Miyahara T, Kakizawa Y, Hongo K: **Investigation of radiofrequency-induced temperature elevation of aneurysm clips in a 3.0-tesla magnetic resonance environment.** *Neurosurgery* 2007, **61(5)**:1062-1065, discussion 1065-1066.
43. ASTM: **American Society for Testing and Materials (ASTM) International. Designation F 2503-05: standard practice for marking medical devices and other items for safety in the magnetic resonance environment.** West Conshohocken, PA: ASTM International; 2005.
44. Shellock FG, Woods TO, Crues JV: **MR labeling information for implants and devices: explanation of terminology.** *Radiology* 2009, **253(1)**:26-30.
45. Shellock FG, Kanal E: **Aneurysm clips: evaluation of MR imaging artifacts at 1.5 T.** *Radiology* 1998, **209(2)**:563-566.
46. Romner B, Olsson M, Ljunggren B, Holtas S, Saveland H, Brandt L, Persson B: **Magnetic resonance imaging and aneurysm clips. Magnetic properties and image artifacts.** *J Neurosurg* 1989, **70(3)**:426-431.
47. Pradilla G, Chaichana KL, Hoang S, Huang J, Tamargo RJ: **Inflammation and cerebral vasospasm after subarachnoid hemorrhage.** *Neurosurgery clinics of North America* **21(2)**:365-379.
48. Nath AR, Beauchamp MS: **Dynamic changes in superior temporal sulcus connectivity during perception of noisy audiovisual speech.** *J Neurosci* 2011, **31(5)**:1704-1714.
49. Ellmore TM, Hood AJ, Castriotta RJ, Stimming EF, Bick RJ, Schiess MC: **Reduced volume of the putamen in REM sleep behavior disorder patients.** *Parkinsonism & related disorders* 2010, **16(10)**:645-649.
50. Khursheed F, Tandon N, Tertel K, Pieters TA, Disano MA, Ellmore TM: **Frequency-specific electrocorticographic correlates of working memory delay period fMRI activity.** *Neuroimage* 2011, **56(3)**:1173-1782.
51. Cox RW: **AFNI: software for analysis and visualization of functional magnetic resonance neuroimages.** *Comput Biomed Res* 1996, **29(3)**:162-173.
52. Dale AM, Fischl B, Sereno MI: **Cortical surface-based analysis. I. Segmentation and surface reconstruction.** *Neuroimage* 1999, **9(2)**:179-194.
53. Fischl B, Sereno MI, Dale AM: **Cortical surface-based analysis. II: Inflation, flattening, and a surface-based coordinate system.** *Neuroimage* 1999, **9(2)**:195-207.
54. Ellmore TM, Beauchamp MS, Breier JI, Slater JD, Kalamangalam GP, O'Neill TJ, Disano MA, Tandon N: **Temporal lobe white matter asymmetry and language laterality in epilepsy patients.** *Neuroimage* 2010, **49(3)**:2033-2044.
55. Ellmore TM, Beauchamp MS, O'Neill TJ, Dreyer S, Tandon N: **Relationships between essential cortical language sites and subcortical pathways.** *J Neurosurg* 2009, **111(4)**:755-766.
56. Sherbondy A, Akers D, Mackenzie R, Dougherty R, Wandell B: **Exploring connectivity of the brain's white matter with dynamic queries.** *IEEE Trans Vis Comput Graph* 2005, **11(4)**:419-430.
57. Catani M, Howard RJ, Pajevic S, Jones DK: **Virtual in vivo interactive dissection of white matter fasciculi in the human brain.** *Neuroimage* 2002, **17(1)**:77-94.
58. Fernandez-Miranda JC, Rhoton AL Jr, Alvarez-Linera J, Kakizawa Y, Choi C, de Oliveira EP: **Three-dimensional microsurgical and tractographic anatomy of the white matter of the human brain.** *Neurosurgery* 2008, **62(6 Suppl 3)**:989-1026, discussion 1026-1028.
59. Fernandez-Miranda JC, Rhoton AL Jr, Kakizawa Y, Choi C, Alvarez-Linera J: **The claustrum and its projection system in the human brain: a microsurgical and tractographic anatomical study.** *J Neurosurg* 2008, **108(4)**:764-774.
60. Forget TR Jr, Benitez R, Veznedaroglu E, Sharan A, Mitchell W, Silva M, Rosenwasser RH: **A review of size and location of ruptured intracranial aneurysms.** *Neurosurgery* 2001, **49(6)**:1322-1325, discussion 1325-1326.
61. Lai HP, Cheng KM, Yu SC, Au Yeung KM, Cheung YL, Chan CM, Poon WS, Lui WM: **Size, location, and multiplicity of ruptured intracranial aneurysms in the Hong Kong Chinese population with subarachnoid haemorrhage.** *Hong Kong medical journal = Xianggang yi xue za zhi/Hong Kong Academy of Medicine* 2009, **15(4)**:262-266
62. Osawa M, Hongo K, Tanaka Y, Nakamura Y, Kitazawa K, Kobayashi S: **Results of direct surgery for aneurysmal subarachnoid haemorrhage: outcome of 2055 patients who underwent direct aneurysm surgery and profile of ruptured intracranial aneurysms.** *Acta Neurochir (Wien)* 2001, **143(7)**:655-663, discussion 663-654.
63. Tuch DS: **Q-ball imaging.** *Magn Reson Med* 2004, **52(6)**:1358-1372.
64. Wedeen VJ, Hagmann P, Tseng WY, Reese TG, Weisskoff RM: **Mapping complex tissue architecture with diffusion spectrum magnetic resonance imaging.** *Magn Reson Med* 2005, **54(6)**:1377-1386.
65. Carter AR, Astafiev SV, Lang CE, Connor LT, Rengachary J, Strube MJ, Pope DL, Shulman GL, Corbetta M: **Resting interhemispheric functional magnetic resonance imaging connectivity predicts performance after stroke.** *Ann Neurol* 2010, **67(3)**:365-375.

Automated vs manual delineations of regions of interest- a comparison in commercially available perfusion MRI software

Ivana Galinovic[1*], Ann-Christin Ostwaldt[2], Carina Soemmer[3], Helena Bros[1], Benjamin Hotter[1], Peter Brunecker[1] and Jochen B Fiebach[1]

Abstract

Background: In perfusion magnetic resonance imaging a manual approach to delineation of regions of interest is, due to rater bias and time intensive operator input, clinically less favorable than an automated approach would be. The goal of our study was to compare the performances of these approaches.

Methods: Using Stroketool, PMA and Perfscape/Neuroscape perfusion maps of cerebral blood flow, mean transit time and Tmax were created for 145 patients with acute ischemic stroke. Volumes of hypoperfused tissue were calculated using both a manual and an automated protocol, and the results compared between methods.

Results: The median difference between the automatically and manually derived volumes was up to 210 ml in Perfscape/Neuroscape, 123 ml in PMA and 135 ml in Stroketool. Correlation coefficients between perfusion volumes and radiological and clinical outcome were much lower for the automatic volumes than for the manually derived ones.

Conclusions: The agreement of the two methods was very poor, with the automated use producing falsely exaggerated volumes of hypoperfused tissue. Software improvements are necessary to enable highly automated protocols to credibly assess perfusion deficits.

Keywords: Magnetic resonance imaging, Perfusion MRI, Acute ischemic stroke

Background

The increased use of the perfusion imaging (PI) – diffusion-weighted imaging (DWI) mismatch hypothesis [1] in studies of acute ischemic stroke (AIS) and clinical practice [1,2] is raising demands from software packages developed for volumetric calculations of hypoperfusion. Typically these programs offer the possibility to delineate a region of interest (ROI) manually but also, to a varying extent, automatically. Manual approaches to delineation are biased and require time intensive operator input. Therefore a mostly automated procedure, if accurate, would be preferred in clinical practice. The goal of our study was comparing the automated approach to the manual approach while using a number of different software packages.

* Correspondence: ivana.galinovic@charite.de
[1]Center for Stroke Research Berlin, Charité-Universitätsmedizin Berlin, Campus Benjamin Franklin, Hindenburgdamm 30, 12200 Berlin, Germany
Full list of author information is available at the end of the article

Methods

The study design and cohort characteristics have been previously reported [3]. Briefly, using Stroketool (Digital Image Solutions, Germany, http://www.digitalimagesolutions.de), PMA (v3.2.0.4, ASIST, Japan, http://asist.umin.jp/index-e.htm) and Perfscape/Neuroscape (Olea Medical SAS, France, http://www.olea-medical.com) perfusion maps of cerebral blood flow (CBF), mean transit time (MTT) and Tmax were calculated for 145 patients imaged within 24 hours of AIS. The inclusion criteria were: clinically and radiologically confirmed AIS, hypoperfusion on the initial PI examination (assessed by the attending neuroradiologist) and availability of a follow-up MRI scan. For each parameter map, three thresholds were applied. The Tmax thresholds were 4, 6 and 8 seconds of delay [4] and the MTT thresholds were 5, 6 and 8 seconds. As no uniform CBF scale was available, the three CBF thresholds were different across software. Both MTT and CBF thresholds were chosen empirically using a

Table 1 Difference of ROI volumes between the automated and the manual protocol

Program	Perfscape/Neuroscape	PMA	PMA with filtering *	Stroketool	Stroketool with filtering *
	Median	Median	Median	Median	Median
	IQR	IQR	IQR	IQR	IQR
Parameter					
Tmax 4 s	25.80	123.68	64.91	122.89	37.50
	12.8–66.1	75.2–206.8	27.3–138.1	75.6–176.5	14.9–75.3
Tmax 6 s	12.74	29.48	4.83	53.18	7.75
	4.1–34.4	16.4–67.8	1.0–22.4	34.0–82.6	1.8–18.3
Tmax 8 s	8.05	23.16	2.68	31.78	1.67
	2.6 - 28.1	13.5 – 55.4	0.4 – 15.8	16.1 – 50.1	0.2 – 6.5
MTT 5 s	186.78	35.12	11.59	129.35	58.74
	151.4–248.5	17.8–87.8	3.4–44.1	82.5–225.7	21.8–130.5
MTT 6 s	154.40 114.8–207.0	16.76 8.4–49.0	4.34 0.9–18.4	80.18 49.1–143.6	26.51 8.0–63.7
MTT 8 s	94.24	7.36	0.77	33.82	6.07
	55.0–143.3	3.8–17.4	0.3–3.9	20.9–57.6	1.6–18.8
CBF highest threshold	209.92	54.35	23.05	134.50	67.28
	160.0–262.8	27.5–107.9	7.6–64.4	89.9–193.0	39.0–110.2
CBF medium threshold	151.93	36.14	10.51	87.28	35.27
	97.6–212.2	18.6–65.9	3.7–36.5	59.4–134.0	18.1–61.7
CBF lowest threshold	63.66	23.40	4.33	53.95	12.73
	39.6–119.4	13.3–39.3	1.4–15.3	37.2–83.0	6.6–28.4

CBF indicates cerebral blood flow; MTT mean transit time; IQR interquartile range. All values are in ml.
* Values indicate volumes after additional CSF filtering in SPM8.

random sample of acute stroke patients. ROI volumes were calculated using a manual and an automated protocol. In the automated protocol, once the thresholds have been applied, no further post-processing was done. Maps created in PMA and Stroketool also underwent a second post-processing step in SPM8 (Wellcome Trust Centre for Neuroimaging, UK) to cut away scalp and spaces filled with cerebrospinal fluid (CSF). This was not necessary for Perfscape/Neuroscape due to the program's implemented filtering. In the manual protocol a human rater excluded, from the thresholded maps, areas unlikely to reflect credible hypoperfusion.

Radiological outcome was defined as the final lesion volume on follow-up FLAIR images. Clinical outcome was defined as the National Institute of Health Stroke Scale (NIHSS) score at the time of hospital discharge. All statistics were done in PASW Statistics 18. Analyses of correlations were performed using the Spearman signed-ranks correlation test.

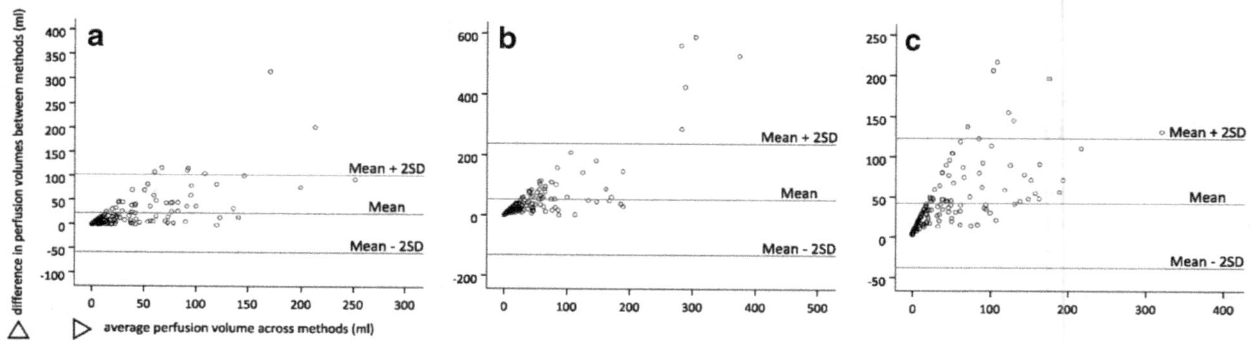

Figure 1 Bland-Altman plots for the top performing automatic map and threshold, without additional CSF filtering for PMA and Stroketool a- Perfscape/Neuroscape; b- PMA and c- Stroketool. The mean and the limits of agreement (mean +/−2 standard deviations) are shown as solid lines. The difference in perfusion volumes was calculated as the manually derived volume subtracted from the automated one.

Results

The median final lesion volume was 6.55 ml (IQR 0.8 – 31.6 ml). The median difference between the automatically and manually derived volumes was up to 210 ml (between 90% and 386%) in Perfscape/Neuroscape, 123 ml (between 192% and 1415%) in PMA and 135 ml (between 357% and 815%) in Stroketool. (Table 1). Bland-Altman plots for agreement of methods are shown in Figure 1. All correlation coefficients between volumes of perfusion deficit and radiological and clinical outcome were considerably lower for the automatic volumes than for the manually derived ones. The top performing automated map was Tmax in all three programs. With additional filtering applied to automated volumes calculated in PMA and Stroketool the median difference between the automatically and manually derived volumes dropped down to a maximum of 64.91 ml (between 44% and 238%) and 67.28 ml (between 33% and 369%), respectively (Table 1).

Discussion

The median volume of the perfusion deficit varied greatly based on the map and threshold and even across software for the same map and threshold. This discrepancy could in part be explained through the different choice of AIFs, the use of different deconvolution techniques, different implementations of the same calculation algorithm as well as differences in motion correction across different programs [5-7]. Our group had already conducted a study on a group of patients with no ischemia, using the same three software packages, and observed the presence of numerous artifacts; typically the cortex proximal to the skull and infratentorial cerebral and cerebellar tissue [8]. Programs without implemented CSF filtering also suffered from arti facts such as ventricles, eyeballs and scalp [8]. As expected, the same artifacts were present in our current patient cohort. This explains the weaker correlation coefficients and overshoot of the automated delineations as compared to the manual ones. Although most of the values on the Bland-Altman difference plot fall within the limits of agreement (Figure 1), these are much too broad with regards to the cohort's median lesion volumes and the fact that, based on location, even a lesion of a few ml can be clinically significant. Additional CSF filtering greatly reduced the differences between the automatic and the manual volumes, pointing to a need for implemented filtering.

Conclusion

In conclusion, current automated use of the here evaluated programs would lead to falsely exaggerated volumes of hypoperfused tissue in patients with AIS. However a number of improvements, such as algorithms for judging perfusion asymmetry between hemispheres and allowing selection of the vessel territory of expected hypoperfusion, could aid automated protocols in credibly assessing perfusion deficits.

Competing interests

The authors have no conflicts of interest to declare. All vendors provided software free of charge, no author received grants or fees from any of the involved software right owners and companies.

Authors' contributions

IG gathered the patient cohort, partly analyzed the imaging data, performed statistical analysis and drafted the manuscript. ACO participated in the analysis of the imaging data. CS participated in the analysis of the imaging data. HB participated in the analysis of the imaging data. BH participated in the gathering of the patient cohort and the drafting of the manuscript. PB performed the automated segment of data analysis. JBF was responsible for supervision and co-drafted the final version of the manuscript with IG. All authors read and approved the final manuscript.

Acknowledgements

No acknowledgements.

Sources of funding

The research leading to these results has received funding from the Federal Ministry of Education and Research via the grant Center for Stroke Research Berlin (01 EO 0801).

Author details

[1]Center for Stroke Research Berlin, Charité-Universitätsmedizin Berlin, Campus Benjamin Franklin, Hindenburgdamm 30, 12200 Berlin, Germany.
[2]International Graduate Program Medical Neurosciences, Charite-Universitätsmedizin, Berlin, Luisenstrasse 56, 10117 Berlin, Germany.
[3]Charité-Universitätsmedizin, Berlin, Charitéplatz 1, 10117 Berlin, Germany.

References

1. Hacke W, Albers G, Al-Rawi Y, Bogousslavsky J, Davalos A, Eliasziw M, *et al*: **The Desmoteplase in Acute Ischemic Stroke Trial (DIAS): a phase II MRI-based 9-hour window acute stroke thrombolysis trial with intravenous desmoteplase.** *Stroke* 2005, **36**:66–73.
2. Kohrmann M, Juttler E, Fiebach JB, Huttner HB, Siebert S, Schwark C, *et al*: **MRI versus CT-based thrombolysis treatment within and beyond the 3 h time window after stroke onset: a cohort study.** *Lancet Neurol* 2006, **5**:661–667.
3. Galinovic I, Ostwaldt AC, Soemmer C, Bros H, Hotter B, Brunecker P, *et al*: **Search for a map and threshold in perfusion MRI to accurately predict tissue fate: a protocol for assessing lesion growth in patients with a persistent vessel occlusion.** *Cerebrovasc Dis* 2011, **32**:186–193.
4. Olivot JM, Mlynash M, Thijs VN, Kemp S, Lansberg MG, Wechsler L, *et al*: **Optimal Tmax threshold for predicting penumbral tissue in acute stroke.** *Stroke* 2009, **40**:469–475.
5. Kosior RK, Kosior JC, Frayne R: **Improved dynamic susceptibility contrast (DSC)-MR perfusion estimates by motion correction.** *J Magn Reson Imaging* 2007, **26**:1167–72.
6. Kim J, Leirab EC, Callison RC, Ludwiga B, Moritani T, Magnotta VA, Madsen MT: **Toward fully automated processing of dynamic susceptibility contrast perfusion MRI for acute ischemic cerebral stroke.** *Comput Methods Programs Biomed* 2010, **98**:204–213.
7. Yamada K, Wu O, Gonzalez RG, Bakker D, Copen WA, Weisskoff RM, Rosen BR, Yagi K, Nishimura T, Sorensen AG: **Magnetic resonance perfusion-weighted imaging of acute cerebral infarction: effect of the calculation methods and underlying vasculopathy.** *Stroke* 2002, **33**(1):87–94.
8. Galinovic I, Brunecker P, Ostwaldt AC, Soemmer C, Hotter B, Fiebach JB: **Fully automated postprocessing carries a risk of substantial overestimation of perfusion deficits in acute stroke magnetic resonance imaging.** *Cerebrovasc Dis* 2011, **31**:408–413.

28

Reduction of claustrophobia during magnetic resonance imaging: methods and design of the "CLAUSTRO"

Judith Enders[1†], Elke Zimmermann[1†], Matthias Rief[1], Peter Martus[2], Randolf Klingebiel[3], Patrick Asbach[1], Christian Klessen[1], Gerd Diederichs[1], Thomas Bengner[4], Ulf Teichgräber[1], Bernd Hamm[1], Marc Dewey[1*]

Abstract

Background: Magnetic resonance (MR) imaging has been described as the most important medical innovation in the last 25 years. Over 80 million MR procedures are now performed each year and on average 2.3% (95% confidence interval: 2.0 to 2.5%) of all patients scheduled for MR imaging suffer from claustrophobia. Thus, prevention of MR imaging by claustrophobia is a common problem and approximately 2,000,000 MR procedures worldwide cannot be completed due to this situation. Patients with claustrophobic anxiety are more likely to be frightened and experience a feeling of confinement or being closed in during MR imaging. In these patients, conscious sedation and additional sequences (after sedation) may be necessary to complete the examinations. Further improvements in MR design appear to be essential to alleviate this situation and broaden the applicability of MR imaging. A more open scanner configuration might help reduce claustrophobic reactions while maintaining image quality and diagnostic accuracy.

Methods/Design: We propose to analyze the rate of claustrophobic reactions, clinical utility, image quality, patient acceptance, and cost-effectiveness of an open MR scanner in a randomized comparison with a recently designed short-bore but closed scanner with 97% noise reduction. The primary aim of this study is thus to determine whether an open MR scanner can reduce claustrophobic reactions, thereby enabling more examinations of claustrophobic patients without incurring the safety issues associated with conscious sedation. In this manuscript we detail the methods and design of the prospective "CLAUSTRO" trial.

Discussion: This randomized controlled trial will be the first direct comparison of open vertical and closed short-bore MR systems in regards to claustrophobia and image quality as well as diagnostic utility.

Background

Magnetic resonance (MR) imaging has been described as the most important medical innovation in the last 25 years [1]. There has been an enormous increase in the use of this modality in the clinical setting. Over 80 million MR procedures are now performed each year worldwide. For an MR scan, patients typically have to be placed in a long, narrow tube [2]. Thus, claustrophobia preventing MR imaging is a common problem. Between 1% and 15% of all patients scheduled for MR imaging suffer from claustrophobia and cannot be imaged, or they require sedation to complete the scan (mean: 2.3%; 95% confidence interval: 2.0% to 2.5%) [3]. Thus it can be estimated that worldwide approximately 2,000,000 MR procedures cannot be performed or are prematurely terminated due to claustrophobia. At an average cost of € 500 per MR imaging, this is equal to a loss of productivity of € 1 billion, which is an important financial loss for the health care system. Therefore, claustrophobia is not only a common problem that prevents many patients from benefiting from the findings obtained with MR imaging but also represents an important socioeconomic issue for the health care system.

* Correspondence: marc.dewey@charite.de
† Contributed equally
[1]Departments of Radiology, Charité, Medical School, Humboldt Universität zu Berlin and Freie Universität Berlin, Germany
Full list of author information is available at the end of the article

Patients with claustrophobic anxiety are more likely to be frightened and experience a feeling of confinement or being closed in during MR imaging [4,5]. Those anxious patients have been reported to experience claustrophobia in up to 35% of all cases [6]. In these patients conscious sedation and additional sequences (after sedation) may be necessary to complete the examinations. This situation involves significant risks of adverse events [7-9] and is associated with extra costs because it reduces workflow, limits patient acceptance, and wastes valuable scanning time. Improving comfort during MR imaging (mainly reduction of noise and sensations of confinement by a fairly panoramic view) appears to be essential to avoid claustrophobic reactions [10,11]. The positive effect of noise reduction and improved patient-centered design (short and wide bore) has recently been shown in a large cohort study in over 55,000 patients using a newly designed closed MR unit (with 97% noise reduction and cylindrical CT-like appearance) with 1.5-T field and up to 45 mT/m gradient strength [3]. However, even on such recent scanners, claustrophobic patients cannot undergo MR imaging without potentially life-threatening sedation.

A more open vertical scanner configuration might be an alternative, but until recently such systems operated at rather low field strengths (0.2 T), resulting in poor image quality especially in imaging of the brain [12]. Thus, recently introduced open MR scanners with an all-around view and both high field (1.0 T) and high gradient strength (up to 26 mT/m) might be a valuable clinical alternative to further reduce claustrophobia while maintaining diagnostic image quality and diagnostic accuracy [13,14]. The more all-around view from the inside of open MR scanners is likely to reduce the incidence of claustrophobia. However, new closed MR scanners with patient-centered design (short and wide bore) and noise reduction have also been shown to greatly reduce claustrophobic reactions by a factor of up to 3 [3]. Nevertheless, no direct comparison of these two scanner types in regards to claustrophobia and image quality as well as diagnostic utility has been performed thus far. Therefore, it is unclear whether an open vertical or a closed short-bore MR design is more effective in reducing claustrophobia that prevents MR imaging. Moreover, by itself the design of open MR scanners cannot guarantee a reduction in claustrophobia or an improvement in patient outcome. The most decisive evidence for judging the efficacy of diagnostic tests comes from randomized comparisons in which the controlled design eliminates the biases of observational studies [15,16]. Randomized trials are needed to define the clinical role of such open MR scanners in patients with claustrophobic anxiety. Also no study has addressed which specific scanner design patients would prefer for imaging. Therefore, this study is designed to determine whether an open vertical or a closed short-bore MR design is more effective in alleviating claustrophobic anxiety preventing MR imaging and which further improvements might be necessary to reduce claustrophobia during MR imaging.

Methods/Design

Primary and secondary objectives

We propose to analyze the rate of claustrophobic reactions and clinical utility of an open MR scanner in a randomized comparison with a recently designed short-bore but closed scanner with 97% noise reduction. This trial will be the first to appraise the potential for claustrophobia reduction and clinical relevance of open MR scanners in claustrophobic patients with a clinical indication for MR imaging. Furthermore, this trial will analyze and compare the cost-effectiveness of the two MR scanners, which is important in view of the enormous annual loss of healthcare productivity due to claustrophobia during MR imaging. Also, patient preferences and image quality will be analyzed. Thus, this randomized trial may have the potential to influence both the clinical and economical utilization of MR imaging. If an open MR scanner can be shown to reduce claustrophobia in a randomized comparison it might be justified to recommend this approach for routine clinical application in certain high-risk anxiety patients or in certain imaging centers.

The primary aim of this study is thus to determine the ability of an open MR scanner to reduce claustrophobic reactions, thereby expanding the use of MRI in patients with claustrophobic anxiety. To achieve this, claustrophobic reactions (while entering the scanner room or during the MR procedure) that prevent MR imaging without sedation will be compared in the two randomized study groups. Thus, the question to be answered by this project is whether an open vertical or a short-bore MR design will alleviate claustrophobia that prevents MR imaging to a greater extent. The main secondary aims are the correlation of patients' scores in several validated psychological self-report questionnaires with the occurrence of claustrophobic events, the duration of MR imaging in the two groups, and to systematically analyze if and what further design improvements might be necessary to reduce claustrophobia during MR imaging in the future. Therefore, patient preferences concerning MR scanner design will be determined (Figure 1, Table 1). These insights are important to be able to define which further improvements by vendors might be necessary to reduce claustrophobic reactions during MR imaging.

Further secondary aims are the influence of MR imaging results on clinical management in the two groups, cost-effectiveness of the two scanners, image quality achieved in claustrophobic patients using the two

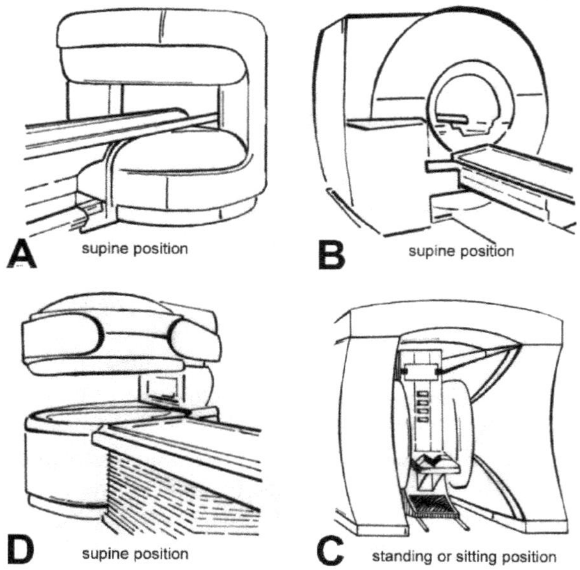

Figure 1 Drawings of four MR scanners which will be used in the custom-made questionnaire to assess which specific MR scanner design is evaluated to be the most attractive. Patients will be asked to rank the four MR scanner types according to their preferences. First, this assessment will be done assuming equal diagnostic utility of the MR scanners, and second, assuming for scanner **A** good, for scanner **B** very good, for scanner **C** moderate and for scanner **D** adequate diagnostic utility. **Panel A** shows the open MR scanner with a vertical magnetic field design and 1-T field strength (Panorama, Philips). **Panel B** shows the closed MR scanner with a short- and wide-bore design and 1.5-T field strength (Magnetom Avanto, Siemens). **Panel C** shows an open MR scanner with a one column design and a 0.4-T vertical magnetic field. **Panel D** shows a MR scanner with a 0.6-T horizontal magnetic field and a top/front-open design which allows upright positioning of the patient, while patients have to be examined in supine position on the scanners **A-C**. This information will allow defining which further improvements by the vendors might be necessary to reduce claustrophobic reactions during MR imaging.

scanners, patient acceptance and preference in regards to the diagnostic procedure in the two randomized study groups, and the development of patients' anxiety during 4 to 6 weeks and 7 months after MR imaging.

Design

This is a randomized controlled trial of patients with reported claustrophobia during prior MR imaging or with the inability to undergo MR imaging in conventional scanners. Eligible patients will be randomly assigned to one of the following study groups. 1) The open MR scanner: imaging will be performed in a state-of-the-art scanner with a vertical magnetic field and 360° open design and 1-T field strength (Panorama, Philips, Figure 2A) [14], and 2) A state-of-the-art MR scanner (control group) without an open design but significant noise reduction of 97% (to below 99 dB(A)) and patient-centered design (short and wide bore) with 1.5-T field strength, which has already been shown to reduce claustrophobia by a factor of 3 compared with conventional MR scanners (Magnetom Avanto, Siemens, Figure 2B) [3]. The study design is shown in Figure 3.

In order to improve patient acceptance, patients who are assigned to imaging in one MR scanner but cannot bear this procedure due to claustrophobia will not be sedated (with conscious sedation according to the standards of the American Society of Anesthesiology) [17], but will be cross-referred to imaging in the other scanner in order to preclude adverse events associated with sedation (Figure 3) [7-9]. This will also allow direct comparison of the two options in those patients as an ancillary study, which would otherwise be unethical. If patients cannot tolerate imaging in the first MR scanner in which they are assigned without claustrophobic reactions, this will be categorized as an event for the primary hypothesis of this project. In case patients cannot undergo imaging in either of the two scanners, conscious sedation according to the standards of the American Society of Anesthesiology will be performed (using Dormicum IV) to enable imaging [17].

Anxiety will be measured using different validated psychological self-report questionnaires such as the Spielberger State-Trait Anxiety Inventory [STAI] [18], the "Fragebogen zu körperbezogenen Ängsten, Kognitionen und Vermeidung [AKV]" [19], the Fear Survey Schedule [FSS-III] [20], and the Claustrophobia Questionnaire [CLQ] [21].

This randomized study has been approved by the local institutional review board at Charité. The clinical experiments will be performed according to the DECLARATION OF HELSINKI - Ethical Principles for Medical Research Involving Human Subjects and the Medizinproduktgesetz (German Medicinal Products Law).

This is an investigator-sponsored industry-independent study.

Patients

Patients with reported claustrophobia during MR imaging or with inability to undergo MR imaging in conventional scanners because of claustrophobic anxiety will be eligible for the study and subsequent randomization if they have a clinical indication for MR imaging of the head, spine, or shoulder. Patients must not have any absolute or relative contraindication to MR imaging for safety reasons [22], must not have a body weight of more than 200 kg (maximum table weight), will be primarily examined without conscious sedation, and have to be at least 18 years old. Patients must have at least moderate levels of anxiety towards claustrophobic situations as determined using the Claustrophobia Questionnaire [CLQ] [21] (an arithmetic mean of at least 1.0

Table 1 Summary of the items addressed in the custom-made questionnaire to assess satisfaction with the MR scan and preferences concerning MR scanner design

Item	Range
Preparation and information	Excellent/Good/Satisfactory/Fair/Poor
Concern	Not at all/Very little/Little/High/Very high
Comfort	Excellent/Good/Satisfactory/Fair/Poor
Feeling helpless/embarrassed	Not at all/Little/Moderate/Strong/Very strong
Anxiety	Horizontal visual analogue scale of 10 cm (0-100)
Noise	Horizontal visual analogue scale of 10 cm (0-100)
Pain	Horizontal visual analogue scale of 10 cm (0-100)
Complications	Yes/No/If yes, which complications
Reasons for premature termination (if applicable)	Free text
Reasons for successful completion (if applicable)	Free text
Willingness to undergo future examinations on the MR scanner	Yes/No/Maybe
General satisfaction with the MR scan	Excellent/Good/Satisfactory/Fair/Poor
Summary	
Advantages/Disadvantages of the respective MR scanner	Free text
Ranking of four MR scanners of different design assuming equal diagnostic utility (Figure 1)	1 to 4
Ranking of four MR scanners assuming different diagnostic utility (Figure 1)	1 to 4
Ranking of the two MR scanners used in the study (Figure 2)	1 to 2
Advantages/Disadvantages of the two MR scanners used in the study	Free text

must be reached by rating anxiety on a scale from 0 to 4 for each of 26 items). All patients will have to give written informed consent before randomization.

Sample size and statistical analysis

We expect claustrophobia rates in this high-risk patient cohort of 20% in the control group (recent closed short-bore MR imaging) and 5% in the intervention group (open MR imaging). With 82 evaluable patients per group we will achieve the desired power of 80%. Conservatively taking into account an expected drop-out rate of 5%, a total of 174 patients, 87 per group, have to be allocated.

The assumed claustrophobia rates are based on 1) all previous publications on claustrophobia during MR imaging as summarized [3], 2) an expected prevalence of claustrophobic reactions in conventional MR scanners in the study population of at least 60%, and 3) the ability of both open and the recently designed short-bore but closed MR scanners to significantly reduce claustrophobia preventing MR imaging to approximately 5 and 20%, respectively, as indicated in recent nonrandomized pilot studies [3,13,14].

The primary endpoint, claustrophobia that prevents MR imaging, will be evaluated in the intention-to-treat population using a χ^2 test. Secondary endpoints will be evaluated by parametric or nonparametric analysis of variance or Mantel-Haenszel tests according to scaling. Appropriate parameters of effect size (e.g., odds ratios) with confidence intervals will be calculated. Subgroups (e.g., sex, age groups, direction of scanning [head-first vs. feet-first]) will be analyzed exploratively.

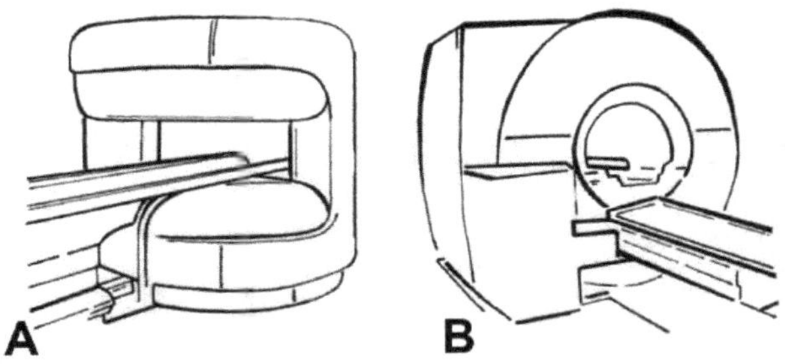

Figure 2 Drawings of the two MR scanners to which patients will be randomized in the study. Panel A shows the open MR scanner with a vertical magnetic field with 1.0-T field strength (Panorama, Philips), up to 26 mT/m gradient strength, acoustic scanner noise of maximum 150 dB(A), and a 0.45 m high and 1.6 m wide patient aperture (0.7 m wide patient table). **Panel B** shows the closed MR scanner with 1.5-T field strength, up to 45 mT/m gradient strength, 97% noise reduction to below 99 dB(A), and a conical shaped wide (0.6 m) and short (1.5 m) bore resembling the gantry of a computed tomography scanner, which has been shown to reduce claustrophobia by a factor of 3 (Magnetom Avanto, Siemens).

Validated questionnaires, MR imaging and need for further improvements

Validated written self-report questionnaires addressing anxiety in general and anxiety related to MR imaging will be used. These include the following: the Spielberger State-Trait Anxiety Inventory [STAI] [18], the "Fragebogen zu körperbezogenen Ängsten, Kognitionen und

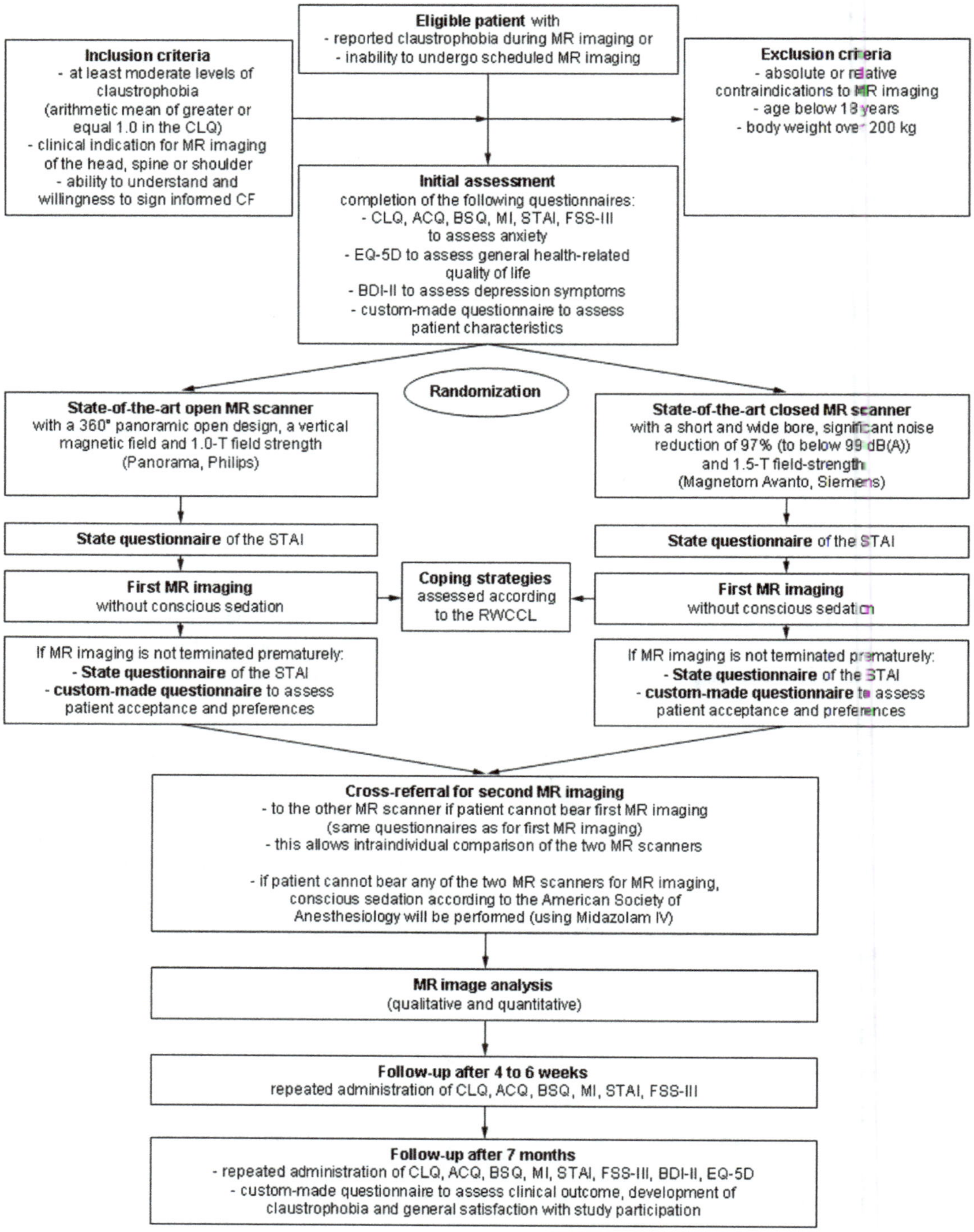

Figure 3 Chart of CLAUSTRO study design. The diagram depicts the randomization procedure, patient flow, and data analysis. **Abbreviations:** AKV = Fragebogen zu körperbezogenen Ängsten, Kognitionen und Vermeidung [19]. BDI-II = Beck Depression Inventory II [24]. CF = Consent Form. CLQ = Claustrophobia Questionnaire [21]. FSS-III = Fear Survey Schedule III [20]. RWCCL = Revised Ways of Coping Checklist [29]. STAI = State-Trait Anxiety Inventory [18].

Vermeidung" [AKV] [19], the Fear Survey Schedule [FSS-III] [20], and the Claustrophobia Questionnaire [CLQ] [21]. Also further nonvalidated custom-designed questionnaires will be used to address patient preferences concerning MR scanner design and which specific scanner design they consider most attractive (Figure 1, Table 1). This information is important to be able to define which further improvements by vendors might be necessary to reduce claustrophobia during MR imaging. Furthermore, patient characteristics, patient satisfaction, clinical outcome, and development of claustrophobia will be addressed (Table 2 and 3). All patients will be asked to again complete some of the questionnaires 4-6 weeks and 7 months after MR imaging. Patients can send back the completed questionnaires to the study coordinator using prepaid envelopes that are sent together with the questionnaires.

Initial assessment

Immediately after enrollment, patients will complete the above-mentioned questionnaires (German versions of STAI [18], AKV [19], FSS-III [20], and CLQ [21]; and a custom-made questionnaire addressing patient characteristics, Table 2). As depression has been shown to influence anxiety-coping in phobic patients [23], and anxiety can be a symptom of depressive disorders, depression symptoms will be explored using the revised Beck Depression Inventory [BDI-II] [24]. General health-related quality of life will be assessed using the EuroQol questionnaire [EQ-5D] [25]. All questionnaires which will be used for initial assessment are described below.

The Claustrophobia Questionnaire [CLQ] [21]

The German version of the Claustrophobia Questionnaire consists of 26 items which assess two separate but related fears hypothesized to comprise claustrophobia: the fear of suffocation (e.g., "having a bad cold and finding it difficult to breathe through your nose") and the fear of restriction (e.g., "locked in a small dark room without windows for 15 min"). For each item anxiety is rated on a scale from 0 (not at all anxious) to 4 (extremely anxious). Summary test scores range from 0 (no anxiety) to 104 (maximum anxiety). The CLQ will be used to determine patients' levels of anxiety toward claustrophobic situations. As an inclusion criterion patients must reach an arithmetic mean of at least 1.0 in the CLQ (equal to a summary score of at least 26) to be eligible for randomization.

The Spielberger State-Trait Anxiety Inventory [STAI] [18]

The German version of the Spielberger State-Trait Anxiety Inventory is based on two questionnaires (State

Table 2 Summary of items addressed in the custom-made questionnaire for initial assessment

Item	Range
School graduation	German secondary schools (Hauptschule, Realschule, Gesamtschule)/Grammar school/ GDR schools (EOS, POS)
Leaving school after grade	Free text
Last or current profession	If not employed: Pensioner/Unemployed
Gross family income per month	€0-500/500-1000/1000-1500/1500-2000/2000-2500/2500-3000/3000-4000/4000-5000/> 5000
Marital status	Single/Living with partner/Married/Divorced/Living apart/Single mother or father/ Widowed
Number of Children/Number of children under 18 years	Free text
Current extent of claustrophobia	Horizontal visual analogue scale of 10 cm (0-100)
Claustrophobia during MR imaging in the past	Yes/No/If yes description
Claustrophobia preventing prior scheduled MR imaging	Yes/No/If yes description
When did claustrophobic anxiety occur for the first time	Free text
Ideas or strategies to cope with anxiety before and during MR imaging	Yes/No/If yes description*
Belief in successful completion of MR imaging (self-efficacy)	Yes/No/Maybe
Fear of diagnostic findings by MR imaging	Yes/No
Medication	Yes/No/If yes which drugs and dosage
Psychosomatic or psychiatric diseases	Yes/No/If yes which diseases
Previous or current psychotherapy	Yes/No/If yes what kind and how long

*Coping strategies will be categorized according to the Revised Ways of Coping Checklist (RWCCL) [29].

Abbreviations:

EOS = "Erweiterte Oberschule".

GDR = German Democratic Republic.

POS = "Polytechnische Oberschule".

Table 3 Summary of items addressed in the custom-made follow-up questionnaire

Item	Range
Examination, Result, Treatment	
MR findings have revealed the reason for current medical condition (from patients' point of view)	Yes/No
The diagnostic findings obtained by MR imaging have already been known	Yes/No
The diagnostic findings have led to consequences in treatment	Yes/No/If Yes: Conservative treatment/Surgery/Other (patients are asked to add the medical report or the name of the attendant doctor/hospital)
Additional diagnostic findings by other examinations	Yes/No/If yes, which diagnoses (patients are asked to add the medical report or the name of the attendant doctor/hospital)
Improvement of medical condition during the last 7 months	Yes/No/If yes: Without treatment/After treatment/After another measure
Claustrophobia	
Current extent of claustrophobia	Horizontal visual analogue scale of 10 cm (0-100)
Attempts to alleviate claustrophobia during the last 7 months	Yes/No/If yes: Psychotherapy/Drugs/Own problem-solving methods
Willingness to start therapy if possible	Yes/No
Time willing to investigate in ambulant or stationary therapy	Nothing/Up to how much time per month/year
Money willing to investigate in therapy (in addition to health insurance contribution)	Nothing/Up to how much money per month/year
Satisfaction	
Initial assessment and information about the study	Very good/Good/Satisfactory/Fair/Not at all
Option to see the MR scanners prior to imaging	Very good/Good/Satisfactory/Fair/Not at all
Information about MR imaging	Very good/Good/Satisfactory/Fair/Not at all
MR imaging	Very good/Good/Satisfactory/Fair/Not at all
Delivery of diagnostic findings	Very good/Good/Satisfactory/Fair/Not at all
Further MR imaging	Yes/No/If Yes, of which anatomical region and why
Hypothetical willingness to take part in the study again	Yes/No
Willingness to undergo another MR imaging at the Department of Radiology at Charité Berlin	Yes/No
Would you recommend others to have a scheduled MR imaging at the Department of Radiology at Charité Berlin	Yes/No
Requests, comments, criticism	Free text

and Trait), each with 20 items to be rated on a scale from 1 (almost never) to 4 (very much so). The items are short statements, e.g., "I feel nervous and restless". The State questionnaire consists of 10 positive and 10 negative items which assess the current state of anxiety. The Trait questionnaire consists of 13 positive and 7 negative items assessing the general state of anxiety. Summary test scores range from 20 (no anxiety) to 80 (maximum anxiety).

The Fear Survey Schedule [FSS-III] [20]

The Fear Survey Schedule was originally developed to assess change in phobic behavior and generalized anxiety in conditioning therapy. The revised and extended FSS-III has been designed for clinical use. The version of the FSS-III used here consists of 78 items measuring fear, phobic behavior, and generalized anxiety. Each item is a phrase of 2-6 words (e.g., "Being in an elevator") for which a person rates anxiety on a scale from 1 (not at all) to 4 (very much). There are 6 subclassifications of fear in the FSS-III: animal fears (9 items), social and interpersonal fears (18 items), fears of tissue damage, illness, death and their associations (19 items), noise fears (4 items), other classical phobias (20 items), and miscellaneous fears such as strange places, falling, failure, imaginary creatures, strange shapes, feeling angry, dull weather, or making mistakes (8 items). According to Lukins et al. 9 items of the FSS reflect a range of aversive characteristics of the MR imaging procedure: vacuum cleaner noise, being alone, loud noises, being in an elevator, enclosed places, and journeys by airplane [26]. Summary fear scores range from 0 to 312.

The „Fragebogen zu körperbezogenen Ängsten, Kognitionen und Vermeidung [AKV]" [19]

The AKV is the German version of the Body Sensations Questionnaire (BSQ), the Agoraphobic Cognitions Questionnaire (ACQ), and the Mobility Inventory (MI) of Chambless et al. [27]. The AKV consists of three systems for the diagnosis of anxiety and somatoform disorders. Each system assesses different symptoms of anxiety and somatoform disorders:

- The "Fragebogen zur Angst vor körperlichen Symptomen" (BSQ, German version) explores the fear of body sensations as internal triggers of anxiety. The questionnaire consists of 17 items (e.g., "heart palpitations") for which anxiety is rated on a scale from 1 (not at all) to 5 (extremely). Summary scores range from 17 to 85. Patients will be asked to report which three of the 17 body sensations occur most frequently when they are anxious or nervous.
- The "Fragebogen zu angstbezogenen Kognitionen" (ACQ, German version) explores the tendency to catastrophizing cognitions and apprehensions which can come along with body sensations. There are two subscales: the "loss of control" subscale (e.g., "I am going to go crazy") and the "physiological consequences" subscale (e.g., "I will have a heart attack"), each with 7 items. For all items occurrence in situations of anxiety is rated on a scale from 1 (never) to 5 (always). Summary scores range from 14 to 70. Patients will be asked to report which three of the 14 cognitions occur most frequently when they are anxious or nervous.
- The "Mobilitätsinventar" (MI, German version) explores the extent and complexity of phobic avoidance behavior referring to external triggers of anxiety. The questionnaire consists of 27 items describing the most important agoraphobic situations (e.g., "elevators"). For each item avoidance is rated twice for "being alone" and "in company" on a scale from 1 (never) to 5 (always). Summary scores range from 54 to 270.

The Beck Depression Inventory (BDI-II) [24]

The Beck Depression Inventory is one of the most widely used self-report measures of depression. The German version of the revised Beck Depression Inventory (BDI-II) consists of 21 items comprising the diagnostic criteria for Major Depressive Disorder according to the Diagnostic and Statistical Manual of Mental Disorders [28]. Patients have to rate how they have been feeling for the past two weeks. Each of the 21 items corresponds to a symptom of depression (e.g., concentration difficulty, loss of energy). On 19 items there are 4 statements assessing different severity codes of a symptom (ranging from 0-3). On two items (16 and 18) there are 7 options (though ranging from 0-3) to assess an increase or decrease of appetite and sleep. A summary score of 0-13 is considered minimal depression, 14-19 mild depression, 20-28 moderate depression, and 29-63 severe depression.

The EuroQol (EQ-5D) [25]

The EuroQol is a generic non-disease-specific instrument for valuing general health-related quality of life. The questionnaire includes single item measures of five health dimensions: mobility, self-care, daily activities, pain and discomfort, anxiety and depression. Each item has three response options (no problem, some or moderate problems, extreme problems) to rate patients' perceived health status. In addition, the EuroQol includes a vertical visual analogue scale ranging from 0 (worst imaginable) to 100 (best imaginable) to rate the current state of health.

Custom-made questionnaire for initial assessment

The custom-made questionnaire for initial assessment addresses patient characteristics such as marital status, gross family income, and claustrophobia during previous MR imaging. The items addressed here are summarized in Table 2.

MR imaging and image analysis

MR imaging

MR imaging will be performed in the supine position using phased-array coils. On the open MR scanner the following coils will be used: a large body coil for imaging of the spine, a small flex coil for imaging of the shoulder, and, to alleviate the feeling of confinement, the neck coil will be used for imaging of the head (in an upside-down position) making use of the elliptical coil design available. If the neck coil is not tolerated for head imaging on the open MR scanner, a multipurpose flex coil can be used as a second alternative. On the closed short-bore MR scanner the spine-array coils that are integrated into the table will be used for imaging of the spine, a small 1-channel circular polarized flex coil will be used for imaging of the shoulder, and a 12-channel bird-cage head coil will be used for imaging of the head. For imaging of the cervical spine, the shoulder, and the head, patients will be examined head-first on both scanners because feet-first imaging, which alleviates claustrophobia by a factor of more than 10 [3], is not possible for these diagnostic questions. For lumbar spine imaging, a feet-first approach can and thus will be utilized on both scanners. Contrast-enhanced sequences will only be obtained if clinically indicated. On the following pages the MR sequences and their characteristics are listed allowing a convenient comparison of the sequence approaches used on both MR scanners for imaging of the head, spine (cervicothoracic, and thoracolumbar), and shoulder (Tables 4, 5, 6, and 7). For detailed information on the sequence characteristics see Additional files 1, 2, 3, and 4. The primary aim of the sequence setup is to obtain a voxel size that is as similar as possible on both scanners. Differences in acquisition time might result from this aim due to different field strengths and gradients.

To assess patients' anxiety before and during MR imaging the State questionnaire of the State-Trait Anxiety Inventory will be used directly before and after MR imaging. The questionnaire which will be used after imaging

Table 4 Head MR imaging sequences*

	Magnetom Avanto	Panorama
Basic Sequences		
Generic sequence name	T1w SE axial	
Vendor sequence name	T1 SE tra	T1w SE
Resulting voxel size (mm)	0.9 × 0.9 × 5.0	0.9 × 0.9 × 5.0
Acquisition time (min:sec)	3:48	4:13
Generic sequence name	PD+T2w TSE axial	
Vendor sequence name	PD+T2 TSE tra	Dual TSE
Resulting voxel size (mm)	0.9 × 0.9 × 5.0	0.9 × 1.0 × 5.0
Acquisition time (min:sec)	3:50	4:15
Generic sequence name	TIRM axial	
Vendor sequence name	T2 TIRM tra dark-fl	T2w FLAIR
Resulting voxel size (mm)	0.9 × 0.9 × 5.0	0.9 × 1.0 × 5.0
Acquisition time (min:sec)	3:38	6:36
Optional Sequences**		
Generic sequence name	DWI axial	
Vendor sequence name	Ep2 D diff3 scan trace	DWI
Resulting voxel size (mm)	1.8 × 1.8 × 5.0	1.9 × 1.9 × 5.0
Acquisition time (min:sec)	0:48	0:58
Generic sequence name	T2w Star axial	
Vendor sequence name	T2 fl2 D tra hemo	T2w FFE
Resulting voxel size (mm)	0.9 × 0.9 × 5.0	0.9 × 0.9 × 5.0
Acquisition time (min:sec)	3:01	5:08
Generic sequence name	T1w MPRAGE post contrast agent	
Vendor sequence name	T1 fl3Dsag	T1w 3 D FFE
Resulting voxel size (mm)	0.9 × 0.9 × 1.0	1.0 × 1.2 × 1.0
Acquisition time (min:sec)	6:49	7:44

*For further information on the sequence characteristics see Additional file 1.

**These sequences will only be acquired if a clinical indication (e.g., for contrast-enhanced T1-weighted sequences) exists. In all patients, however, the basic sequences listed above will be obtained.

Abbreviations:

Dual = Double Echo.

DWI = Diffusion-Weighted Imaging.

EPI = Echo Planar Imaging.

FFE = Fast Field Echo.

FLAIR = FLuid Attenuation Inversion Recovery.

MPRAGE = Magnetization Prepared RApid Gradient Echo.

PD = Proton Density.

Sag = sagittal.

SE = Spin Echo.

T1w = T1-weighted.

T2w = T2-weighted.

TIRM = Turbo Inversion Recovery Measurement.

Tra = transverse.

TSE = Turbo Spin Echo.

Table 5 Cervicothoracic spine MR imaging sequences*

	Magnetom Avanto	Panorama
Basic Sequences		
Generic sequence name	T2w sagittal	
Vendor sequence name	T2 TSE rst sag	T2w TSE
Resulting voxel size (mm)	0.9 × 1.0 × 3.0	1.1 × 1.1 × 3.0
Acquisition time (min:sec)	3:25	5:09
Generic sequence name	T1w sagittal	
Vendor sequence name	T1 TSE sag	T1w TSE
Resulting voxel size (mm)	1.0 × 1.5 × 3.0	1.1 × 1.5 × 3.0
Acquisition time (min:sec)	4:01	4:15
Generic sequence name	T2w axial	
Vendor sequence name	T2 me2 D tra	3 D mFFE
Resulting voxel size (mm)	1.0 × 1.0 × 3.0	1.0 × 1.0 × 3.0
Acquisition time (min:sec)	6:53	7:38
Optional Sequences**		
Generic sequence name	TIRM	
Vendor sequence name	TIRM	STIR TSE
Resulting voxel size (mm)	1.2 × 1.5 × 3.0	1.2 × 1.7 × 3.0
Acquisition time (min:sec)	5:42	5:56
Generic sequence name	T1w sagittal post contrast agent	
Vendor sequence name	T1 TSE sag	T1w TSE
Resulting voxel size (mm)	1.5 × 1.0 × 3.0	1.1 × 1.5 × 3.0
Acquisition time (min:sec)	4:01	4:15
Generic sequence name	T1w axial post contrast agent	
Vendor sequence name	T1 TSE tra	T1w TSE
Resulting voxel size (mm)	1.0 × 1.2 × 3.0	1.0 × 1.2 × 3.0
Acquisition time (min:sec)	2:16	4:12

*For further information on the sequence characteristics see Additional file 2.

**These sequences will only be acquired if a clinical indication (e.g., for contrast-enhanced T1-weighted sequences) exists. In all patients, however, the basic sequences listed above will be obtained.

Abbreviations:

FFE = Fast Field Echo.

Me = medic.

Sag = sagittal.

STIR = Short T1 Inversion Recovery.

T1w = T1-weighted.

T2w = T2-weighted.

TIRM = Turbo Inversion Recovery Magnitude.

Tra = transverse.

TSE = Turbo Spin Echo.

is reworded in the past tense to assess patients' anxiety during the MR scan. This questionnaire will not be administered if the MR procedure is terminated before starting the scan (Figure 3).

Patients' strategies to cope with their anxiety will be assessed according to the Revised Ways of Coping Checklist (RWCCL) [29]. The RWCCL is a self-report measure of coping which is based on Lazarus' transactional model of stress [30]. The questionnaire consists of five scales: problem-focused coping (15 items, e.g., "made a plan of action and followed it"), wishful thinking (8 items, e.g., "daydreamed or imagined a better time or place than the one I was in"), seeks social support (6 items, e.g.,"talked to others and accepted their sympathy"), avoidance (10 items, e.g., "tried to make myself feel better by eating, drinking, smoking, taking medications") and blamed self (3 items, e.g., "blamed yourself). The RWCCL will not be used as a self-report measure, but instead coping strategies will be assessed by a study assistant, who will not influence interactions between patients and radiology technicians

Table 6 Thoracolumbar spine MR imaging sequences*

	Magnetom Avanto	Panorama
Basic Sequences		
Generic sequence name	T2w sagittal	
Vendor sequence name	T2 TSE rst sag	T2w TSE
Resulting voxel size (mm)	0.9 × 1.0 × 3.0	1.1 × 1.1 × 3.0
Acquisition time (min:sec)	3:25	5:09
Generic sequence name	T1w sagittal	
Vendor sequence name	T1 TSE sag	T1w TSE
Resulting voxel size (mm)	1.0 × 1.5 × 3.0	1.1 × 1.5 × 3.0
Acquisition time (min:sec)	4:01	4:15
Generic sequence name	T2w axial	
Vendor sequence name	T2 TSE rst tra	T2w TSE
Resulting voxel size (mm)	0.6 × 0.8 × 4.0	0.7 × 0.8 × 4.0
Acquisition time (min:sec)	2:23	2:45
Optional Sequences**		
Generic sequence name	TIRM sagittal	
Vendor sequence name	TIRM sag	STIR TSE
Resulting voxel size (mm)	1.2 × 1.5 × 3.0	1.2 × 1.7 × 3.0
Acquisition time (min:sec)	5:42	5:56
Generic sequence name	T1w sagittal post contrast agent	
Vendor sequence name	T1 TSE sag	T1w TSE
Resulting voxel size (mm)	1.0 × 1.5 × 3.0	1.1 × 1.5 × 3.0
Acquisition time (min:sec)	4:01	4:15
Generic sequence name	T1w axial post contrast agent	
Vendor sequence name	T1 TSE tra	T1w TSE
Resulting voxel size (mm)	1.0 × 1.2 × 4.0	1.0 × 1.2 × 4.0
Acquisition time (min:sec)	3:22	3:30

*For further information on the sequence characteristics see Additional file 3.

**These sequences will only be acquired if a clinical indication (e.g., for contrast-enhanced T1-weighted sequences) exists. In all patients, however, the basic sequences listed above will be obtained.

Abbreviations:

Sag = sagittal.

STIR = Short T1 Inversion Recovery.

T1w = T1-weighted.

T2w = T2-weighted.

TIRM = Turbo Inversion Recovery Magnitude.

Tra = transverse.

TSE = Turbo Spin Echo.

Table 7 Shoulder MR imaging sequences*

	Magnetom Avanto	Panorama
Basic Sequences		
Generic sequence name	T1w axial	
Vendor sequence name	T1 tra	T1w TSE
Resulting voxel size (mm)	0.9 × 0.7 × 3.5	0.7 × 0.9 × 3.5
Acquisition time (min:sec)	2:17	2:47
Generic sequence name	T2w axial	
Vendor sequence name	T2 me2 D tra	3 D mFFE WATS
Resulting voxel size (mm)	0.7 × 1.0 × 3.5	0.7 × 1.0 × 3.5
Acquisition time (min:sec)	3:19	7:11
Generic sequence name	TIRM coronal	
Vendor sequence name	T1 TIRM cor	STIR
Resulting voxel size (mm)	0.6 × 0.8 × 4.0	0.6 × 0.9 × 4.0
Acquisition time (min:sec)	5:15	6:36
Generic sequence name	PD+T2w TSE coronal	
Vendor sequence name	PD+T2 TSE cor	Dual dr tsetse
Resulting voxel size (mm)	0.6 × 0.8 × 4.0	0.6 × 0.8 × 4.0
Acquisition time (min:sec)	4:16	5:59
Generic sequence name	T2w TSE parasagittal	
Vendor sequence name	T2 TSE rst fs parasag	T2 TSE SPIR
Resulting voxel size (mm)	0.7 × 0.9 × 4.0	0.7 × 0.9 × 4.0
Acquisition time (min:sec)	4:04	4:52

*For further information on the sequence characteristics see Additional file 4.

Abbreviations:

Cor = coronal.

Dual = Double echo.

FFE = Fast Field Echo.

Me = medic.

Parasag = parasagittal.

PD = Proton Density.

Sag = sagittal.

SPIR = Spectral Presaturation Inversion Recovery.

STIR = Short T1 Inversion Recovery.

T1w = T1-weighted.

T2w = T2-weighted.

TIRM = Turbo Inversion Recovery Magnitude.

Tra = transverse.

TSE = Turbo Spin Echo.

WATS = WATer only Selection.

(radiographers). Items not conforming to MR imaging will be excluded from this questionnaire.

Furthermore, a study assistant will record important information in an MR imaging questionnaire: scan duration, claustrophobic events, the anatomical region examined, the use of optional sequences and/or contrast agent, the names of all staff members interacting with the patient, assistance by the staff, any complications or interruption during the scan, the kind of ear protection (headphones, earplugs or none on the noise-reduced MR scanner) as well as sedation information.

MR image analysis

MR images will be analyzed by two blinded readers on a workstation (Centricity PACS Workstation RA 1000, GE Healthcare). Details of the MR image analysis can be found in the image analysis forms (Additional files 5, 6, and 7).

Qualitative image analysis will be performed via grading from 1 to 5. The scale will be 1 = optimal, 2 = good, 3 = moderate, 4 = poor, 5 = nondiagnostic to rate contrast, contour sharpness, and overall image quality and 1 = none, 2 = minimal, 3 = moderate, 4 = major, 5 = nondiagnostic to rate artifacts and noise. Artifacts will be classified as being due to motion, pulsation, metal, noise, or other. In shoulder imaging the fatty infiltration grade of cuff muscles will be determined on a scale from 0 to 4 (0 = no fat, 1 = a few streaks of fat, 2 = more muscle than fat, 3 = as much muscle as fat, 4 = more fat than muscle) according to Goutallier et al. [31], and the grade of muscle atrophy of cuff muscles will be determined on a scale from 0 to 4 (0 = none, 2 = mild, 3 = moderate, 4 = severe) according to Warner et al. [32]. In addition, the permitted diagnostic quality of assessment of rotator cuff muscles and their ligaments (coronal imaging) and the glenoid labrum (axial imaging) will be determined via grading from 0 to 5 (1 = optimal, 2 = good, 3 = moderate, 4 = poor and 5 = nondiagnostic).

Quantitative image analysis will be performed via measurements of signal intensities (SI) in circular regions of interest (ROI) ranging in size from 0.02 up to 0.4 cm^2 standardized according to the anatomy. Mean values and standard deviations will be calculated for each measurement in each standard sequence of either head, spine, or shoulder MR imaging. Standard deviations (SD) of the ROI signals will be used to measure noise, and signal-to-noise and contrast-to-noise ratios were calculated as recently described [33]. Furthermore, contour clarity will be analyzed as recently described [34], using ImageJ http://rsbweb.nih.gov/ij/. Contour clarity in head imaging will be distinguished between corticospinal fluid, caudate nucleus, and genu of corpus callosum. In spine imaging, contour clarity will be determined for gray and white matter of the spinal cord, corticospinal fluid, and vertebral body. In shoulder imaging, it will be determined for joint fluid and glenoid labrum (axial images), for fat and muscle (deltoideus), and for bone marrow (humerus head).

Need for further improvements

A custom-made questionnaire will be used to track certain features of the MR procedure (e.g., pain and noise) and patient preferences concerning MR scanner design and which specific scanner design patients consider most attractive (Figure 1). This information is important to be able to define which further improvements by vendors might be necessary to reduce claustrophobic reactions during MR imaging. In Table 1 we have summarized the main objectives addressed in this questionnaire.

Follow-up after 4 to 6 weeks

At the initial follow-up, the STAI [18], AKV [19], FSS-III [20], and CLQ [21] questionnaires will be repeated. The State questionnaire of the STAI will be repeated in two versions assessing the current state of anxiety and the state of anxiety during MR imaging (if accomplished without sedation).

Follow-up after 7 months

At the final follow-up, the STAI [18], AKV [19], FSS-III [20], CLQ [21], BDI-II [24], and EuroQol [25] questionnaires will be repeated. The State questionnaire of the STAI will be repeated in two versions assessing the current state of anxiety and the state of anxiety during MR imaging (if accomplished without sedation). Moreover, a custom-made questionnaire will be administered to assess clinical outcome, development of claustrophobic anxiety, and general satisfaction with the study participation. The items addressed here are summarized in Table 3.

Discussion

Patients with claustrophobic anxiety, who are more likely to be frightened during MR imaging, have been reported to experience claustrophobia in up to 35% of all examinations [6]. To complete the scan, conscious sedation and additional sequences (after sedation) may be necessary in these patients. This situation involves significant risks of adverse events [7-9] and is associated with additional costs because it reduces workflow, limits patient acceptance, and wastes valuable scanning time and thus induces costs. On the other hand, prematurely terminated scans as well mean an important financial loss for the health care system. Improved patient comfort during MR imaging (mainly reduction of noise and sensation of confinement) appears to be essential to avoid claustrophobic reactions [10,11].

A more patient-centered design of closed MR systems is one effective approach to make MR imaging more comfortable for patients. Few studies have investigated patient acceptance and the potential to reduce claustrophobic anxiety of recent closed MR scanners with noise reduction and short- and wide-bore design in comparison to conventional MR scanners.

In a large cohort study of 55,734 outpatients, Dewey et al. assessed the potential to reduce claustrophobia of a recent 1.5-T MR scanner with 97% noise reduction and a short- and wide-bore design [3]. Patients were examined on either the recent or a conventional MR scanner. The recent MR scanner was shown to reduce claustrophobia by a factor of 3, although there were more head-first examinations on that scanner. Intraindividual comparisons of patients who underwent imaging on both MR units showed similar results with a claustrophobia rate of below 1% [3].

In a retrospective study on the occurrence of claustrophobia in 5,682 patients examined on either a 1.5-T closed MR scanner or a 0.5-T noise-reduced MR scanner with a short and wide bore Dantendorfer et al. found no significant difference between the two MR units [35]. However, there was a selection bias because staff was referring highly anxious patients to the recent MR scanner. Thus, the authors conclude that the short-bore MR scanner may in fact reduce claustrophobia [35]. In a later study by Dantendorfer et al., 297 patients without MR imaging experience were randomly examined on either a 1.5-T closed MR scanner or a recent

0.5-T noise-reduced MR scanner with a short and wide bore [36]. Anxiety before and after the scan was among others assessed using the State questionnaire of the STAI. Although patients felt more at ease in the recent MR scanner (concerning noise and confinement), there was no significant difference in patient acceptance and occurrence of motion artifacts. Interestingly, there was no correlation between STAI scores and motion artifacts, but patients who were more concerned about the technical apparatus had more motion artifacts [36].

Another approach to improve patient acceptance of MR imaging is a more open vertical scanner configuration, although until recently such systems operated at rather low field strengths (0.2 T), resulting in poor image quality.

Heuck et al. compared two high-field closed MR systems operating at 1.5-T and 1.0-T with an open whole-body scanner and a dedicated extremity MR system, both operating at 0.2-T [37]. In 40 patients examined on each system (160 total) they found a mainly positive condition and acceptance for all MR scanners. However, patients who were examined on the open MR scanners felt significantly more confident and calm, despite longer examination durations. Patients' suggestions for improvement of the high-field closed MR systems mainly concerned reduction of noise and enlargement of the bore. Nevertheless, these authors concluded that the necessary technical conditions and not differences in patient preference should be crucial for the choice of an MR system [37].

In a recent pilot study Bangard et al. have examined 36 claustrophobic and 36 non-claustrophobic patients on a recently introduced open MR scanner with high-field strength (1.0 T) [14]. Anxiety was assessed using validated questionnaires (STAI, CLQ, MRI FSS [26]). In the claustrophobic patients scan termination rate was reduced to 8% compared to 58.3% in previous examinations on conventional MR systems, and 91.7% preferred the open MR scanner. Furthermore, claustrophobia did not reduce image quality by motion artifacts [14].

A 0.5-T interventional MR scanner with a vertical gap in the bore of the magnet ("double donut") was used in a study by Spouse et al. [13]. 96% of 50 claustrophobic patients who were unable to complete a conventional MR scan successfully underwent MR imaging on the interventional scanner. Patients reported less anxiety than during their previous MR imaging and felt significantly better informed about the procedure. However, friends or relatives were allowed to stay in the magnet room and many patients indicated that this, beside the scanner design, had helped them considerably [13].

In contrast to the above mentioned studies, the CLAUSTRO trial will directly compare an open MR scanner with a vertical 1.0-T magnetic field, and a closed noise-reduced MR scanner with a short- and wide-bore design and 1.5-T field strength in regards to claustrophobia and image quality as well as influence on further clinical management in a randomized controlled trial. Patients included will have at least moderate levels of claustrophobic anxiety, experienced claustrophobia during a prior MR imaging or rejected a current scheduled MR imaging due to claustrophobia, and will have a clinical indication for MR imaging and will thus be at high risk to experience claustrophobia during the MR scan. Anxiety will be assessed before and after MR imaging as well as 4-6 weeks and 7 months after the scan in order to address the development of claustrophobia. Increase of claustrophobic anxiety has been found if the scan is terminated prematurely or high anxiety is tolerated [26,38-40]. On the other hand, there are reports of decreased anxiety after completed MR imaging [40,41]. Long-term alleviation of claustrophobia after completed MR imaging might support the potential of exposure therapy to treat claustrophobia [42,43]. To perform the comparison of image quality as reliable as possible the anatomical regions to be examined will be limited to head, spine and shoulder, and equal sequences on both scanners with comparable voxel sizes will be utilized. Diagnostic utility and clinical outcome will be assessed 7 months after MR imaging which is an appropriate time-frame to detect an influence on clinical management. Of course this will be mediated through the patients and referring physicians' response to MR results. Furthermore, the study will address which specific scanner design is evaluated by patients to be the most attractive and which further improvements in designing MR scanners should be followed by manufacturers. Randomization will be done as the most decisive evidence for judging the efficacy of diagnostic tests comes from randomized comparisons in which the controlled design obviates the biases of observational studies [15,16]. Patients who are assigned to imaging in one MR scanner but cannot bear this procedure due to claustrophobic anxiety will be cross-referred to imaging in the other scanner in order to preclude adverse events associated with sedation [7-9]. This will also allow direct comparison of the two options in those patients as an ancillary study. Due to its design this trial will also be able to analyze and compare the cost-effectiveness of the two MR scanners.

Study limitations

Anxiety during MR imaging can occur due to several other psychosomatic or psychiatric disorders than claustrophobia e.g., panic disorder, adjustment disorder with anxious mood, or major depression [10]. Within the limits of the study, claustrophobia will not be diagnosed according to ICD-10 or DSM-IV criteria [28,44].

Furthermore, there are several features of MR imaging and the patient which can contribute to anxiety beyond confinement by the MR scanner. Such features may be pain, loud noise, the unknown, concerns about diagnostic findings, having to lie still, the examination duration, uncomfortable temperature or the MR scanner itself [5,11,45-47]. Several studies have shown that especially pain is correlated with anxiety during the scan and premature termination [11,38,40]. However, claustrophobia will be assessed using the CLQ [21], and reaching a specific score is an inclusion criterion (an arithmetic mean of greater or equal 1.0 must be reached by rating anxiety on a scale from 1 to 4 for each of 26 items). Furthermore, a custom-made questionnaire addressing prior claustrophobic events before or during scheduled MR imaging and first occurrence of claustrophobia will be fulfilled by a study assistant in the manner of a structured interview. Further questionnaires will help to examine generalized anxiety, patients' health status (including pain) and depression symptoms. The pain and noise levels which patients experience during MR imaging will be assessed directly after the scan by using horizontal visual analogue scales and patients will be asked to report whether they are afraid of diagnostic findings in MR imaging. Claustrophobia as part of e.g., a panic disorder is no exclusion criterion. However, patients will be asked to report whether they have known psychosomatic or psychiatric disorders. In general, in the majority of articles addressing anxiety leading to premature termination of MR imaging, anxiety is referred to as "claustrophobia" [5]. For the assessment of anxiety during MR imaging it is also important to know whether patients take any anxiolytic or sedative drugs or other psychotropics which will thus be examined. Different examination times (due to different sequence duration, anxiety or complications) and different coils will also be assessed.

Another feature of MR imaging whose influence on patients' condition will be difficult to measure is the support by nursing stuff, radiographers and physicians. Several studies have shown the importance of social support and the appreciation of a caring attitude of others by anxious patients [13,47-49]. It might yet influence patients to know that staff is aware of their anxiety and the staff may act more caring because of this awareness. However, patients' seeking social support will be assessed by evaluating coping strategies and patients will be asked to report what did particularly help them to cope with their anxiety. Furthermore, the staff will be instructed not to be "overprotective" and not to suggest coping strategies to the patients. Of course, patients will experience more attendance than in clinical routine. To keep the influence as constant as possible, patients will mainly be attended by two female staff members throughout the study and there will be a limited number of physicians and radiographers who perform MR imaging.

With regard to the comparison of image quality, the primary aim of the sequence set-up is to obtain a voxel size that is as similar as possible on both MR scanners. Thus, compromises have to be made concerning the best possible image quality still providing comparability. Motion artifacts due to anxiety might also play a role [45,50] but should be obviated by the high number of patients and randomization.

Concerning the closed MR scanner with short- and wide-bore design which will be used in this study, it should be mentioned that there are scanners with even shorter and wider bores like the Siemens Magnetom Espree with 0,7 m diameter and 1,25 m length of the scanner bore. However, this improvement in scanner design affects the image quality which can be achieved with this MR scanner.

Conclusions

This randomized controlled trial will be the first direct comparison of open vertical and closed short-bore MR systems in regards to claustrophobia and image quality as well as diagnostic utility. If an open MR scanner can be shown to reduce claustrophobia in a randomized comparison it might be justified to recommend this approach for routine clinical application in certain high-risk anxiety patients or in certain imaging centers. Furthermore, it is the first study to address which specific scanner design is evaluated by patients to be the most attractive for imaging. This knowledge is important to be able to define which further improvements by the vendors might be necessary to reduce claustrophobic reactions. Accordingly, this randomized trial has the potential to influence both the clinical and economical utilization and impact of MR imaging.

Additional material

Additional file 1: Appendix Table S1. Further information on head MR imaging sequences used.

Additional file 2: Appendix Table S2. Further information on cervicothoracic spine MR imaging sequences used.

Additional file 3: Appendix Table S3. Further information on thoracolumbar spine MR imaging sequences used.

Additional file 4: Appendix Table S4. Further information on shoulder MR imaging sequences used.

Additional file 5: Appendix Figure S1. MR image analysis form for quantitative and qualitative analysis of head imaging.

Additional file 6: Appendix Figure S2. MR image analysis form for quantitative and qualitative analysis of spine imaging.

Additional file 7: Appendix Figure S3. MR imaging analysis form for quantitative and qualitative analysis of shoulder imaging.

Author details

[1]Departments of Radiology, Charité, Medical School, Humboldt Universität zu Berlin and Freie Universität Berlin, Germany. [2]Departments of Biostatistics and Clinical Epidemiology, Charité, Medical School, Humboldt Universität zu Berlin and Freie Universität Berlin, Germany. [3]Divisions of Neuroradiology, Charité, Medical School, Humboldt Universität zu Berlin and Freie Universität Berlin, Germany. [4]Departments of Clinical Psychology, Charité, Medical School, Humboldt Universität zu Berlin and Freie Universität Berlin, Germany.

Authors' contributions

JE, EZ, and MD drafted the manuscript and participated in the design of the study and its coordination. MR participated in the design of the study and its coordination and helped to draft the manuscript. PM provided statistical expertise and participated in the design of the study. RK, PA, CK, GD, TB, UT, and BH gave administrative, technical, or logistic support and critically revised the article for important intellectual content. MD conceived the study. All authors read and approved the final manuscript.

Competing interests

Dr. Dewey reported receiving grant support from GE Healthcare, Bracco, Guerbet, the European Funds for Regional Development (EFRE), the German Heart Foundation/German Foundation of Heart Research, and Toshiba Medical Systems and lecture fees from Toshiba Medical Systems, Cardiac MR Academy Berlin, Guerbet, and Bayer-Schering; he is also a consultant for Guerbet. Dr. Rief reported receiving travel reimbursement from CMC contrast. Dr. Teichgräber reported grant support from the Technology Foundation Berlin, Philips Medical Systems, and EFRE. Prof. Hamm reported receiving grant support from GE Healthcare, Schering, Siemens Medical Solutions, and Toshiba Medical Systems, and lecture fees from Siemens Medical Solutions and Bayer-Schering. Furthermore, there are institutional master research agreements with Philips Medical Systems, Siemens Medical Solutions, and Toshiba Medical Systems. These funding sources had no role in the collection, analysis, or interpretation of the data or in the decision to submit the manuscript for publication. The other authors reported no financial disclosures.

References

1. Fuchs VR, Sox HC Jr: **Physicians' views of the relative importance of thirty medical innovations.** *Health Aff (Millwood)* 2001, **20**:30-42.
2. Hailey D: **Open magnetic resonance imaging (MRI) scanners.** *Issues Emerg Health Technol* 2006, 1-4.
3. Dewey M, Schink T, Dewey CF: **Claustrophobia During Magnetic Resonance Imaging: Cohort Study in Over 55,000 Patients.** *J Magnet Reson Imag* 2007, **26**:1322-27.
4. Kortepeter MG: **MRI: my resonant image.** *Ann Intern Med* 1991, **115**:749-50.
5. Melendez JC, McCrank E: **Anxiety-related reactions associated with magnetic resonance imaging examinations.** *JAMA* 1993, **270**:745-7.
6. Brennan SC, Redd WH, Jacobsen PB, Schorr O, Heelan RT, Sze GK, Krol G, Peters BE, Morrissey JK: **Anxiety and panic during magnetic resonance scans.** *Lancet* 1988, **2**:512.
7. Bluemke DA, Breiter SN: **Sedation procedures in MR imaging: safety, effectiveness, and nursing effect on examinations.** *Radiology* 2000, **216**:645-52.
8. Malviya S, Voepel-Lewis T, Eldevik OP, Rockwell DT, Wong JH, Tait AR: **Sedation and general anaesthesia in children undergoing MRI and CT: adverse events and outcomes.** *Br J Anaesth* 2000, **84**:743-8.
9. Berlin L: **Sedation and analgesia in MR imaging.** *AJR Am J Roentgenol* 2001, **177**:293-6.
10. Flaherty JA, Hoskinson K: **Emotional distress during magnetic resonance imaging.** *N Engl J Med* 1989, **320**:467-8.
11. Katz RC, Wilson L, Frazer N: **Anxiety and its determinants in patients undergoing magnetic resonance imaging.** *J Behav Ther Exp Psychiatry* 1994, **25**:131-4.
12. Merl T, Scholz M, Gerhardt P, Langer M, Laubenberger J, Weiss HD, Gehl HB, Wolf KJ, Ohnesorge I: **Results of a prospective multicenter study for evaluation of the diagnostic quality of an open whole-body low-field MRI unit. A comparison with high-field MRI measured by the applicable gold standard.** *Eur J Radiol* 1999, **30**:43-53.
13. Spouse E, Gedroyc WM: **MRI of the claustrophobic patient: interventionally configured magnets.** *Br J Radiol* 2000, **73**:146-51.
14. Bangard C, Paszek J, Berg F, Eyl G, Kessler J, Lackner K, Gossmann A: **MR imaging of claustrophobic patients in an open 1.0T scanner: Motion artifacts and patient acceptability compared with closed bore magnets.** *Eur J Radiol* 2007, **64**:152-7.
15. Moher D, Jones A, Lepage L: **Use of the CONSORT statement and quality of reports of randomized trials: a comparative before-and-after evaluation.** *Jama* 2001, **285**:1992-5.
16. Friedman LM, Furberg CD, DeMets DL: **Fundamentals of clinical trials.** St. Louis: Mosby; 1985.
17. **Practice guidelines for sedation and analgesia by non-anesthesiologists. A report by the American Society of Anesthesiologists Task Force on Sedation and Analgesia by Non-Anesthesiologists.** *Anesthesiology* 1996, **84**:459-71.
18. Spielberger CD: **Manual for the State-Trait Anxiety Inventory (STAI).** Palo Alto, CA: Consulting Psychologists Press; 1983.
19. Ehlers A, Margraf J: **Fragebogen zu körperbezogenen Ängsten, Kognitionen und Vermeidung (AKV). Manual (2., überarb. und neunormierte Auflage).** Göttingen: Beltz Test GmbH; 2001.
20. Wolpe J, Lang PJ: **Manual for the Fear Survey Schedule (rev. ed.).** San Diego, CA: Education and Industrial Testing Service; 1977.
21. Radomsky AS, Rachman S, Thordarson DS, McIsaac HK, Teachman BA: **The Claustrophobia Questionnaire.** *J Anxiety Disord* 2001, **15**:287-97.
22. Dewey M, Schink T, Dewey CF: **Frequency of referral of patients with safety-related contraindications to magnetic resonance imaging.** *Eur J Radiol* 2007, **63**:124-7.
23. Vitaliano PP, DeWolfe DJ, Maiuro RD, Russo J, Katon W: **Appraised Changeability of a Stressor as a Modifier of the Relationship Between Coping and Depression: A Test of the Hypothesis of Fit.** *J Pers Soc Psychol* 1990, **59**:582-592.
24. Hautzinger M, Keller F, Kühner C: **Das Beck Depressionsinventar II. Deutsche Bearbeitung und Handbuch zum BDI II.** Frankfurt a. M.: Harcourt Test Services; 2006.
25. Group E: **EuroQol - A new facility for the measurement of health-related quality of life.** *Health Policy* 1990, **16**:199-208.
26. Lukins R, Davan IG, Drummond PD: **A cognitive behavioural approach to preventing anxiety during magnetic resonance imaging.** *J Behav Ther Exp Psychiatry* 1997, **28**:97-104.
27. Chambless DL, Caputo GC, Bright D, Gallagher R: **Assessment of fear in agoraphobics: the body sensations questionnaire and the agoraphobic cognitions questionnaire.** *J Consult Clin Psychol* 1984, **52**:1090-7.
28. **Diagnostic and Statistical Manual of Mental Disorders.** Washington, DC: American Psychiatric Association, 4 2000.
29. Vitaliano PP, Russo J, Carr JE, Maiuro RD, Becker J: **The Ways of Coping Checklist: Revision and Psychometric Properties.** *Multivar Behav Res* 1985, **20**:3-26.
30. Folkman S, Lazarus RS: **An analysis of coping in a middle-aged community sample.** *J Health Soc Behav* 1980, **21**:219-39.
31. Goutallier D, Postel JM, Bernageau J, Lavau L, Voisin MC: **Fatty muscle degeneration in cuff ruptures. Pre- and postoperative evaluation by CT scan.** *Clin Orthop Relat Res* 1994, **304**:78-83.
32. Warner JJ, Higgins L, Parsons IMt, Dowdy P: **Diagnosis and treatment of anterosuperior rotator cuff tears.** *J Shoulder Elbow Surg* 2001, **10**:37-46.
33. Waugh SA, Ramkumar PG, Gandy SJ, Nicholas RS, Martin P, Belch JJ, Struthers AD, Houston JG: **Optimization of the contrast dose and injection rates in whole-body MR angiography at 3.0T.** *J Magn Reson Imaging* 2009, **30**:1059-67.
34. Rodenwaldt J, Kopka L, Meyer HJ, Vosshenrich R, Funke M, Grabbe E: **Determination of contour clarity in contrast-enhanced MR angiography: definition and clinical evaluation exemplified by ECG-triggered imaging of the thoracic aorta.** *Rofo* 1998, **169**:616-21.
35. Dantendorfer K, Wimberger D, Katschnig H, Imhoff H: **Claustrophobia in MRI scanners.** *Lancet* 1991, **338**:761-2.
36. Dantendorfer K, Amering M, Bankier A, Helbich T, Prayer D, Youssefzadeh S, Alexandrowicz R, Imhof H, Katschnig H: **A study of the effects of patient anxiety, perceptions and equipment on motion artifacts in magnetic resonance imaging.** *Magn Reson Imaging* 1997, **15**:301-6.
37. Heuck A, Bonél H, Huber A, Müller-Lisse GU, Sittek H, Reiser M: **Akzeptanz von Hochfeld-Ganzkörper-MR-Geräten, offenem MR-System und**

dediziertem Extremitätenscanner durch die Patienten. *Radiologe* 1997, **37**:778-784.

38. Fishbain D, Goldberg H, Labbé E, Zacher D, Steele-Rosomoff R, Rosomoff H: MR imaging as a trigger for persistent claustrophobia. *AJR Am J Roentgenol* 1989, **152**:653.
39. Rachman S: The conditioning theory of fear-acquisition: a critical examination. *Behav Res Ther* 1977, **15**:375-87.
40. Kilborn LC, Labbé EE: Magnetic resonance imaging scanning procedures: development of phobic response during scan and at one-month follow-up. *J Behav Med* 1990, **13**:391-401.
41. Harris LM, Robinson J, Menzies RG: Evidence for fear of restriction and fear of suffocation as components of claustrophobia. *Behav Res Ther* 1999, **37**:155-9.
42. Quirk ME, Letendre AJ, Ciottone RA, Lingley JF: Evaluation of three psychologic interventions to reduce anxiety during MR imaging. *Radiology* 1989, **173**:759-62.
43. Booth R, Rachman S: The reduction of claustrophobia–I. *Behav Res Ther* 1992, **30**:207-21.
44. International Statistical Classification of Diseases and Health Related Problems (ICD-10). Geneva: World Health Organization; 2004.
45. Quirk ME, Letendre AJ, Ciottone RA, Lingley JF: Anxiety in patients undergoing MR imaging. *Radiology* 1989, **170**:463-6.
46. Nazemi H, Dager SR: Coping strategies of panic and control subjects undergoing lactate infusion during magnetic resonance imaging confinement. *Compr Psychiatry* 2003, **44**:190-7.
47. Granet RB, Gelber LJ: Claustrophobia during MR imaging. *N J Med* 1990, **87**:479-82.
48. Törnqvist E, Mansson A, Larsson EM, Hallström I: It's like being in another world - Patients' lived experience of magnetic resonance imaging. *J Clin Nurs* 2006, **15**:954-61.
49. Carter MM, Hollon SD, Carson R, Shelton RC: Effects of a safe person on induced distress following a biological challenge in panic disorder with agoraphobia. *J Abnorm Psychol* 1995, **104**:156-63.
50. MacKenzie R, Sims C, Owens RG, Dixon AK: Patients' perceptions of magnetic resonance imaging. *Clin Radiol* 1995, **50**:137-43.

Permissions

All chapters in this book were first published in MI, by BioMed Central; hereby published with permission under the Creative Commons Attribution License or equivalent. Every chapter published in this book has been scrutinized by our experts. Their significance has been extensively debated. The topics covered herein carry significant findings which will fuel the growth of the discipline. They may even be implemented as practical applications or may be referred to as a beginning point for another development.

The contributors of this book come from diverse backgrounds, making this book a truly international effort. This book will bring forth new frontiers with its revolutionizing research information and detailed analysis of the nascent developments around the world.

We would like to thank all the contributing authors for lending their expertise to make the book truly unique. They have played a crucial role in the development of this book. Without their invaluable contributions this book wouldn't have been possible. They have made vital efforts to compile up to date information on the varied aspects of this subject to make this book a valuable addition to the collection of many professionals and students.

This book was conceptualized with the vision of imparting up-to-date information and advanced data in this field. To ensure the same, a matchless editorial board was set up. Every individual on the board went through rigorous rounds of assessment to prove their worth. After which they invested a large part of their time researching and compiling the most relevant data for our readers.

The editorial board has been involved in producing this book since its inception. They have spent rigorous hours researching and exploring the diverse topics which have resulted in the successful publishing of this book. They have passed on their knowledge of decades through this book. To expedite this challenging task, the publisher supported the team at every step. A small team of assistant editors was also appointed to further simplify the editing procedure and attain best results for the readers.

Apart from the editorial board, the designing team has also invested a significant amount of their time in understanding the subject and creating the most relevant covers. They scrutinized every image to scout for the most suitable representation of the subject and create an appropriate cover for the book.

The publishing team has been an ardent support to the editorial, designing and production team. Their endless efforts to recruit the best for this project, has resulted in the accomplishment of this book. They are a veteran in the field of academics and their pool of knowledge is as vast as their experience in printing. Their expertise and guidance has proved useful at every step. Their uncompromising quality standards have made this book an exceptional effort. Their encouragement from time to time has been an inspiration for everyone.

The publisher and the editorial board hope that this book will prove to be a valuable piece of knowledge for researchers, students, practitioners and scholars across the globe.

List of Contributors

Jian-Min Shen, Xian-Wu Xia, Wu-Gen Kang, Jian-Jun Yuan and Liang Sheng
Department of Medical imaging, Taizhou municipal hospital, Taizhou Medical College, Taizhou 318000, PR China

Andrei Lebovici, Silviu A Sfrangeu and Diana Feier
Radiology Department, Emergency County Hospital, "Iuliu Hatieganu" University of Medicine and Pharmacy, Cluj-Napoca, Romania

Cosmin Caraiani
Department of Imaging, Regional Institute of Gastroenterology and Hepatology, "Iuliu Hatieganu" University of Medicine and Pharmacy, Cluj-Napoca, Romania

Mihai Suciu, Florin Elec and Ciprian Lucan
Department of Urology, Clinical Institute of Urology and Kidney Transplant, "Iuliu Hatieganu" University of Medicine and Pharmacy, Cluj-Napoca, Romania

Gheorghita Iacob
Department of Pathology, Clinical Institute of Urology and Kidney Transplant, "Iuliu Hatieganu" University of Medicine and Pharmacy, Cluj-Napoca, Romania

Mircea Buruian
Department of Radiology, County Emergency Hospital Mures, University of Medicine and Pharmacy, Targu-Mures, Romania

Kristina Imeen Ringe, Dagmar Hartung, Christian von Falck, Frank Wacker and Hans-Jürgen Raatschen
Department of Diagnostic and Interventional Radiology, Hannover Medical School, Carl-Neuberg Str. 1, Hannover 30625, Germany

Owen J Arthurs, Martin J Graves, Andrea D Edwards, Ilse Joubert, Pat AK Set and David J Lomas
Department of Radiology, Cambridge University Hospitals NHS Foundation Trust, Cambridge CB2 0QQ, UK

Owen J Arthurs
Department of Radiology, Great Ormond Street Hospital for Children NHS Foundation Trust, London, UK

Owen J Arthurs
UCL Institute of Child Health, London, UK

Luigi Cormio, Giuseppe Di Fino, Oscar Selvaggio, Paolo Massenio and Giuseppe Carrieri
Department of Urology and Renal Transplantation, University of Foggia, Via Luigi Pinto, 71122 Foggia, Italy

Carmen Scavone and Luca Macarini
Department of Radiology, University of Foggia, Foggia, Italy

Francesca Sanguedolce
Department of Pathology, University of Foggia, Foggia, Italy

Laura Merlini and Mehrak Anooshiravani
Unit of Pediatric Radiology Geneva University Hospital HUG, 6 Willy-Donzé, Geneva 1205, Switzerland

Dimitri Ceroni
Unit of Pediatric Orthopedics, University Hospital, Geneva, Switzerland

Stefan Buchner, Kurt Debl and Andreas Luchner
Klinik und Poliklinik für Innere Medizin II, Universitätsklinikum Regensburg, Franz-Josef-Strauss-Allee 11, 93042 Regensburg, Germany

Behrus Djavidani
Institut für Röntgendiagnostik, Universitätsklinikum Regensburg, Regensburg, Germany

Franz-Xaver Schmid
Klinik und Poliklinik für Herz-, Thorax- und herznahe Gefäßchirurgie, Universitätsklinikum Regensburg, Regensburg, Germany

Keita Miyazaki, Hidetada Fukushima, Kazunobu Norimoto and Kazuo Okuchi
Department of Emergency and Critical Care Medicine, Nara Medical University, Shijo-cho, 840, Kashihara City, Nara, Japan

Youhei Kogeichi
Department of Neurosurgery, Nara Medical University, Shijo-cho, 840, Kashihara City, Nara, Japan

Tomoo Watanabe
Department of Neurosurgery, Nara Prefecture General Medical Center, Hiramatsu, 1-30-1, Nara City, Nara, Japan

Toshiaki Taoka
Department of Radiology, Nara Medical University, Shijo-cho, 840, Kashihara City, Nara, Japan

Andre Rudolph, Florian von Knobelsdorff-Brenkenhoff, Julius Traber, Johannes Schüler, Ralf Wassmuth and Jeanette Schulz-Menger
Working Group CMR, Experimental and Clinical Research Center, a joint cooperation between the Charité Medical Faculty and the Max-Delbrück Center for Molecular Medicine, Lindenberger Weg 80, 13125 Berlin, Germany

Andre Rudolph, Florian von Knobelsdorff-Brenkenhoff, Julius Traber, Johannes Schüler, Ralf Wassmuth and Jeanette Schulz-Menger
Dept. of Cardiology and Nephrology, HELIOS-Kliniken Berlin Buch, Schwanebecker Chaussee 50, 13125 Berlin, Germany

Daniel Messroghli
Department of Congenital Heart Disease and Pediatric Cardiology, Deutsches Herzzentrum Berlin, Berlin, Germany

Johannes Schüler, Ralf Wassmuth, Jeanette Schulz-Menger, Julius Traber, Andre Rudolph and Florian von Knobelsdorff-Brenkenhoff
Dept. of Cardiology and Nephrology, HELIOS-Kliniken Berlin Buch, Schwanebecker Chaussee 50, 13125 Berlin, Germany

Daniel Messroghli
Department of Congenital Heart Disease and Pediatric Cardiology, Deutsches Herzzentrum Berlin, Berlin, Germany

Alfredo Revenaz and Enrico Fainardi
Unità Operativa di Neuroradiologia, Dipartimento di Neuroscienze e Riabilitazione, Azienda Ospedaliero-Universitaria of Ferrara, Arcispedale S. Anna, Via Aldo Moro 8, 44124 Cona, Ferrara, Italy

Massimiliano Ruggeri
Consiglio Nazionale delle Ricerche, 44124 Ferrara, Italy

Marcella Laganà and Niels Bergsland
MR Research Laboratory, IRCCS Don Gnocchi Foundation ONLUS, Milan, Italy

Niels Bergsland
Buffalo Neuroimaging Analysis Center, Department of Neurology, University at Buffalo SUNY, Buffalo, NY, USA

Elisabetta Groppo
Sezione di Neurologia, Dipartimento di Scienze Biomediche e Chirurgico Specialistiche, Università di Ferrara, Ferrara, Italy

Marco Rovaris
Unità Operativa di Sclerosi Multipla, Fondazione Don Gnocchi ONLUS, IRCCS S. Maria Nascente, 20148 Milano, Italy

Ansgar Espeland, Nils Vetti and Jostein Kråkenes
Department of Radiology, Haukeland University Hospital, Jonas Liesvei 65, 5021, Bergen, Norway
Department of Surgical Sciences, University of Bergen, Bergen, Norway

Gert Reiter
Siemens Healthcare, Graz, Austria

Gabriel Adelsmayr, Michael Fuchsjäger and Ursula Reiter
Division of General Radiology, Department of Radiology, Medical University of Graz, Auenbruggerplatz 9/P, A-8036 Graz, Austria

Gabor Kovacs and Horst Olschewski
Division of Pulmology, Department of Internal Medicine, Medical University of Graz, & LBI for Lung Vascular Research Graz, Graz, Austria

Andreas Greiser and Aurelien F. Stalder
Siemens Healthcare, Erlangen, Germa

Michael Fiechter, Tobias A Fuchs, Catherine Gebhard, Julia Stehli, Bernd Klaeser, Robert Manka, Oliver Gaemperli and Philipp A Kaufmann
Department of Radiology, Cardiac Imaging, University Hospital Zurich, Zurich, Switzerland

Costantina Manes, Barbara E Stähli, Felix C Tanner, Oliver Gaemperli and Robert Manka
Department of Cardiology, Cardiovascular Center, University Hospital Zurich, Zurich, Switzerland

Felix C Tanner, Philipp A Kaufmann and Michael Fiechter
Zurich Center for Integrative Human Physiology (ZIHP), University of Zurich, Zurich, Switzerland

David S Wack, Michael G Dwyer, Niels Bergsland, Deepa Ramasamy, Carol Di Perri, Sara Hussein, Christopher Magnano and Robert Zivadinov
Buffalo Neuroimaging Analysis Center, Department of Neurology, School of Medicine and Biomedical Sciences, University at Buffalo, State University of New York at Buffalo, Buffalo, NY, USA

David S Wack
Department of Nuclear Medicine, University at Buffalo, State University of New York at Buffalo, Buffalo, NY, USA

Laura Ranza
Department of Neuroradiology, IRCCS, C. Mondino, University of Pavia, Pavia, Italy

Robert Zivadinov
MR Imaging Clinical Translational Research Center, School of Medicine and Biomedical Sciences, University at Buffalo, State University of New York, Buffalo, NY, USA

Kevin Seals
School of Medicine and Biomedical Sciences, State University of New York at Buffalo, Buffalo, NY, USA

James M Elliott
Department of Physical Therapy and Human Movement Sciences, Feinberg School of Medicine, Northwestern University, 645 North Michigan Avenue, Suite 1100 room 1139, Chicago, IL 60611, USA

David M Walton
School of Physical Therapy, Western University, London, Ontario, Canada

Alfred Rademaker
Department of Preventive Medicine, Feinberg School of Medicine, Northwestern University, Chicago, IL, USA

Todd B Parrish
Department of Biomedical Engineering, McCormick School of Engineering, Northwestern University, Evanston, IL, USA
Department of Radiology, Feinberg School of Medicine, Northwestern University, Chicago, IL, USA

Anna Gärdin, Torkel B Brismar, Tomas Movin and Adel Shalabi
Department of Clinical Science, Division of Medical Imaging and Technology, Intervention and Technology at Karolinska Institutet, Stockholm SE-141-86, Sweden

Anna Gärdin and Torkel B Brismar
Department of Radiology, Karolinska University Hospital in Huddinge, Stockholm SE-141-86, Sweden

Tomas Movin
Department of Clinical Science, Division of Orthopedics and Biotechnology, Intervention and Technology at Karolinska Institutet, Stockholm SE-141-86, Sweden

Adel Shalabi
Centre for Medical Imaging, Department of Radiology, Oncology and Radiation Sciences Akademiska University Hospital, Uppsala SE-751-85, Sweden

Leo Ai
Department of Biomedical Engineering, University of Iowa, 200 Hawkins Drive C721 GH, Iowa City, IA 52242, USA

Xin Gao
Department of Medical Imaging, Suzhou Institute of Biomedical Engineering and Technology, Suzhou, China

Jinhu Xiong
Department of Radiology, University of Iowa, Iowa, USA

Jane Tufvesson, Marcus Carlsson, Anthony H. Aletras, Henrik Engblom, Håkan Arheden and Einar Heiberg
Department of Clinical Physiology, Skåne University Hospital in Lund, Lund University, Lund, Sweden

Einar Heiberg and Jane Tufvesson
Department of Biomedical Engineering, Faculty of Engineering, Lund University, Lund, Sweden

Anthony H. Aletras
Laboratory of Medical Informatics, School of Medicine, Aristotle University of Thessaloniki, Thessaloniki, Greece

Jean-François Deux
Department of Cardiology, Henri Mondor Hospital, Creteil, France

David Erlinge and Sasha Koul
Department of Cardiology, Lund University, Lund, Sweden

Peder Sörensson and John Pernow
Department of Medicine, Karolinska Institutet, Karolinska University Hospital, Stockholm, Sweden

Dan Atar
Department of Cardiology B, Oslo, University Hospital Ullevål and Faculty of Medicine, University of Oslo, Oslo, Norway

Jingjing Chen, Xianglong Shi, Weiqun Bi and Shi-en Liu
Department of Radiology, The Affiliated Hospital of Qingdao University, Qingdao 266000, Shandong Province, China

Youjiao Si
Department of Radiology, Yantai Affiliated Hospital of Binzhou Medical University, Yantai 264100, Shandong Province, China

Kaikai Zhao
Department of Oncology, Yantai Affiliated Hospital of Binzhou Medical University, Yantai 264100, Shandong Province, China

Hui Hua
Department of Thyroid Surgery, The Affiliated Hospital of Qingdao University, No. 16 Jiangsu Road, Qingdao 266000, Shandong Province, China

Marianna Fontana, Ana Martinez-Naharro, Julian D. Gillmore and Philip N. Hawkins
National Amyloidosis Centre, University College London, Royal Free Hospital, London, UK

James C. Moon, Thomas A. Treibel and Marianna Fontana
Institute of Cardiovascular Science, University College London, London, UK

James C. Moon, Thomas A. Treibel and Stefania Rosmini
Barts Heart Centre, West Smithfield, London EC1A 7BE, UK

Raymond Y. Kwong
Non-Invasive Cardiac Imaging, Cardiovascular Medicine Division, Brigham and Women's Hospital, Harvard Medical School, Boston, MA, USA

Syuichi Tetsuka
Department of Neurology, Hospital of Yuki, 9629-1, Yuki, Yuki-City, Ibaraki 307-0001, Japan

Hiroaki Nonaka
Obstetrics & Gynecology, Hospital of International University of Health and Welfare, 537-3, Iguchi, Nasushiobara, Tochigi 329-2763, Japan

G. S. Gulsin, A. Singh and G. P. McCann
Department of Cardiovascular Sciences, University of Leicester and the NIHR Biomedical Research Centre, Glenfield Hospital, Groby Road, Leicester, UK

Luguang Chen, Qian Zhan, Wenjia Peng, Tao Song, Qi Liu and Jianping Lu
Department of Radiology, Changhai Hospital of Shanghai, The Second Military Medical University, No.168 Changhai Road, Shanghai 200433, China

Ullamari Hakulinen, Antti Brander, Pertti Ryymi, Seppo Soimakallio, Prasun Dastidar and Hannu Eskola
Department of Radiology, Medical Imaging Center of Pirkanmaa Hospital District, Teiskontie 35 PL 2000, 33521, Tampere, Finland

Hannu Eskola and Ullamari Hakulinen
Department of Biomedical Engineering, Tampere University of Technology, Tampere, Finland

Juha Öhman
Department of Neurosurgery, Tampere University Hospital, Tampere, Finland

Prasun Dastidar and Seppo Soimakallio
Tampere Medical School, University of Tampere, Tampere, Finland

Mika Helminen
Science Center of Pirkanmaa Hospital District, Tampere, Finland

Tomoyuki Tajima, Hiroshi Kawaguchi and Atsuhiro Sakamoto
Department of Anesthesiology, Nippon Medical School, Bunkyo-ku, Tokyo, Japan

Keiko Hirakawa
NMR Laboratory and Department of Legal Medicine, Nippon Medical School, Bunkyo-ku, Tokyo, Japan

Faraz Khursheed, Fiona Rohlffs, Dong H Kim and Timothy M Ellmore
The Vivian L. Smith Department of Neurosurgery and Mischer Neuroscience Institute, The University of Texas Medical School at Houston, 6431 Fannin St., Houston TX 77030, USA

Shuichi Suzuki
Department of Diagnostic and Interventional Imaging, The University of Texas Medical School at Houston, 6431 Fannin St., Houston TX 77030, USA
Neurointerventional/Neuro Endovascular, Radiological Sciences, University of California, Irvine, 101 The City Drive South, Rt. 140, South Bldg. 56, Mail Code: 5005, Orange, CA 92868, USA

Ivana Galinovic, Helena Bros, Benjamin Hotter, Peter Brunecker and Jochen B Fiebach
Benjamin Franklin, Hindenburgdamm 30, 12200 Berlin, Germany

Ann-Christin Ostwaldt
International Graduate Program Medical Neurosciences,Charite-Universitätsmedizin, Berlin, Luisenstrasse 56, 10117 Berlin, Germany

Carina Soemmer
Charité-Universitätsmedizin, Berlin, Charitéplatz 1, 10117 Berlin, Germany

Judith Enders, Elke Zimmermann, Matthias Rief, Patrick Asbach, Christian Klessen, Gerd Diederichs, Ulf Teichgräber, Bernd Hamm and Marc Dewey
Departments of Radiology, Charité, Medical School, Humboldt Universität zu Berlin and Freie Universität Berlin, Germany

Peter Martus
Departments of Biostatistics and Clinical Epidemiology, Charité, Medical School, Humboldt Universität zu Berlin and Freie Universität Berlin, Germany

Randolf Klingebiel
Divisions of Neuroradiology, Charité, Medical School, Humboldt Universität zu Berlin and Freie Universität Berlin, Germany

Thomas Bengner
Departments of Clinical Psychology, Charité, Medical School, Humboldt Universität zu Berlin and Freie Universität Berlin, Germany

Index